Springer Japan KK

M. Imamura (Ed.)

Superficial Esophageal Neoplasm

Pathology, Diagnosis, and Therapy

With 90 Figures, Including 7 in Color

Springer

Masayuki Imamura, MD, FACS
Professor and Chairman
Surgery and Surgical Basic Science
Graduate School of Medicine, Kyoto University
54 Kawaharacho, Shogoin, Sakyo-ku, Kyoto 606-8507, Japan

ISBN 978-4-431-67997-4

Library of Congress Cataloging-in-Publication Data

Superficial esophageal neoplasm : patholgy, diagnosis, and therapy / M. Imamura (ed.).
p. ; cm.
Includes bibliographical references and index.
ISBN 978-4-431-67997-4 ISBN 978-4-431-67873-1 (eBook)
DOI 10.1007/978-4-431-67873-1

1. Esophagus—Cancer—Congresses. I. Imamura, Masayuki. II. Kyoto Symposium on Esophageal Cancer (2000)
[DNLM: 1. Esophageal Neoplasma—Congresses. 2. Adenocarcinoma—Congresses. WI 250 S959 2002]
RC280.E8 S87 2002
616.99′432—dc21

2001049711

Printed on acid-free paper

Originally published by Springer-Verlag Tokyo in 2002
Softcover reprint of the hardcover 1st edition 2002

Typesetting: Best-set Typesetter Ltd., Hong Kong

SPIN: 10842624

Foreword

This book, containing the proceedings of the 2000 Kyoto Symposium on Esophageal Cancer, is an important contribution for all types of physicians interested in both squamous and adenocarcinoma of the esophagus. The volume has great legitimacy and relevance. The symposia hosted by Professor Masayuki Imamura brought together the leaders in several disciplines from Japan with other acknowledged authorities from Europe, the United States, Australia, and other parts of Asia. Japan has long been a leader in making advances in understanding the pathology, diagnosis, and treatment of esophageal squamous cell carcinoma, for several decades originally led by Professor Komei Nakayama and his students. It is now clear that Japanese are also beginning to suffer from esophageal adenocarcinoma and Barrett's columnar lined epithelium, thus enabling the Japanese to formulate studies on the pathology, diagnosis, and treatment for the full spectrum of esophageal neoplasms. The authoritativeness of these proceedings is established not only by the long tradition of Japanese leadership in the field but by the contributions of the principal leaders from the Nakayama school participating in the honorary faculty and local scientific committee.

The relevance of this volume and symposium is established by the wise decision to concentrate on the issues concerning superficial esophageal tumors and attempting to achieve an international consensus on the pathological diagnoses as well as approaches to diagnosis, surgical and other types of treatment. Not much has developed in recent years to advance the diagnosis and treatment of more advanced esophageal cancers, but the availability of earlier and more accurate diagnosis for superficial esophageal squamous and adenocarcinoma are changing the approaches to these disorders. This is particularly important because of the rapid increase in the incidence of adenocarcinoma of the esophagus and its relationship to Barrett's epithelium. It is essential to consolidate knowledge about these early tumors to agree on classifications and definitions.

For example, superficial esophageal cancer might be regarded as Stage 1 carcinoma according to the currently employed international staging system. However, Stage 1 classification includes epithelial, mucosal, and submucosal neoplasms which have remarkably different opportunities for therapy affecting the prognosis. Epithelial esophageal cancer, the earliest form of esophageal cancer, has been shown to be curable by local treatments including endoscopic resection and laser-based treatments, whereas Stage 1 cancer also includes tumors penetrating the full thickness of mucosa and even extending to the submucosa. Such cancers have been shown to spread on occasion to regional lymph nodes and may be variable in the thickness of penetration. Clearly local treatment only for these Stage 1 cancers is inappropriate for some patients, and the degree of radicality of the advocated surgery varies widely from center to center. Methods for making certain of the depth of penetration of various Stage 1 cancers become critical to diagnosis and pathological classification. Similarly there is confusion among international centers between epithelial neoplasms described as high-grade or severe dysplasia and those described as carcinoma in situ or mucosal carcinoma. By focusing on these specific aspects for superficial esophageal cancer, the authors of these chapters have made an important contribution to the future of the debate and resolution of controversy.

David B. Skinner, M.D.
President Emeritus
Professor of Cardiothoracic Surgery and Surgery
NewYork-Presbyterian
The University Hospitals of Columbia and Cornell

Former
President and Chief Executive Officer
The New York Hospital

Former
Professor of Surgery
Cornell University Medical College

Preface

This book is a collection of papers from the Kyoto Symposium on Esophageal Cancer, which was held July 28–29, 2000, in Kyoto, Japan. About 200 doctors, including pathologists, physicians, surgeons, and endoscopists, gathered from all parts of the world for discussions aimed at reaching a consensus on the clinicopathological understanding of the diagnosis and treatment of esophageal cancer.

In recent years the detection of early esophageal cancer has become much easier as a result of technical developments in endoscopic observation, bringing about benefits to patients, with complete cure of the disease possible by esophageal mucosal resection with an endoscope. We know that about 50% of patients with esophageal cancer that has invaded the submucosa have metastatic lymph nodes, and the 5-year survival rate of these patients is almost 50%. Thus, pathological diagnosis of superficial esophageal cancer has become a very important issue not only for pathologists but also for clinicians. Another recent concern internationally in esophageal cancer is the rapid increase of adenocarcinoma. Many problems remain unsolved in the development and treatment of adenocarcinoma, including the diagnosis and treatment of reflux esophagitis.

At the Kyoto Symposium productive discussions of these problems were conducted and near-consensus was reached in the area of diagnostic pathology. Discussions on differences in diagnosis of superficial esophageal cancer and various grades of dysplasia were held by pathologists from Australia, Italy, Sweden, Germany, Thailand, France, the United States, and Japan after examining prepared specimens. Through these discussions of pathology, as will be seen in this book, we learned to our surprise that there already existed a basic agreement on the diagnosis of severe dysplasia and/or superficial cancer.

Subsequent discussions were held by young molecular biologists as they considered the molecular basis of the development, invasion, and metastasis of esophageal cancer. Endoscopists, surgeons, and radiologists discussed treatment of early squamous cell carcinoma as well as early adenocarcinoma based on the results of particular treatment modalities. Thoracoscopic esophagectomy for superficial esophageal cancer was also discussed on the basis of international experience. We were pleased that an international study had started collecting evidence of adenocarcinoma or squamous cell carcinoma to find the key to differentiation of dysplasia from early cancer at the molecular level.

The actual discussions are recorded in this book as they took place. These lectures by prominent scientists will be of interest to all doctors who are concerned with esophageal cancer. We strongly hope that this book thus will be a basis for further efforts to establish an international consensus on the diagnosis and treatment of early esophageal cancer.

We would like to thank Dr. Kan Kondo for his excellent transcription of the discussions. Publication of this book was supported by a 2001 Grant-in Aid (No. 135314) for Publication of Scientific Research Results from the Japan Society for the Promotion of Science.

Masayuki Imamura
Editor
Kyoto

Contents

Contributors

Part 1
Current Clinicopathological Topics in Superficial Neoplasm of the Esophagus

Definition of the Stomach and Esophagus

PARAKRAMA CHANDRASOMA

Introduction

It is difficult to believe that the medical community has reached the twenty-first century without a clear and accurate understanding of what the stomach and esophagus are. As with anything that does not have a standard definition, papers on diseases of the esophagus vary considerably in the way the esophagus, stomach, and gastroesophageal junction are defined. The most common definition uses the proximal limit of the gastric rugal folds as defining the gastroesophageal junction [1]. Others use the squamocolumnar junction [2], the lower end of the lower esophageal sphnicter, or the peritoneal reflection [3] to define the junction. These definitions are accepted despite evidence that they are incorrect. For example, it is well known that the squamocolumnar junction moves proximally due to glandular metaplasia of the lower esophagus in patients who have reflux [4]. The lower esophageal sphincter (LES) is commonly shortened in patients who have reflux [5]. Both the squamocolumnar junction and the LES are therefore variable points and cannot be used to define the lower end of the esophagus. The peritoneal reflection is clearly not an appropriate definition of the lower end of the esophagus. In normal patients the LES, which is approximately 5 cm long, has an abdominal length that is usually about 2 cm. The abdominal part of the LES, which is part of the lower esophagus, is normally lined by peritoneum. Despite all these definitions, for most people the esophagus is usually defined as the tubal structure that changes abruptly at the gastroesophageal junction to become the saccular stomach.

It is important to recognize that there is no accepted histologic definition of the esophagus and stomach. The commonly used histologic description of this region recognizes that there is a transitional mucus-secreting epithelium known as cardiac mucosa between the squamous epithelium of the esophagus and the oxyntic acid-secreting mucosa of the stomach. The accepted extent of this epithelium is traceable to Hayward, who in 1961 stated that this cardiac mucosa lines the most distal 2–3 cm of the esophagus and an undefined extent of the proximal stomach [6]. According to

Department of Surgical Pathology, LAC-USC Medical Center, Room 16-905, 1200 N. State Street, Los Angeles, CA 90033, USA

Hayward, this mucus-secreting epithelium was necessary to prevent digestion of the squamous epithelium by gastric acid. This reason is incorrect. We now know that the LES normally performs the function of preventing gastric acid from coming into contact with the squamous epithelium of the esophagus. Hayward's conclusion about the extent of cardiac mucosa was not accompanied by any supporting studies or data. If Hayward's assertion is correct, there is no conclusion about whether this transitional cardiac mucosa lines the stomach, esophagus, or both. The commonly accepted dogma suggests that we believe that cardiac mucosa is present in the most distal 3 cm of the esophagus and an undefined extent of the proximal (or cardiac) region of the stomach. If this is true, the gastroesophageal junction must be somewhere within this cardiac mucosal extent and cannot be accurately defined histologically.

These concepts have significant practical implications, the most important of which relates to the definition of Barrett's esophagus. If one accepts that the most distal 2–3 cm of the esophagus is normally lined by cardiac mucosa, glandular mucosa in the esophagus can be regarded as abnormal only if it is present at a level higher than 3 cm in the tubular esophagus. Long-segment Barrett's esophagus is the occurrence of intestinal metaplasia in glandular mucosa above this 3 cm level in the distal tubular esophagus. For a long time this was the only accepted definition of Barrett's esophagus. Recent realization that intestinal metaplasia can occur in the normally defined extent of cardiac mucosa has resulted in the definition of two other entities: (a) short-segment Barrett's esophagus, which is the presence of intestinal metaplasia in "normal" glandular mucosa in the distal 3 cm of the esophagus; and (b) intestinal metaplasia of the gastric cardia, which is the presence of intestinal metaplasia in cardiac mucosa of the proximal stomach [1]. Short-segment Barrett's esophagus is becoming recognized as a disease associated with reflux and at risk for adenocarcinoma of the esophagus.

When the accepted dogma is used, another anomaly appears. When patients with adenocarcinoma of the stomach and esophagus are evaluated epidemiologically, distal gastric carcinoma separates out as an entity that is different from proximal gastric adenocarcinoma. Proximal gastric adenocarcinoma (defined as occurring within 5 cm of the gastroesophageal junction), has an epidemiology identical to that of adenocarcinoma of the distal esophagus. Both proximal gastric adenocarcinoma and distal esophageal adenocarcinoma are significantly associated with gastroesophageal reflux [2]. It should be recognized that the belief that proximal gastric adenocarcinoma is caused by reflux of gastric juice is absurd.

Study of Normal Histology

We undertook an autopsy study in which we examined 72 retrospective cases from the files of the Los Angeles County—USC Medical Center that had an evaluable longitudinal section across the gastroesophageal junctional region [7]. We classified glandular epithelial types in this region as: (a) cardiac mucosa (CM), defined by the presence of glands that contained mucous cells without parietal cells; (b) oxyntic mucosa (OM), defined by glands that contained parietal and chief cells without mucous cells; (c) oxyntocardiac mucosa (OCM), defined by glands that contained a mixture of mucous cells and parietal cells; and (d) intestinal metaplastic mucosa (IM),

TABLE 1. Epithelial types in the gastroesophageal junctional region

Mucosal type	Paull et al. terminology	Mucous cells	Parietal cells	Goblet cells
Squamous	Squamous	−	−	−
Oxyntic	N/A	−	+	−
Cardiac	Junctional	+	−	−
Oxyntocardiac	Fundic	+	+	−
Intestinal	Specialized	+	−	+

The definition of these mucosal types is based on the types of cells present in the mucosal glands underneath the foveolar region

defined by the presence of goblet cells (Table 1). These definitions are identical to those used by Paull et al. in their classic study of histologic types of columnar-lined esophagus [8], except for the following minor differences: (a) We use the terms "cardiac" and "intestinal" rather than Paull et al.'s terms "junctional" and "specialized" because these terms are more commonly used today; and (b) we use the term "oxyntocardiac mucosa" to describe mucosa where the glands contain a mixture of mucous cells and parietal cells rather than Paull et al.'s "fundic" because "oxyntocardiac mucosa" is purely descriptive without anatomic connotations. The degree of autolysis precluded the accurate evaluation of intestinal metaplasia in this autopsy study.

The study showed that 21 of 72 (29%) patients had only squamous epithelium and OM; 32 of 72 (44%) patients had squamous epithelium, OM, and OCM; and only 19 of 72 (26%) patients had CM (Table 2). When CM or OCM were present, the CM + OCM length, as measured by an ocular micrometer, was less than 0.5 cm in most cases. There was also a tendency for the prevalence of CM and the CM + OCM length to increase with age.

Because a single longitudinal section across the junctional region is not truly representative, we undertook a prospective autopsy study wherein we studied 18 patients more thoroughly [7]. The entire circumference of the junctional region was longitudinally sectioned and examined histologically. Complete examination in this manner showed the presence of OCM in all patients, but CM was absent in 10 of 18 (56%) patients (Table 2). All patients had OCM in some part of the circumference. The length of CM and OCM varied greatly within the circumference; and in 50% of patients some part of the circumference had a direct transition from squamous epithelium to OM without interposed CM or OCM. This study confirmed that, when present, the CM+OCM length was less than 0.5 cm in most patients.

We concluded from these studies that CM is absent from a significant number of people (74% in a limited sample and 56% with complete examination of the junction), the prevalence of CM increases with age, and the maximum CM + OCM length is <0.5 cm in most people and increases with age. Though OCM is present in all patients with complete sampling, its presence is not circumferential in 50% of patients. These conclusions make it highly likely that CM and OCM are abnormal mucosal types. If this is true, the only normal mucosal types in the gastroesophageal junctional region are squamous and OM, which are universally present.

The literature provides support for these data. Kilgore et al. [3], in a careful autopsy study in children under 18 years of age, found that the mean length of cardiac mucosa

TABLE 2. Prevalence of glandular mucosal types at the gastroesophageal junctional region

Study	Population	CM (%)	OCM (%)	CM + OCM (%)	CM + OCM <0.5 cm (%)
Chandrasoma [7]	Normal autopsy (retrospective)	26		71	75
Chandrasoma	Normal autopsy (prospective)	56	100	100	78
Kilgore [3]	Normal autopsy (prospective)	100		100	
Oberg [10]	Normal endoscopy			74	
Jain [11]	Normal endoscopy	35			
Chandrasoma [12]	Severe GERD	96	65	100	

Prospective autopsy studies sample the entire circumference of the gastroesophageal junction; retrospective studies are limited samples

Endoscopic sampling is described as "extensive" and most likely represents three or four biopsies per level. This sampling is closer to limited autopsy sampling than complete sampling

In patients with normal endoscopy, it is likely that the total length of abnormal (CM/OCM) glandular mucosa is <0.5 cm because it is likely that greater lengths are recognized

In this study, endoscopic features were so abnormal as to lead to multiple-level biopsies in the glandular mucosal segment. This likely indicates a CM+OCM length >0.5 cm; 28% of patients in this study had a CM+OCM length >2 cm

The prevalence of CM in patients with severe GERD is significantly (P = <0.001) higher than in "normal" populations

CM, cardiac mucosa; OCM, oxyntocardiac mucosa; GERD, gastroesophageal reflux disease; OM, oxyntic mucosa

All patients have OM (which lines the entire proximal stomach) and stratified squamous epithelium (which lines the esophagus). Definitions of CM and OCM are not uniformly applied in all studies

was 0.18 cm (range 0.1–0.4 cm) (Table 2). In a subsequent extension of this autopsy study, this same group reported that the length of cardiac mucosa increased with age [9].

Extensive sampling of the junctional region in endoscopically normal individuals also lends support to our conclusions. Oberg et al. (I performed the pathologic evaluation for this study) reported that with extensive sampling 26% of patients had no CM or OCM at the junction [10]. Jain et al. [11] reported that 65% of patients had no CM at the junction (Table 2). It is presumed that Jain et al. classified OCM as "fundic" mucosa after Paull's definition. It is striking that the numbers for the presence of CM in Jain et al.'s study (35%) and CM + OCM in Oberg et al.'s study (74%) are similar to the corresponding numbers in our retrospective autopsy study, suggesting that "extensive sampling" at endoscopy is similar to one longitudinal section across the junction at autopsy.

The conclusions that can be drawn from these studies are that cardiac mucosa is frequently absent, its prevalence increases with age, and when present it is frequently found in only part of the circumference of the junctional region. Moreover, its overall length is less than 0.5 cm in most people without reflux.

Study of Patients with Gastroesophageal Reflux Disease

In the study of Oberg et al. [10] from our institution, 246 of 334 (74%) patients who had CM, OCM, or both in biopsy specimens were more likely to have an abnormal 24-h pH test with significantly higher levels of acid exposure than the 88 (26%) patients who did not have CM or OCM in their junctional biopsies. The fact that the presence of CM or OCM (or both) is significantly associated with an abnormal level of acid reflux provides strong evidence that these mucosal types are abnormal and caused by acid reflux.

Chandrasoma et al. reported a series of patients in whom multiple-level biopsies were done on an endoscopically visualized segment of abnormal mucosa [12]. These multiple levels permitted accurate assessment of the CM + OCM length in these patients. Patients with a CM + OCM length >2 cm had markedly greater acid exposure than those with a CM + OCM length of <2 cm.

We also reported a series of 141 consecutive patients who had CM in their biopsies [13]. The incidence of distal gastritis in this group was 21% (30/141), and *Helicobacter pylori* was present in 20 of the 141 (14%). We graded acute and chronic inflammation in CM on a 0–3 scale. All patients with CM had significant chronic inflammation in the CM. In addition, patients with 2+ to 3+ chronic inflammation had more likelihood of an abnormal pH test and a higher level of acid exposure than those with 1+ chronic inflammation. The findings that CM is always inflamed and that patients with severe inflammation have significantly higher acid exposure than those with lesser inflammation strongly support the concept that CM is abnormal mucosa caused by acid reflux.

Clinical Applications of the New Histologic Data

Clinical application of these new histologic data awaits general acceptance of the data. There seems to be no alternative other than to accept that cardiac mucosa is either absent in normal individuals, as concluded by Chandrasoma et al. [7], or that its extent is small (low limit 0.1 cm), as concluded by Kilgore et al. [3]. It is not unreasonable that CM and OCM are present in the junctional region in many people because reflux is an almost universal phenomenon in humans [14]. Because 0.1 cm (1 mm) is such a small length, the discrepancy between the two studies is not significant compared with the presently accepted extent of cardiac mucosa of 3 cm of the distal esophagus and an unspecified extent of the proximal stomach. All definitions of Barrett's esophagus must be altered because these definitions use the old dogma of the normal extent of cardiac mucosa.

It is also important to recognize that histologic examination now provides a means of pathologic diagnosis of reflux disease and assessment of its severity. A normal person is one who has a tubal esophagus that is lined entirely by squamous epithelium that transitions at the gastroesophageal junction to a saccular stomach lined by acid-secreting OM. Biopsy specimens from normal individuals show only squamous epithelium and OM. In patients who have reflux, the distal esophagus becomes damaged, interposing a reflux-damaged lower esophagus between the undamaged esophagus and the stomach. This reflux-damaged esophagus is most accurately identified by the histologic presence of CM and OCM, which are reflux-induced epithelia derived from transformation of squamous epithelium of the lower esophagus. Their presence represents morphologic evidence of reflux [10], and their extent is a measure of the severity of the reflux [12]. Intestinal metaplasia within this abnormal reflux-induced CM is therefore reflux-induced intestinal metaplasia, which is suggested as the appropriate definition of Barrett's esophagus. The diagnosis of Barrett's esophagus becomes purely histologic without the need for endoscopic criteria, which tend to be inaccurate and subject to interobserver variation.

New Definitions for Esophagus and Stomach

These new histologic findings should be correlated with the normal anatomy of this region. In a normal individual the tubal esophagus is lined entirely by squamous epithelium that transitions to OM with its rugal folds at the gastroesophageal junction where the pouch of the stomach begins. The normal esophagus is defined by its lining of squamous epithelium, and the normal stomach is defined by its lining of acid-secreting OM. The gastroesophageal junction in normal people is the squamooxyntic junction. Anatomically, the normal esophagus is entirely tubal, and the normal stomach is entirely saccular. Endoscopically, the gastric rugal folds that characterize gastric mucosa cover the entire proximal stomach, including the anatomic gastric cardia, and extend to the squamous epithelium at the distal end of the tubal esophagus, which is lined by squamous epithelium.

It is important to understand the normal physiologic mechanisms involved here. In the thorax the eosphageal intraluminal pressure is negative and tends to collapse the esophagus and maintain the tubal shape. Below the diaphragm, however, the intraluminal pressure is positive and tends to distend the wall. Retention of the tubal shape of the intraabdominal esophagus is dependent on there being an effective lower esophageal sphincter with a pressure higher than the intraluminal pressure. The distal end of the esophagus is defined by the distal end of the LES. Beyond the LES, the positive intraabdominal pressure causes the stomach to distend into a pouch.

The epithelial lining of this region develops during fetal life from the uncommitted foregut epithelium. This epithelium consists of pluripotent cells that have a wide range of differentiating capability. Many facets of this pluripotent capability are expressed during fetal life, where the epithelium shows a variety of cell types including squamous, mucous, and intestinal. At full term, however, the esophagus is lined almost to its distal end by stratified squamous epithelium and the proximal stomach by pure OM. In the neonate there is frequently a small distance between stratified squamous epithelium and OM that is lined by an uncommitted columnar epithelium devoid of glands. There are few data regarding differentiation during the first year of life. However, the fact that examination of the junctional region in young children shows only squamous epithelium and OM in most patients suggests that the uncommitted epithelium at the junction in the neonate develops into either stratified squamous epithelium or OM. Because the LES develops fully during the first year of life, it would be logical that the uncommitted epithelium is directed toward its final differentiation by exposure to gastric juice. The part of the lining that is protected by the LES becomes squamous and the part below the LES becomes pure OM.

In patients with reflux, a reflux-damaged esophagus is interposed between the normal stomach and the undamaged esophagus. When this is defined by the presence of CM and OCM, as suggested above, one important fact emerges. The gastroesophageal junction (as defined as the proximal limit of pure OM) is frequently located distal to the opening of the tubal part of the esophagus in patients with reflux. The part of the pouch that is lined by CM or OCM (or both) in patients with reflux that lies below the diaphragm is presently called the "proximal stomach" or the "anatomic gastric cardia." This is incorrect according to histologic definition. This part of the foregut that appears anatomically like the proximal stomach must be reflux-damaged esophagus if it is lined by CM and OCM.

The explanation for the pathologic anatomy of reflux relates to changes in the LES. Sphincter abnormalities occur early in patients with reflux. In Oberg et al.'s study of endoscopically normal patients, those who had CM and OCM not only had evidence of reflux but it was associated with a demonstrable decrease in total LES length and the length of the abdominal component of the LES [10]. This appears to indicate that the LES length decreases in patients with reflux, beginning at its distal end and progressing cephalad.

When the abdominal esophagus is not protected by the high resting pressure of the LES, its positive intraluminal pressure causes it to become progressively distended. Over time, this results in the distal esophagus becoming pouch-like and not distinguishable anatomically from the stomach, a process I call "gastricization." The gastricized, dilated, distal esophagus is no longer protected from exposure to gastric contents by the shortened LES, and the original squamous epithelium lining is converted to an abnormal glandular mucosa with histologic characteristics of CM and OCM. The process of gastricization is limited to the abdominal length of the LES, which is 3–4 cm so long as the diaphragm is normal.

Gastricization of the lower esophagus explains several things. First, it recognizes that the pouch-like structure distal to the tubular esophagus is the stomach in normal people but represents gastricized esophagus in patients with reflux. This provides an explanation as to why adenocarcinoma of the "proximal stomach" is associated epidemiologically with gastroesophageal reflux [2]. Adenocarcinoma of the proximal stomach is really adenocarcinoma of the gastricized distal esophagus if reflux has resulted in gastricization of the lower esophagus. This situation can be distinguished from true adenocarcinoma of the proximal stomach by examining the mucosa in the proximal stomach: If the mucosa is pure OM, the structure is stomach; if it is CM or OCM, it is gastricized lower esophagus.

In recent studies on esophagectomy specimens from patients who have Barrett's esophagus with dysplasia (a group known to have reflux disease), we have separated the tubal esophagus from the saccular stomach. Longitudinal sections obtained from the proximal end of the saccular stomach show that there is a variable amount of CM and OCM in the proximal stomach. In this region lined by CM and OCM there are submucosal mucous glands and squamous-lined ducts. These glands are similar to those seen in the esophagus and are never seen in the true stomach lined by OM. These findings strongly support the concept of gastricization of the lower esophagus.

It is hoped that the new histologic definitions of normal esophagus, normal stomach, reflux-damaged esophagus, and Barrett's esophagus will increase our understanding of this region. The importance of such understanding is that reflux disease is one of the most common diseases of humans and the incidence of reflux-induced adenocarcinoma is rapidly increasing in the United States and western Europe [15]. Understanding the pathophysiology of a disease is essential before effective treatment and preventive methods can be undertaken.

References

1. Sampliner RE (1998) Practice guidelines on the diagnosis, surveillance, and therapy of Barrett's esophagus. Am J Gastroenterol 93:1028–1031
2. Lagergren J, Bergstrom R, Lindgren A, Nyren O (1999) Symptomatic gastroesophageal reflux as a risk factor for esophageal adenocarcinoma. N Engl J Med 340:825–831
3. Kilgore SP, Ormsby AH, Gramlich TL, et al (1999) The gastric cardia is not a metaplastic mucosa secondary to gastroesophageal reflux disease (GERD). Gastroenterology 116:A213
4. Csendes A, Maluenda F, Braghetto I, et al (1993) Location of the lower esophageal sphnicter and the squamous columnar mucosal junction in 109 healthy controls and 778 patients with different degrees of endoscopic esophagitis. Gut 34:21–27
5. Stein HJ, DeMeester TR, Naspetti R, et al (1991) Three dimensional imaging of the lower esophageal sphincter in gastroesophageal reflux disease. Ann Surg 214:364–384
6. Hayward J (1961) The lower end of the esophagus. Thorax 16:36–41
7. Chandrasoma PT, Der R, Ma Y-L, et al (2000) Histology of the gastroesophageal junction; an autopsy study. Am J Surg Pathol 24:402–409
8. Paull A, Trier JS, Dalton MD, Camp RC, Loeb P, Goyal RK (1976) The histologic spectrum of Barrett's esophagus. N Engl J Med 295:476–480
9. Ormsby AH, Goldblum JR, Kilgore SP, et al. (1999) The frequency and nature of intestinal metaplasia (IM) of the esophagogastric junction (EGJ): a population based study of 198 consecutive autopsies. Lab Invest 79:7A
10. Oberg S, Peters JH, DeMeester TR, et al (1997) Inflammation and specialized intestinal metaplasia or cardiac mucosa is a manifestation of gastroesophageal reflux disease. Ann Surg 226:522–532
11. Jain R, Aquino D, Harford WV, Lee E, Spechler SJ (1998) Cardiac epithelium is found infrequently in the gastric cardia. Gastroenterology 114:A160
12. Chandrasoma PT, Lokuhetty DM, DeMeester TR, et al (2000) Definition of histologic changes in gastroesophageal reflux disease. Am J Surg Pathol 24:344–351
13. Der R, Tsao-Wei DD, DeMeester T, et al (2001) Carditis: a manifestation of gastroesophageal reflux disease. Am J Surg Pathol (in press)
14. Jamieson JR, Stein HJ, DeMeester TR, et al (1992) Ambulatory 24-H esophageal pH monitoring: normal values, optimal thresholds, specificity, sensitivity, and reproducibility. Am J Gastroenterol 87:1102–1111
15. Blot WJ, Devesa SS, Kneller RW, Fraumeni JF (1991) Rising incidence of adenocarcinoma of the esophagus and gastric cardia. JAMA 265:1287–1289

Q & A after Dr. Chandrasoma's presentation

Dr. Kato (Cancer Institute of Tokyo, Japan): Specialized columnar epithelium is now considered by most pathologists as a kind of intestinal metaplasia. However, I have seen some of what is called SCE that does not show any mucous phenotype but still keeps the gastric mucin phenotype. Do you still think that SCE is a type of intestinal metaplasia?

Dr. Chandrasoma: If you analyze specialized columnar epithelium morphologically, it is actually cardiac mucosa that has developed goblet cells. The way in which cardiac mucosa develops goblet cells is different from gastric intestinal metaplasia based on mucin histochemistry and immunocytochemistry. Specialized columnar epithelium in the esophagus is defined as tissue with one or more goblet cells that prove to be alcian blue-positive and contain acid mucin in what looks like cardiac mucosa. Gastric intestinal metaplasia is different. It occurs in oxyntic mucosa or antral mucosa that has undergone atrophy in the elongated foveolar regions in which goblet cell metaplasia occurs. It occurs in relatively nonproliferative in active epithelium. Immunohistochemically, by using cytokeratins 7 and 20 you can differentiate between gastric intestinal metaplasia and SCE fairly accurately. From a diagnostic standpoint, this is not that important. It is important from the research standpoint, however. From the diagnostic standpoint, only a small number of our patients with cardiac mucosal abnormalities had any abnormalities in the distal stomach. Therefore when we see cardiac mucosa with intestinal metaplasia, wherever it is, we diagnose Barrett's esophagus. There is some suggestion that Barrett's epithelium undergoes specialized columnar epithelial metaplasia, or intestinal metaplasia, it develops colonic epitopes compared with the small intestinal epitopes that characterize gastric intestinal metaplasia. Moreover, there is an antibody called DAS-1, which tends to identify Barrett's epithelium but not gastric intestinal metaplasia. So there are differences between these entities that have not been completely studied.

Dr. Hölscher (University of Cologne, Germany): Regarding your new ideas about pathology of tumors of the gastroesophageal junction, as I understood it you said that subcardial carcinomas are reflux-induced, or are related to reflux. What are the differences from gastric carcinoma? As you know, for Barrett's carcinoma there is a male/female ratio of 8:1, and for subcardial carcinoma it is 2:1. How do you interpret these data?

Dr. Chandrasoma: They are difficult to understand. There are gender differences for cancers in long-segment Barrett's esophagus, which are male-dominated, and cancers in adjacent short-segment Barrett's, which have much lower male dominance. More important epidemiologic analysis is that the incidence of subcardial carcinoma is increasing as true distal gastric adenocarcinomas are decreasing. So are we dealing with two types of cancer (subcardial cancers progressing to Barrett's adenocarcinoma) or three types of cancer with three epidemiologies: distal gastric, subcardial, and carcinomas in the long segment of the Barrett's esophagus? The data are not clear. We are trying to identify the morphologic basis of these lesions. It is true that when you look at intestinal metaplasia that occurs in what looks like the proximal stomach or in the cardiac mucosa in the proximal stomach the gender difference is not as great as for cancers in Barrett's esophagus. We do not have an explanation.

Dr. Itabashi (Ibaragi Prefectural Central Hospital, Tomobe, Japan): I have seen a long fundic gland mucosa lining the lower esophagus. It showed up along cardiac mucosa in the lower esophagus. Do you include such cases with those in Barrett's esophagus or Barrett's epithelium? According to your presentation, you assigned grade III Barrett's esophagus to a group with cardiac mucosa with intestinal metaplasia.

Dr. Chandrasoma: Yes. I don't want to stress this too much because it is controversial, but we believe that cardiac mucosa is the first premalignant lesion in the development of adenocarcinoma. Because it is the first morphologically identified premalignant mucosa we use it to define reflux disease. Oxyntocardiac mucosa, for us, is not the epithelium that develops goblet cells. We have examined thousands of cases and never saw parietal cells and goblet cells in the same gland in the esophagus. So when oxyntic mucosa develops we believe it is a protective mechanism. Moreover, if you identify adenocarcinoma as an end result of the reflux disease, the first morphologically identified abnormality in that sequence is the cardiac mucosa, which we now call reflux disease. We use that information to treat our patients.

Dr. Itabashi: Sometimes it is difficult to determine where the GE junction is from the histological slides. I am a pathologist, and I identify the esophageal wall if I can see esophageal glands in the submucosa. What are your histological criteria for the esophageal wall?

Dr. Chandrasoma: The problem with using esophageal glands and squamous lined ducts is that they are not present consistently or throughout the esophagus. About 14% of our biopsies that have cardiac mucosa have squamous lined ducts, which clearly indicates that cardiac mucosa is in the esophagus. However, because glands are not present right to the end of the esophagus in all our cases, you can't use this criterion to identify where the esophagus ends. Therefore, you are left with criteria you must deduce rather than absolute criteria. I wish I had some method of differentiating the muscle of the esophagus as it becomes gastric muscle; and I wish I could say "this is esophagus" and "this is stomach." I think that submucosal glands and squamous lined ducts are accurate in a positive sense in that when you see them you know that you are in the esophagus. When you don't see them, though, it's not particularly useful because there are areas of the esophagus with no such glands.

Dr. Sarbia (University of Düsseldorf, Germany): As you pointed out, your definition of reflux esophagitis changes from clinical to pathological. According to your definition, I estimate that about one-half to one-third of the population has reflux esophagitis. Could you comment on this point?

Dr. Chandrasoma: The problem of reflux esophagitis is finding a control population. In the United States in a group such as this audience, if I measure the pH of the lower esophagus with a pH meter I will find that everyone has reflux. So reflux is present in virtually everyone other than people with achalasia. When Jamieson and DeMeester did the original study to determine the quantitative level of reflux that produces symptoms, they found it to be exposure of the lower esophagus to a pH of less than 4 for more than 4.5% of the 24-h period, which amounts to 64 minutes. Therefore you must have acid in the lower esophagus detected by a pH meter for 64 minutes every day before symptoms of reflux appear. Because the entire population has some element of reflux, it should not be surprising to have one-third to one-half of the population with evidence of reflux disease. In fact, I am surprised that it's not more. Actually, if you look at the morphologic evidence of reflux disease including oxyntocardiac mucosa, a small amount can be found in virtually everybody. We are developing a method for histologically identifying subclinical reflux. It should not surprise anyone that morphologic changes of subclinical disease are associated with universal reflux.

Histopathology of Early Neoplasia in Barrett's Esophagus

Jeremy R. Jass

Introduction

The evolution of early epithelial neoplasia in the lower esophagus occurs in three principal stages. Inflammation and ulceration due to chemical irritation caused by gastroesophageal reflux results in replacement of the squamous epithelium of the lower esophagus by a columnar epithelium showing intestinal differentiation. The columnar epithelial lining, or Barrett's esophagus, is classified as the long type when the segment is ≥3 cm or the short type when the length is <3 cm. The second stage is the development of focal or multifocal intraepithelial neoplasia (dysplasia) within Barrett's esophagus. The final stage is the emergence of an invasive (malignant) subclone spreading sequentially into lamina propria, muscularis mucosae, and submucosa. From the diagnostic perspective, critical issues are the diagnosis of Barrett's esophagus, the distinction between reactive change and unequivocal intraepithelial neoplasia, and the recognition of high-grade intraepithelial neoplasia requiring surgical intervention.

Barrett's Esophagus

Barrett's esophagus is lined by columnar epithelial cells that resemble the foveolar and surface mucous cells of gastric mucosa and a smaller, scattered population of intestinal-type goblet cells. The columnar cells secrete mainly neutral mucin, whereas the goblet cells secrete acid mucin, staining magenta and purple, respectively, with alcian blue-diastase periodic acid-Schiff (PAS). Paneth cells are absent or sparse. The hybrid gastrointestinal or "specialized" phenotype is confirmed by immunostaining with antibodies to mucin core proteins, as both gastric mucin MUC5AC and intestinal mucin MUC2 are expressed [1, 2]. Barrett's mucosa is therefore identical to incomplete intestinal metaplasia of gastric mucosa. As in the stomach, subtypes secreting sulfomucin may show a more selective association with neoplasia [3]. Carditis may be associated with *Helicobacter pylori* infection or gastroesophageal reflux. Complete

Department of Pathology, University of Queensland School of Medicine, Herston, Queensland 4006, Australia

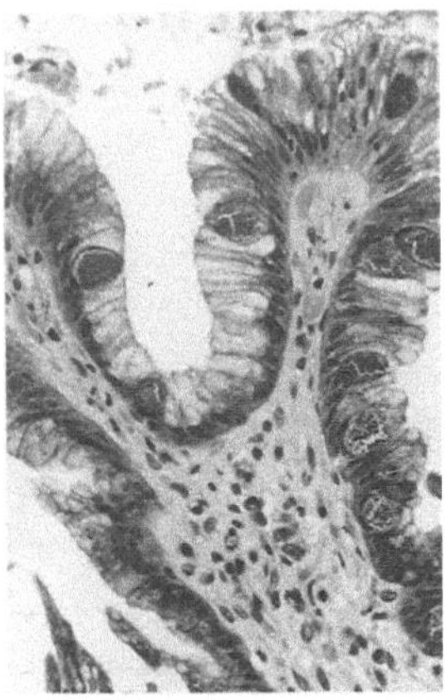

FIG. 1. Barrett's epithelium at high magnification showing columnar mucous cells and goblet cells covering villi. (H&E, ×400)

intestinal metaplasia in the cardia is a marker for *H. pylori* infection, whereas incomplete intestinal metaplasia is associated with reflux [4]. Therefore, it is the specific subtype of intestinal metaplasia rather than the simple demonstration of goblet cells that serves as a biomarker for gastroesophageal reflux disease.

Barrett's mucosa is recognized in hematoxylin and eosin-stained sections not only by the combination of columnar mucous cells and interposed goblet cells but by architectural changes including low villosity and an irregular crypt architecture comprising loss of parallelism, tortuosity, and branching. Squamous islands and ducts of submucosal esophageal glands (when present) confirm the esophageal site of biopsied columnar epithelium [5]. The lamina propria may be replaced by fibromuscular tissue, and surgical specimens reveal distinct splitting of the muscularis mucosae into two layers [6]. Mucin stains (alcian blue-diatase PAS) assist in diagnosing or confirming the presence of goblet cells, but scattered goblet cells are not pathognomonic of Barrett's esophagus. It is the overall architecture of the partially intestinalized (specialized) mucosa that allows the diagnosis to be achieved (Fig. 1).

Neoplasia in Barrett's Esophagus: Definitions in East and West

Genetic or epigenetic changes initiate Barrett's esophagus. The recent demonstration of abnormal methylation of multiple genes in large contiguous fields suggests either a concerted methylation change or clonal expansion of cells with methylated genes [7]. Based on cytokeratin phenotypes, it has been argued that Barrett's esophagus is not the result of upward spread by gastric mucosa but occurs through transformation of stem cells in the ducts of submucosal esophageal glands [8]. Despite these interesting genetic insights, the diagnosis of neoplasia is restricted to focal lesions characterized by abnormal differentiation, cytology, and architecture. Two terms have been used to describe early or noninvasive neoplasia in the gastrointestinal tract: adenoma and dysplasia. Adenoma refers to a well circumscribed, often polypoid lesion. Adenomatous cells show maturation arrest, and the cytoplasm is amphophilic owing to an abundance of RNA. Nuclei are crowded, elongated, pseudostratified, and darkly staining. Proliferative activity is maintained within superficial epithelium. Growth occurs mainly by crypt fission. Dysplasia arises in a background of chronic inflammation and refers to a flat, poorly circumscribed lesion in which the morphological changes range from those typical of adenoma to a variety of patterns (Fig. 2). Growth occurs by a combination of crypt fission and lateral intraepithelial spread.

The recognition of flat adenoma by Japanese endoscopists and pathologists blurs the distinction between adenoma and dysplasia. Many Japanese pathologists have little or no use for the term dysplasia. Lesions diagnosed as dysplasia in the West can instead be accommodated by three alternatives: (1) reactive or regenerative change; (2) adenoma (sessile and raised, flat, or depressed); and (3) intraepithelial carcinoma. Adenoma is regarded as an uncommon lesion in Barrett's esophagus [9], though a case might be made for interpreting circumscribed patches of adenomatous dysplasia as flat adenoma. Low-grade dysplasia (intraepithelial neoplasia) is still overdiagnosed though probably less frequently now than in the past. Most Western pathologists recognize an appearance that is clearly not reactive, falls short of carcinoma, and is unlike adenoma (Fig. 3). This lesion may be termed dysplasia or intraepithelial neoplasia, though many Japanese pathologists interpret high-grade intraepithelial neoplasia (and some low-grade intraepithelial neoplasia) as mucosal adenocarcinoma. Given the fact that the same treatment (surgical ablation) is required for high-grade dysplasia and intraepithelial carcinoma (carcinoma in situ), differences between Western and Japanese pathologists can be resolved by combining these terms

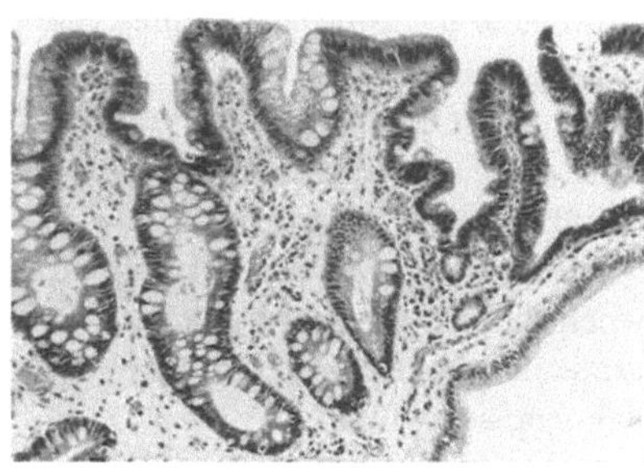

FIG. 2. Low-grade villiform intraepithelial neoplasia (dysplasia) in Barrett's esophagus. (H&E, ×100)

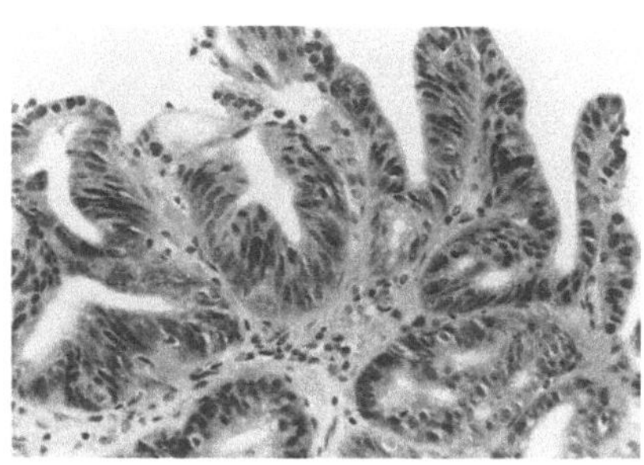

FIG. 3. High-grade intraepithelial neoplasia (dysplasia) in Barrett's esophagus. (H&E, ×200)

as high-grade noninvasive neoplasia [10]. Ironically, the more aggressive diagnosis (intraepithelial carcinoma) is treated by endoscopic mucosal resection in Japan, whereas surgical resection is the usual treatment in the West for a diagnosis of high-grade dysplasia.

Reactive versus Neoplastic Change

The distinction between reactive and neoplastic change in Barrett's esophagus can be difficult or even impossible in the presence of severe inflammation or erosion [11]. Intraepithelial neoplasia is an uncommon lesion, even in subjects with long-segment Barrett's esophagus, and may be overdiagnosed. It is generally unwise to diagnose intraepithelial neoplasia in the presence of active inflammation, acute erosion, and immature granulation tissue (Fig. 4). Reactive nuclei are enlarged and may be uniformly hyperchromatic or vesicular with some nucleolar prominence. Nuclear pleomorphism is not seen. Coarsening of the nuclear membrane, irregular chromatin clumping, marked nucleolar enlargement, and nuclear stratification are more suggestive of neoplastic change. With reactive change there is expansion of the proliferative zone, but cytoplasmic maturation, marked by the presence of apical mucin droplets, occurs superficially, and mitotic activity ceases. With neoplasia, maturation arrest and mitotic activity are seen superficially and in the crypt base. A particularly useful diagnostic criterion for neoplasia is an abrupt transition between neoplastic and non-neoplastic intestinalized crypts in which atypical and nonatypical cells are side by side. By contrast, reactive changes blend gradually with columnar epithelium with a clearly innocent appearance. Neoplastic change is accompanied by irregular budding and branching of crypts or deeper glands opening into the crypt base, generating crowded or back-to-back tubules. Gland branching is less marked in reactive or regenerating epithelium.

Special stains may be helpful for distinguishing reactive and neoplastic change. In reactive epithelium, mucin is demonstrated in the intracytoplasmic theca and is mainly neutral. In neoplasia mucin is acidic and expressed within the glycocalyx. Nuclear staining for p53 is rarely observed in nonneoplastic mucosa (Fig. 5) (except when there is associated neoplasia), but it occurs in 33% of biopsies showing low-grade intraepithelial neoplasia and 87% of biopsies showing high-grade intraepithelial neoplasia [12].

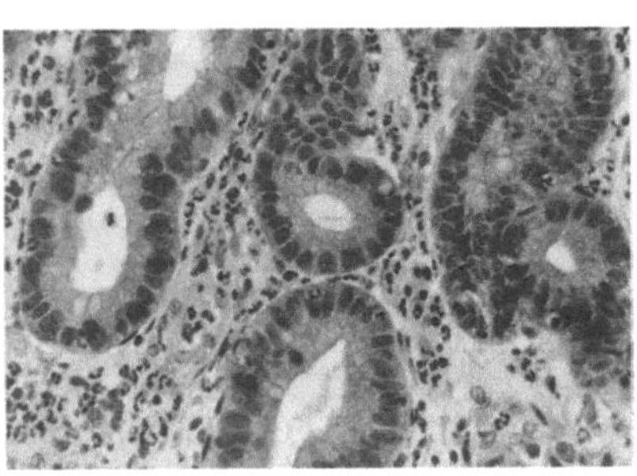

FIG. 4. Reactive epithelial changes in Barrett's esophagus. Neutrophils are conspicuous. (H&E, ×200)

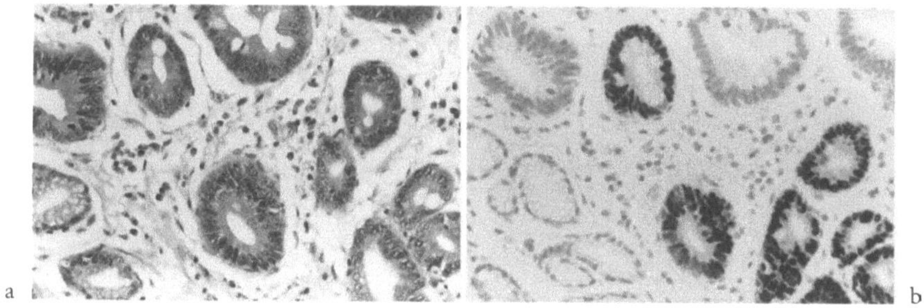

FIG. 5. Barrett's esophagus showing nuclear p53 expression in nondysplastic glands (adjacent to cancer—not shown). (**a**: H&E. **b**: p53 immunostaining, ×400)

Intraepithelial Neoplasia (Dysplasia) versus Carcinoma

Whereas the distinction between reactive and neoplastic change is a problem of histopathological interpretation that has important management implications, the distinction between intraepithelial neoplasia and carcinoma is more conceptual and semantic; difficulties can be minimized by careful clinicopathological correlation. Clearly a diagnosis of neoplastic change in a patient with unremarkable Barrett's esophagus has implications that are different from those of the same diagnosis in a patient with an ulcerated mass in the lower esophagus. With experience, the endoscopist may be able to target some early neoplastic changes by observing an ill-defined area of slight mucosal elevation with a velvety surface (a lesion that is midway between dysplasia and flat adenoma).

One conceptual difficulty with intraepithelial neoplasia rests on its uncertain clinical behavior. An intraepithelial neoplasm presenting as a circumscribed lesion or adenoma may progress to cancer over a period of years or not at all. Nevertheless, local excision of a circumscribed neoplasm is the usual practice if the procedure can be achieved with minimal risk of complications. Intraepithelial neoplasia occurring as a poorly circumscribed or multifocal change in flat mucosa is generally viewed as a more ominous lesion, particularly if the changes are graded as high. Levels of interobserver agreement for high-grade intraepithelial neoplasia are not perfect [13] but can be fine-tuned by consensus [12]. Confirmation of the diagnosis is an indication for surgical ablation on the basis that the likelihood of subsequent progression to invasive and potentially incurable malignancy is unacceptably high.

The surgical treatment of neoplasia attempts to balance the threat posed by the disease and the risks of surgical intervention. Radical surgery has traditionally followed a definitive diagnosis of cancer, and the main criterion for a diagnosis of gastrointestinal cancer has (in the West) been the demonstration of invasion. Adenocarcinoma in Barrett's esophagus is diagnosed when there is invasion of the lamina propria. Fibromuscular proliferation in the lamina propria is associated with glandular distortion that may mimic malignancy, particularly if glands are dysplastic [14]. In the absence of obvious infiltration by noncohesive cells, the distinction between high-grade intraepithelial neoplasia and intramucosal carcinoma can sometimes be difficult or impossible. To meet the semantic differences between East and West and

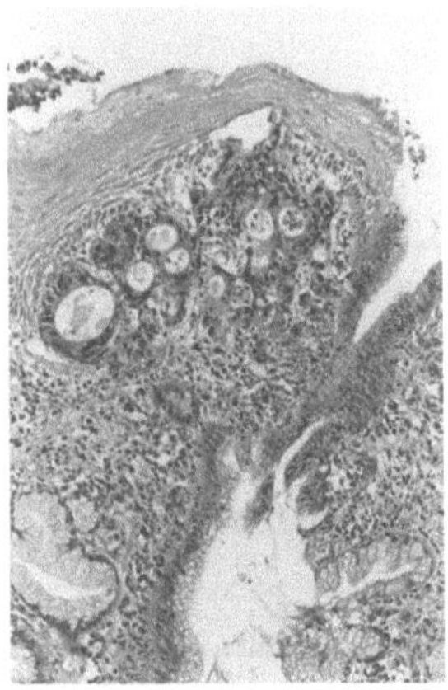

FIG. 6. Adenocarcinoma in Barrett's esophagus invading the squamous epithelium. (H&E, ×100)

the subjectivity associated with a diagnosis of early invasion, it has been suggested that the term "mucosal high-grade neoplasia" be introduced to encompass (1) high-grade intraepithelial neoplasia; (2) noninvasive or intraepithelial carcinoma (carcinoma in situ); (3) changes suspicious for invasive cancer; and (4) intramucosal carcinoma. Ablation (endoscopic mucosal resection or surgical resection) is required for all four categories of mucosal lesion, and the procedure of choice depends on the size of the lesion, the endoscopic or radiological assessment of the depth of invasion, the age and health of the patient, and local expertise [15].

By the time submucosal invasion has occurred, diagnosis by endoscopy, imaging, or pathology is relatively straightforward. Invasive adenocarcinoma is distinguished by the breakdown of normal architectural patterns, intraluminal necrosis or mucin (or both), stromal desmoplasia, and the cytological appearance of neoplasia, described above (Fig. 6).

References

1. Endo T, Tamaki K, Arimura Y, et al (1998) Expression of sulfated carbohydrate chain and core peptides of mucin detected by monoclonal antibodies in Barrett's esophagus and esophageal adenocarcinoma. J Gastroenterol 33:811–815
2. Labouvie C, Machado JC, Carneiro F, et al (1999) Differential expression of mucins and trefoil peptides in native epithelium, Barrett's metaplasia and squamous cell carcinoma of the oesophagus. J Cancer Res Clin Oncol 125:71–76
3. Jass JR (1981) Mucin histochemistry of the columnar epithelium of the oesophagus: a retrospective study. J Clin Pathol 34:866–870
4. Voutilainen M, Färkkilä M, Juhola M, et al (1999) Complete and incomplete intestinal metaplasia at the oesophagogastric junction: prevalences and associations with endoscopic erosive oesophagitis and gastritis. Gut 45:644–648
5. Takubo K, Nixon JM, Jass JR (1995) Ducts of esophageal glands proper and Paneth cells in Barrett's esophagus: frequency in biopsy specimens. Pathology 27:315–317
6. Takubo K, Sasajima K, Yamashita K, et al (1991) Double muscularis mucosae in Barrett's esophagus. Hum Pathol 22:1158–1161
7. Eads CA, Lord RV, Kurumboor SK, et al (2000) Fields of aberrant CpG island hypermethylation in Barrett's esophagus and associated adenocarcinoma. Cancer Res 60:5021–5026

8. Ormsby AH, Goldblum JR, Rice TW, et al (1999) Cytokeratin subsets can reliably distinguish Barrett's esophagus from intestinal metaplasia of the stomach. Hum Pathol 30:288–294
9. Thurberg BL, Duray PH, Odze RD (1999) Polypoid dysplasia in Barrett's esophagus: a clinicopathologic, immunohistochemical, and molecular study of five cases. Hum Pathol 30:745–752
10. Schlemper RJ, Itabashi M, Kato Y, et al (1997) Differences in diagnostic criteria for gastric carcinoma between Japanese and Western pathologists. Lancet 349:1725–1729
11. Lewin KJ, Appelman HD (1996) Atlas of Tumor Pathology. Tumors of the Esophagus and Stomach. AFIP, Washington, DC
12. Khan S, Do K-A, Kuhnert P, et al (1998) Diagnostic value of p53 immunohistochemistry in Barrett's esophagus: an endoscopic study. Pathology 30:136–140
13. Reid BJ, Weinstein WM, Lewin KJ, et al (1988) Endoscopic biopsy can detect high-grade dysplasia or early adenocarcinoma in Barrett's esophagus without grossly recognizable neoplastic lesions. Gastroenterology 94:81–90
14. Rubio CA, Riddell R (1988) Musculo-fibrous anomaly in Barrett's mucosa with dysplasia. Am J Surg Pathol 12:885–889
15. Schlemper RJ, Kato Y, Stolte M (2000) Diagnostic criteria for gastrointestinal carcinomas in Japan and Western countries: proposal for a new classification system of gastrointestinal epithelial neoplasia. J Gastroenterol Hepatol 15(suppl):C52–C60

Q & A after Dr. Jass's presentation

Dr. Rubio (Karolinska Institute, Sweden): Many years ago I worked with Professor Riddell, who described 29 patients with this type of desmoplastic stroma who underwent esophagectomy. They had high-grade dysplasia but no carcinoma. If we compare these data with yours, the incidence of desmoplastic stroma was about the same as what we see in the solitary rectal ulcer in the rectum. Even normal glands, which are surrounded by desmoplastic stroma, resemble highly differentiated carcinoma.

Dr. Jass: What you say may be correct because there is obviously going to be scarring in this condition where intense inflammation is driving these changes. One must test this possibility with samples we agree contain cancer and some that contain dysplasia falling short of cancer. It would be interesting to determine if such a study is useful. I found desmoplasia to be extremely useful in other conditions, particularly colorectal cancer, for distinguishing adenoma from dysplasia. It is a highly specific and sensitive marker, although it may not be in this situation. I am not aware of the details of the publication you described, but it is a question of testing these things. Until we test them in a large series of many observers, we cannot know their status.

Dr. Shimoda (National Cancer Center Hospitals, Japan): If the biopsy specimen taken from the esophagus contains squamous epithelium, it is easy to define the invasion. If squamous epithelium is replaced by Barrett's epithelium or columnar epithelium, however, can we define the invasion?

Dr. Jass: That is an important question. Can we actually diagnose invasion? What do we mean by invasion? It is quite obvious when there is very irregular architecture where many small groups of cells are moving into the lamina propria or the connective tissue; but when one has more differentiated glands, it is difficult to say if it is invasive or noninvasive. Although in the West we put invasion as the number one feature, in fact we do not have good criteria for determining if it is invasive or noninvasive. We rely on other criteria, such as cytology and architecture.

Dr. Shimoda: I think that in desmoplastic reactions we find the cancer exposure to the surface, but the cancer may not ulcerate the epithelium and mucosa. If the biopsy is obtained in this condition, we cannot define the desmoplastic reaction, but the cancer is invading the submucosa. How about the fact that desmoplastic reaction cannot be found in the cancer invading the submucosa, which maintains the overlying mucosa?

Dr. Jass: One has to test desmoplasia, and I think that it is not useful in the nonulcerating forms of early cancer. In fact, I would say that it is of no use, but I haven't tested it myself, so I don't know. It is just one of the features I would put on a list we might want to use to distinguish between reactive and neoplastic epithelium. It may not be useful for the lesions you mentioned.

Superficial Carcinoma of the Esophagus in Japan: Curable Lesion

Kaiyo Takubo[1], Tomio Arai[2], Motoji Sawabe[2], Koji Sasajima[3], and Ken-ichi Mafune[4]

About 20 years ago superficial carcinoma of the esophagus was rare, and reports of only single cases were presented at medical society meetings or in medical journals in Japan. Today superficial carcinoma has become much more common. We therefore describe recent clinicopathological findings for esophageal carcinomas in Japan, focusing especially on superficial lesions.

Esophageal carcinoma is the sixth most common cause of death due to malignant neoplasms in Japanese men, the rate being 4.5%; and in women esophageal carcinoma ranks eleventh among the common causes of death, although the rate is only 1.3%. In terms of incidence, the male/female ratio in Japan is about 5:1.

Guidelines for Clinical and Pathologic Studies on Carcinoma of the Esophagus and the Japanese Society for Esophageal Diseases

The book *Guidelines for Clinical and Pathologic Studies on Carcinoma of the Esophagus*, 9th edition, by the Japanese Society for Esophageal Diseases (JSDE) [1] describes how to handle fresh surgical materials, macroscopic and microscopic classification of esophageal carcinomas, definitions of the locations of carcinomas and the numbering of regional lymph nodes, group classification of lymph nodes based on the location of the primary carcinoma, staging of esophageal carcinomas, and clinical and histological criteria for assessing the effects of irradiation and anticancer chemotherapy. The Guidelines provide descriptions of the depth of tumor invasion, infiltrative

[1]Department of Clinical Pathology, Tokyo Metropolitan Institute of Gerontology, 35-2 Sakaecho, Itabashi-ku, Tokyo 173-0015, Japan
[2]Department of Pathology, Tokyo Metropolitan Geriatric Hospital, 35-2 Sakaecho, Itabashi-ku, Tokyo 173-0015, Japan
[3]First Department of Surgery, Nippon Medical School, 1-1-5 Sendagi, Bunkyo-ku, Tokyo 113-8603, Japan
[4]Department of Gastrointestinal Surgery, University of Tokyo Graduate School of Medicine, 7-3-1 Hongo, Bunkyo-ku, Tokyo 113-8655, Japan

growth pattern, absence or presence of intraepithelial spread, lymphatic and vascular permeation, intramural metastasis, lymph node metastasis, and multiple carcinoma. In most hospitals in Japan the clinical and pathological findings of patients with esophageal carcinomas are routinely recorded according to these Guidelines. This allows a comparison of detailed findings among institutions. An English version of the Guidelines was planned for 2001.

Comprehensive Registry of Esophageal Cancer in Japan (1988–1994)

The First English edition of the *Comprehensive Registry of Esophageal Cancer in Japan (1988–1994)* was issued by the Registration Committee for Esophageal Diseases of the JSDE (Chairperson H. Ide, Tokyo Women's Medical University) [2]. Both English (2000) and Japanese (1998) versions of this report have now been published. A total of 13 180 cases were registered from 1988 to 1994 from 166 institutions in Japan, and registration from these same institutions is continuing. For this book, analyses of clinical and pathologic findings of patients with esophageal carcinoma were performed on the basis of data recorded according to the JSDE Guidelines.

The incidence of the various histological types of primary esophageal malignant tumor among Japanese surgical cases was reported about two decades ago by Suzuki and Nagayo (1980). In Japan, among a total of 11 783 cases there were then 11 527 squamous cell carcinomas (accounting for 97.8%) and 256 other malignant tumors (2.2%) [3]. No reports on the histological classification of primary esophageal malignancies have described an incidence of squamous cell carcinoma any lower than 94%. Thus in Japan it is unusual to encounter esophageal carcinomas that include adenocarcinomas among the squamous cell carcinomas. Table 1 summarizes data for the reported incidence of adenocarcinoma among primary esophageal malignancies.

Table 1. Reported incidence of adenocarcinoma among primary esophageal malignancies

Study	% Adenocarcinomas
1988 Nagayo and Suzuki (Japan)	0.5 (surgical)–1.7 (Autopsied)
1991 Takubo et al. (Japan)	1.6
1991 Wang et al. (Taiwan)	1.6
1988 JSED (Japan)	1.2
1989 JSED (Japan)	1.5
1990 JSED (Japan)	0.8
1991 JSED (Japan)	1.1
1992 JSED (Japan)	1.4
1993 JSED (Japan)	2.2
1994 JSED (Japan)	1.6
1988 Yang & Dabis (USA, white men)	19.5
1991 Blot et al. (USA)	17.0

JSED, data from the Comprehensive Registry of Esophageal Cancer in Japan (1988–1994), 1st edn. Japanese Society for Esophageal Diseases, 2000

From 1988 to 1994, data from the Comprehensive Registry of Esophageal Cancer (JSDE) [2] showed an incidence of adenocarcinoma ranging from 0.8% to 2.2% in Japan. Taiwan reported similar data. In contrast, in Western countries the incidence of adenocarcinoma has recently been increasing and is now high, with occasional reports of more than 50%.

As to the outcome of esophageal carcinomas, Fig. 1 shows an analysis of crude survival following esophagectomy for 8321 patients with esophageal carcinoma, separated into five groups by the UICC-TNM classification according to disease stage, registered over the 5 years from 1988 to 1994 by the Registration Committee for Esophageal Diseases of the JSDE. Of the 8321 patients for whom follow-up data were available, 232 were stage 0, 1163 were stage I, 1918 were stage IIA, 1614 were stage IIB, 2381 were stage III, and 1003 were stage IV. The 5-year survival for stage 0 patients was 72.3%, stage I 63.1%, stage IIA 49.2%, stage IIB 32.1%, stage III 18.2%, and stage IV 12.1%. Stage 0 and stage I cancers are mucosal or submucosal carcinomas (i.e., superficial carcinoma) without lymph node metastasis using the previous definition of "early carcinoma" of the esophagus in Japan.

Definitions of Superficial and Early Carcinoma of the Esophagus

Figure 2 presents a schema for the definition of superficial carcinoma. Superficial carcinoma of the esophagus is defined in the Guidelines as carcinoma in situ or carcinoma involving the mucosa or submucosa (or both) regardless of the presence or

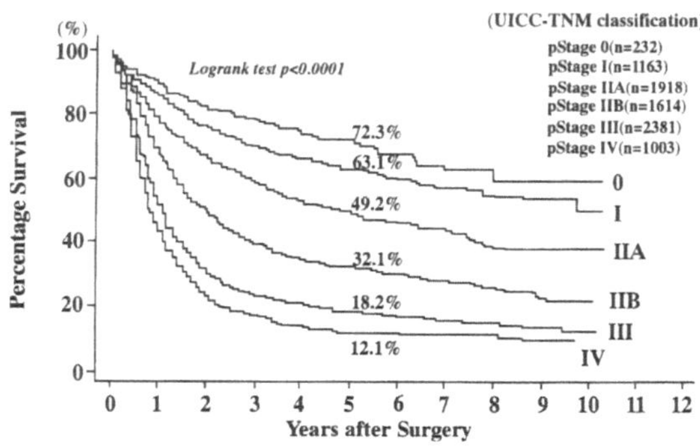

FIG. 1. Survival of patients treated by esophagectomy in relation to p stage. (Data from the Comprehensive Registry of Esophageal Cancer in Japan (1988–1994), 1st edn. The Japanese Society for Esophageal Disease, 2000)

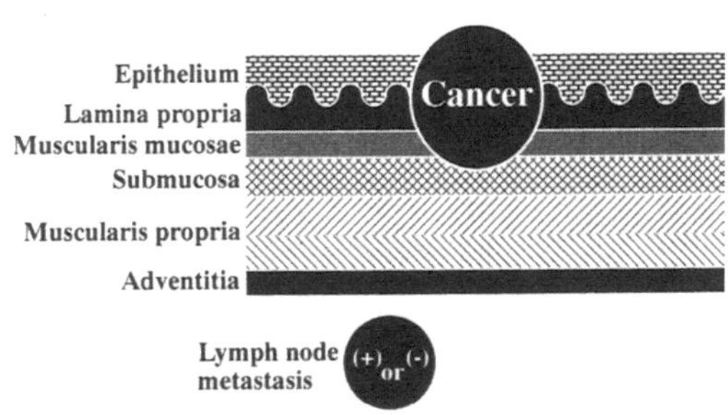

FIG. 2. Definition of superficial carcinoma in the *Guidelines for Clinical and Pathologic Studies on Carcinoma of the Esophagus*

absence of lymph node metastasis [1]. Superficial carcinoma can occasionally be distinguished from advanced carcinoma by macroscopic observation of the cut surface of the tumor or by determining whether a superficial tumor is fixed to the muscularis propria. If the tumor is not fixed, it slides over the muscularis propria when slight force is applied parallel to the mucosa [4].

The previous definition of early carcinoma in the Guidelines (8th edition, 1992) was defined as carcinoma in situ or carcinoma involving the mucosa or submucosa (or both) without lymph node metastasis; that is, the previous definition was superficial carcinoma without lymph node metastasis. Figure 3 shows the new definition of early carcinoma in the 9th edition of the Guidelines (1999). "Early carcinoma" of the esophagus is now defined as carcinoma in situ or invasive intramucosal carcinoma without nodal metastases, that is, intramucosal carcinoma without metastasis including carcinoma in situ [1].

Table 2 shows the incidence of superficial carcinoma among all surgically resected carcinomas in Japan from the Comprehensive Registry of Esophageal Cancer in Japan (1988–1994) [2]. In 1988 superficial carcinomas accounted for about 20% of all esophageal carcinomas, and in 1994 it was about 30%. The incidence of intraepithelial carcinoma (carcinoma in situ) was relatively constant, ranging from 2.0% to 3.9% between 1988 to 1994. The rate for carcinomas invading the mucosa (invasive mucosal carcinomas) has been increasing, from 2.8% in 1988 to 8.1% in 1994. The rate for carcinomas invading the submucosa has also been increasing.

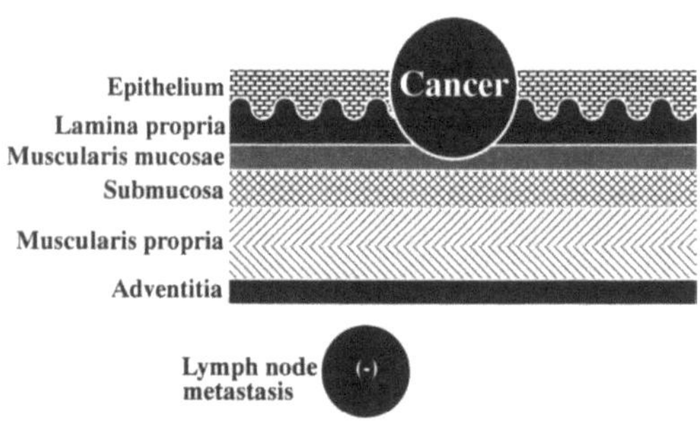

Fig. 3. New definition of early carcinoma. (From the *Guidelines for Clinical and Pathologic Studies on Carcinoma of the Esophagus*, 9th edn. Kanehara, Tokyo, 1999)

Table 2. Incidence of superficial carcinomas among surgically resected carcinomas in Japan

Year	Intraepithelial carcinoma (%)	Invasive mucosal carcinoma (%)	Carcinoma invading submucosa (%)	All superficial carcinomas (%)
1988	2.2	2.8	15.3	20.3
1989	3.7	5.1	14.7	23.5
1990	3.0	4.7	16.4	24.1
1991	3.9	7.5	17.3	28.7
1992	2.5	7.1	20.1	29.7
1993	2.4	8.2	17.8	28.4
1994	2.0	8.1	21.5	31.6

From the Comprehensive Registry of Esophageal Cancer in Japan (1988–1994), 1st edn. Japanese Society for Esophageal Diseases, 2000

Subclassification of Superficial Carcinomas of the Esophagus

Because of the mode of lymph node metastasis, superficial carcinomas have been divided into six groups according to the depth of tumor cell invasion in a proposal by a JSDE committee. In this proposal, the intramucosal carcinomas are divided into three groups: m1, m2, and m3.

m1: intraepithelial noninvasive carcinoma (i.e., carcinoma in situ)
m2: carcinoma invading the lamina propria
m3: carcinoma attached to, or invading the muscularis mucosae

The submucosal carcinomas (carcinomas invading the submucosa) are also divided into three groups: sm1, sm2, and sm3.

sm1: carcinoma invading the upper one-third of the submucosa
sm2: carcinoma invading the middle one-third of the submucosa
sm3: carcinoma invading the lower one-third of the submucosa

Table 3 shows the relations among the depth of invasion, vessel invasion, and lymph node metastasis for superficial carcinomas reported by Makuuchi et al. of Tokai University School of Medicine [5]. In Table 3, m1, m2, m3, sm1, sm2, and sm3 are the subclassifications in the proposal described above. Seventeen patients with carcinoma in situ had no vessel invasion or lymph node metastasis. Fifteen patients with carcinoma invading only the lamina propria and not extending to the muscularis mucosa also had no lymph node metastasis. One patient with carcinoma invasion to the muscularis mucosa had lymph node metastasis. There has been some debate about the latter category. Some pathologists (S. Ishiguro and M. Mano, Osaka Medical Center for Cancer and Cardiovascular Diseases, 2000, personal communication) think that there are problems associated with cutting after fixation in cases of carcinoma invading the muscularis mucosae and having lymph node metastasis. They believe that if the carcinoma were to be cut more carefully, it would reveal submucosal invasion.

Patients with carcinoma invading the upper one-third of the submucosa (sm1) may have lymph node metastasis, and this is the case for about 50% of those with carcinoma invasion of the middle one-third (sm2) or lower one-third (sm3) of the submucosa. Thus mucosal squamous cell carcinomas of the esophagus usually do not

Table 3. Relations among depth of invasion, vessel invasion, and lymph node metastasis in superficial carcinomas

Depth	No. of cases	Vessel invasion	Lymph node metastasis
m1	17	0	0
m2	15	0	0
m3	11	6 (55%)	1 (9%)
sm1	8	8 (62%)	2 (15%)
sm2	20	16 (80%)	8 (40%)
sm3	34	28 (82%)	15 (44%)

From Makuuchi H. et al. [5], with permission

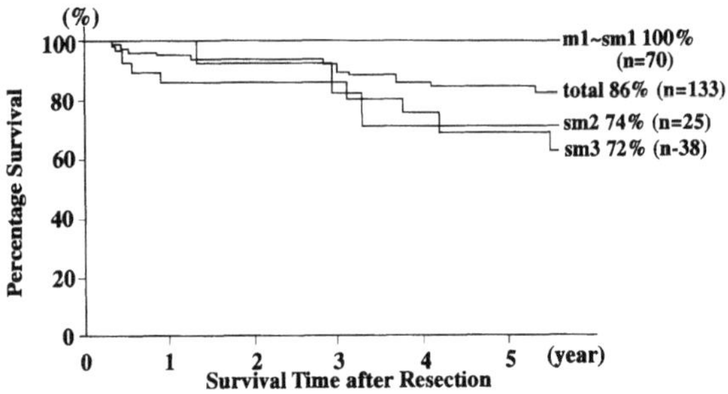

FIG. 4. Survival of patients with superfifical carcinoma of the esophagus treated by esophagectomy. (From Makuuchi et al. [5])

have lymph node metastasis. Reports from Japan giving similar results on the relation between depth of invasion and lymph node metastasis are appearing with some frequency. Therefore m1, m2, and m3 carcinomas are usually treated by endoscopic mucosal resection. Histological differentiation between m1 and m2 (carcinoma in situ or carcinoma invading the lamina propria) is not important clinically because neither carcinoma has lymph node metastasis and both are curable by endoscopic mucosal resection alone.

Figure 4 shows an analysis of the survival curve following esophagectomy in patients with esophageal superficial carcinoma, separated according to the subclassification of the depth of tumor invasion, reported by Makuuchi et al. [5]. All of the 70 patients with m1, m2, m3, or sm1 cancers survived more than 5 years. The 5-year survival rates for patients with sm2 and sm3 cancers were 74% and 72%, respectively. Yoshida (Tokyo Metropolitan Komagome Hospital) [6] has also reported that 111 patients with intramucosal carcinoma survived more than 5 years. Moreover, several groups from Japan have described many patients with intramucosal carcinomas surviving more than 5 years. Early carcinomas of the esophagus are now defined as carcinoma in situ or invasive intramucosal carcinoma without nodal metastases. Thus, early carcinoma by the new definition can be considered completely curable.

Conclusions

Carcinomas of the esophagus in Japan are usually of squamous cell type histologically. Other types of carcinoma, including adenocarcinoma, account for less than 3%. "Superficial carcinoma" has come to represent about 30% of all resected esophageal carcinomas in Japan.

Since 1999 "early carcinoma" has been defined as intramucosal carcinoma without metastasis in the Guidelines for Clinical and Pathologic Studies on Carcinoma of the Esophagus. By the new definition, early carcinoma accounts for about 10% of all resected esophageal carcinomas in Japan.

Among superficial carcinomas, most intramucosal carcinomas have no lymph node or distant metastasis, although lymphatic or venous permeation is observed. Intramucosal carcinomas can be considered curable by endoscopic mucosal resection alone. Major surgery is not necessary for patients with this type of carcinoma.

References

1. Japanese Society for Esophageal Diseases (1999) Guidelines for the clinical and pathologic studies on carcinoma of the esophagus, 9th edn. Kanehara, Tokyo, pp 1–58
2. Registration Committee for Esophageal Cancer of The Japanese Society for Esophageal Diseases (2000) Comprehensive registry of esophageal cancer in Japan (1988–1994), 1st edn. Japanese Society for Esophageal Diseases, Chiba, pp 19–39
3. Suzuki H, Nagayo T (1980) Primary tumors of the esophagus other than squamous cell carcinoma; histological classification and statistics in the surgical and autopsied materials in Japan. Int Adv Surg Oncol 3:73–109
4. Takubo K (2000) Pathology of the esophagus. Educa, Tokyo, pp 131–168
5. Makuuchi H, Shimada H, Chino O, et al (1997) Prognosis of early esophageal cancer; prognosis according to macroscopic and microscopic types. Rinsho Shokakinaika 12:1749–1756 (in Japanese)
6. Yoshida M (1997) Definition of early esophageal cancer. In: Makuuchi H, Yoshida M, Kouzu T (eds) Handbook of endoscopy on early esophageal carcinoma. Chugai-Igakusha, Tokyo, pp 34–37 (in Japanese)

Q & A after Dr. Takubo's presentation

Dr. Nakajima (Kyoto University Hospital, Japan): From the standpoint of the general surgical pathologist, it is difficult to divide the submucosa into three regions. I generally prefer to divide the submucosal layer into two portions: the superifical layer and the deep layer. That is more practical for me; and according to the clinical data, there is no difference between sm2 and sm3, so my impression is that it is clinically more relevant to divide the sm layer into two sublayers rather than three. What is your opinion on this point?

Dr. Takubo: We have offered a proposal, not a decision, so if you prefer to work with two layers, I see no problem. Could you show us the data on the depth of invasion into the submucosal layer when you divide it into two sublayers? Do you have data on the percentage of lymph node metastasis, for example?

Dr. Nakajima: My opinion is mainly based on your data.

Dr. Takubo: Oh, I see. Dr. Ishiguro measured the submucosal invasion by microscopy. Was it 0.4 or 0.2 mm? Dr. Ishiguro, could you tell us the definition of sm1?

Dr. Ishiguro (Osaka Medical Center for Cancer and Cardiovascular Diseases, Japan): Some pathologists in our country measured directly, with a few hundred micrometers defined as sm1. There are many definitions now, and we have yet to determine what is suitable.

Dr. Rubio (Karolinska Institute, Sweden): Talking about sm1, how many sections do you examine before you say that this is not sm2 or sm3? How many sections do you examine before discarding a diagnosis of deeper invasion?

Dr. Takubo: Usually we cut the specimen into 5-mm thickness, but the specimen for endoscopic mucosal resection is only about 2–3 mm. We cut the latter more carefully.

Dr. Chiba (Kyoto University, Japan): How many sections, generally speaking, do you look at to decide whether it is sm1 or sm2?

Dr. Takubo: You mean exact number? Usually we cut the surgical specimen into more than 100 sections. The materials from endoscopic esophagectomy are usually cut into more than 10 sections.

Part 2
Barrett's Esophagus and Adenocarcinoma

Histocytologic Criteria of Adenocarcinoma In Situ of the Esophagus

Carlos A. Rubio

Introduction

Nearly 200 years ago Schmidt [1] reported the occurrence of aberrant foci of gastric mucosa in the esophagus. In 1897 Rüdinger [2] also referred to several publications on aberrant gastric mucosa in the esophagus in the American, English, and German literature; and about 60 years ago, in 1941, Rector and Connelly [3] found aberrant gastric mucosa in 11.8% (n = 118) of 1000 esophaguses at autopsy. Thus, aberrant gastric mucosa and probably aberrant intestinal mucosa of the esophagus have been known for quite some time.

In later years adenocarcinomas originating in the so-called Barrett's mucosa have experienced a dramatic increased incidence in many Western countries [4]. The cause for that augmentation remains elusive. Enigmatically, a parallel increase has not occurred in Asian countries, including Japan.

Increasing Frequency of Esophageal Adenocarcinomas in Sweden

Sweden is a good example for the increased frequency in Western countries. In fact, of all esophageal carcinomas reported to the Swedish National Cancer Registry during a 6-year period (1975–1980), 17.8% (270/1512) were adenocarcinomas. Notably, 19 years later, of all esophageal carcinomas reported to the Swedish National Cancer Registry during a recent 6-year period (1993–1998) 31.3% (607/1942) were adenocarcinomas. When only the last year with available data (1998) was considered, esophageal adenocarcinomas accounted for 37.3% of all esophageal carcinomas in Sweden (129/346).

Between those two 6-year periods (1975–1980 and 1993–1998) the number of squamous carcinomas increased by only 93 cases, whereas the number of esophageal adenocarcinomas increased by 337 cases. Obviously, the increased number of esophageal

Gastrointestinal and Liver Pathology Research Laboratory, Karolinska Institute, 171 76 Stockholm, Sweden

carcinomas in Sweden during the latter 19 years has been mainly due to a dramatic rise in the number of adenocarcinomas.

Esophageal Adenocarcinoma In Situ in Sweden

Whereas in Japan pathologists consider adenocarcinoma in situ as carcinoma, Western pathologists regard high-grade dysplasia and adenocarcinoma in situ of the esophagus as similar lesions. Recently van Sandick et al. [5] postulated that "by definition, high grade dysplasia includes carcinoma in situ." That view probably summarizes the notion of many Western pathologists.

Against that background, it is understandable that much discussion has centered around the different histologic criteria applied by Western and Japanese pathologists [6] to differentiate dysplasia, carcinoma in situ, and adenocarcinoma. In the Western literature, low-grade dysplasia, high-grade dysplasia, and invasive adenocarcinomas are usually defined as "cellular morphologic changes and tissue architecture using previously established criteria" [5]. A review of the cited references indicates that neoplastic lesions were divided into low-grade dysplasia, high-grade dysplasia, and invasive adenocarcinoma. No reference is given to adenocarcinoma in situ (i.e., intraepithelial carcinoma) [4, 5, 7].

As stated above, a total of 129 patients developed adenocarcinoma of the esophagus in Sweden in 1998. Of those, 10.1% (13/129) were adenocarcinomas in situ. Interestingly, no adenocarcinomas in situ were reported between 1975 and 1980.

Criteria to Diagnose Esophageal Adenocarcinoma In Situ

The criteria used to diagnose adenocarcinoma in situ (i.e., intraepithelial carcinoma) of the esophagus at this hospital are presented. The diagnosis is based on several microscopic alterations. The characteristics of those alterations may be grouped into three main categories: architectural alterations of the crypts; intercellular epithelial alterations; and intracellular alterations.

Architectural Alterations of the Crypts

Alterations are found at the luminal or intraluminal aspects of the crypts. The most common architectural distortion of the luminal aspect of the crypts is the occurrence of papillary, villiform, or serrated structures. Those irregularities at the surface aspect are easily detected at endoscopic examination. The usual architectural alteration of the luminal aspect of the crypts is the occurrence of intraglandular bridging, resulting in cribriform crypts. Agglutinated, proliferating crypts usually display a back-to back arrangement.

Intercellular Aberrations

Intercellular aberrations are characterized by abnormal cell maturation (i.e., replacement of normal columnar epithelium by large immature neoplastic cells). Those cells

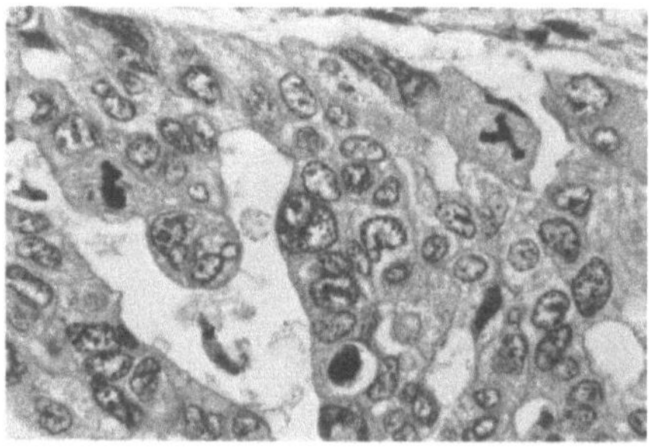

FIG. 1. Intercellular changes include large immature neoplastic cells, nuclear pleomorphism (anisocytosis, anisokaryosis, anisochromatosis), abnormal nuclear polarity, and focal increased number of mitotic figures in the superficial layers. Individual nuclear aberrations include large, irregular eosinophilic or basophilic (due to nucleolus-associated chromatin) nucleoli, irregular chromocenters in the nuclear area or along the nuclear membrane, chromatin bridges, and irregular nuclear membranes. (H&E, ×50)

also display pleomorphism. The latter is recognized by anisocytosis (cells of varying size), anisokaryosis (nuclei of varying size) and anisochromatosis (nuclear chromatin deposits varying among cells) (Fig. 1).

Normally, the maximal nuclear diameter of the nuclei is oriented at right angles to the epithelial–lamina propria mucosal border. This is connoted as normal nuclear polarity. In adenocarcinoma in situ, many nuclei (but not all) have lost their normal polarity (Fig. 1). We prefer the term nuclear polarity to cell polarity, as the cell boundaries are often difficult to identify in esophageal adenocarcinomas in situ. In addition, there is a focal increased number of mitotic figures that encompass the superficial layers of the aberrant epithelium (Fig. 1).

Nuclear Aberrations

The nuclear changes may vary in individual cells (Fig. 1). They usually include large, irregular single or multiple eosinophilic nucleoli or irregular single or multiple basophilic nucleoli (due to nucleolus-associated chromatin), irregular chromatin deposits (chromocenters) in the nuclear area or along the nuclear membrane, chromatin bands connecting those irregular chromocenters to each other (including those along the nuclear membrane) or to the nucleolus-associated chromatin.

The nuclear membrane is often irregular, jagged, and indented. Atypical mitoses are usually present in each of the five phases: prophase, prometaphase, metaphase (Fig. 2), anaphase, and telophase.

Other Alterations

Other alterations include glandular retention cysts (Fig. 3) due to obstruction of the outlet of the glands by proliferating neoplastic cells [8] and a musculofibrous anomaly [9] (Fig. 4), which is the result of the replacement of lamina propria mucosae by muscularis mucosae. That anomaly evolves following prolapse of the esophageal mucosa and leads to secondary fibrosis of the lamina propria mucosae. In small biopsy

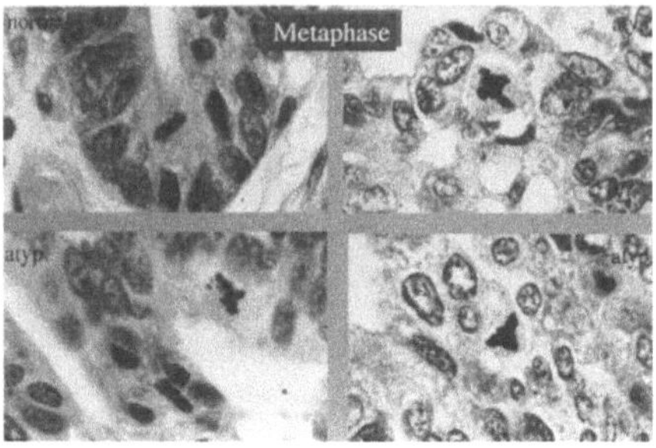

FIG. 2. Metaphases in Barrett's adenocarcinoma in situ. **Top left** Normal metaphase plate. The plate is at a right angle with the basement membrane. **Other quadrants** Note the atypical metaphases: four-polar with lagging chromosomes and tripolar. (H&E, ×125)

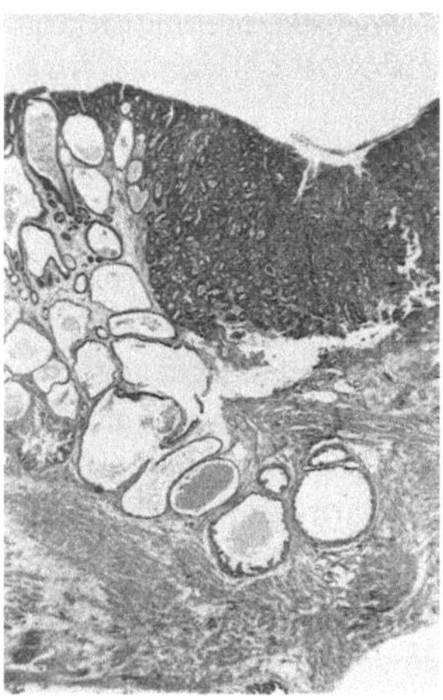

FIG. 3. Glandular retention cysts due to obstruction of the outlet of the glands by adenocarcinoma in situ cells at the top. (H&E, ×5)

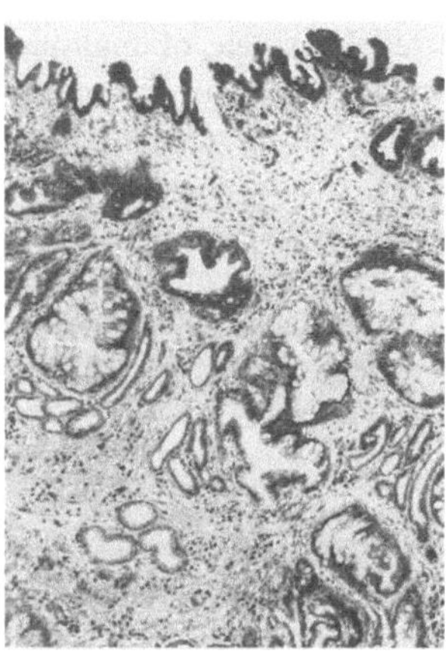

FIG. 4. "Trapped" glands surrounded by a musculofibrous anomaly. The latter is due to replacement of the lamina propria mucosae by the muscularis mucosa. Chronicity leads to secondary fibrosis of the lamina propria mucosae In small biopsies from a Barrett's esophagus, metaplastic glands, glands with dysplasia, or glands with adenocarcinoma in situ surrounded by that musculofibrous anomaly may erroneously be interpreted as invasive carcinoma [9]. (H&E, ×20)

specimens from a Barrett's esophagus, metaplastic glands, glands with dysplasia, or glands with adenocarcinoma in situ surrounded by that musculofibrous anomaly may erroneously be interpreted as invasive carcinoma [9]. A similar phenomenon has been described in the rectum as "solitary ulcer of the rectum."

Conclusions

Adenocarcinoma in situ of the esophagus is characterized histologically by architectural distortion of the crypts and intercellular and intracellular epithelial alterations. Atypical mitoses may be found at all phases of the mitotic cycle. Those changes distinguish adenocarcinoma in situ from high-grade glandular dysplasia. Other changes that may be found are large retention cysts and replacement of the lamina propria mucosae by the muscularis mucosae with secondary fibrosis.

In the recently published Vienna classification of epithelial neoplasias of the gastrointestinal tract, both high-grade dysplasia and adenocarcinoma in situ of the esophagus were listed in the same group (category 4) [6]. This was done because it was considered practical for management of the lesions. Category 4, however, was subdivided into category 4.1 high-grade dysplasia, category 4.2 carcinoma in situ, and category 4.3 suspicion of invasive carcinoma. Notwithstanding, the distinction between those neoplastic lesions is important if we aim in the future to correlate molecular events with the cascade of histocytomorphologic changes that take place in Barrett's mucosa during carcinogenesis.

Acknowledgment. Thanks are due to Mr. Mats Talbäck from the Center of Epidemiology, Cancer Registry, National Board of Health and Welfare, Stockholm.

References

1. Schmidt (1805) De mammalium oesophago atque ventriculo. Inaugural dissertation, in off. Bätheana
2. Rüdinger (1897) Beiträge zur Morphologie des Gaumensegels und des Verdauunsgsapparattes. Stuttgart, p 27
3. Rector LE, Connelly ML (1941) Aberrant mucosa in the esophagus in infants and in children. Arch Pathol 31:285–294
4. Muñoz N, Day NE (1996) Esophageal cancer. In: Schottenfeld D, Fraumeni JG Jr (eds) Cancer Epidemiology and Prevention. Oxford University Press, Oxford, pp 681–692
5. Van Sandick JW, van Lanschott JJ, ten Kate FJ, Offerhaus GJ, Fockens P, Tygat GN, Obertop H (2000) Pathology of early invasive adenocarcinoma of the esophagus or esophagogastric junction: implications for therapeutic decision making. Cancer 88:2429–2437
6. Schlemper R, Dawsey S, Itabshi M, Iwashita A, Kato Y, Koike M, Lewin K, Riddell R, Shimoda T, Sipponen P, Stolte M, Watanabe H (2000) Differences in diagnostic criteria for esophgeal squamous cell carcinomas between Japanese and Western pathologists. Cancer 88:996–1006
7. Reid BJ, Haggitt RC, Rubin CE, Roth G, Surawicz CM, van Belle G, Lewin K, Weinstein WM, Antonioli DA, Goldman H, MacDonald W, Owen D (1988) Observer variations in the diagnosis of dysplasia in Barrett's eophagus. Hum Pathol 19:166–178
8. Rubio CA, Riddell RH (1989) Mucosal cysts in the Barrett's mucosa with dysplasia. APMIS 97:297–301

9. Rubio CA, Riddell RH (1988) Musculo-fibrous anomaly in Barrett's mucosa with dysplasia. Am J Surg Pathol 12:885–889

Q & A after Dr. Rubio's presentation

Dr. Nakajima (Kyoto University Hospital, Japan): As I understand it, your histologic criteria for diagnosing esophageal adenocarcinoma in Barrett's esophagus are similar to those for adenocarcinoma for the stomach or other areas of the gastrointestinal tract. Is that correct?

Dr. Rubio: I think so. That's why I am quite anxious to hear what Dr. Kato is going to say about adenocarcinomas of the esophagus to see if we are in agreement.

Barrett Carcinoma and Esophagus: Experience in Japan, an Area of Low Incidence

Yo Kato[1], Hisanobu Tomimatsu[1], Akio Yanagisawa[1], Toshiki Matsubara[2], and Hiroshi Matsushita[3]

Introduction

The incidence of adenocarcinoma among cases of esophageal carcinoma is more than 30% in the USA and several European countries, and recently the incidence of Barrett carcinoma (BCa) in U.S. Caucasians appears to be increasing together with that of cardiac adenocarcinoma [1]. However, according to our search for resected esophageal carcinomas registered with the Japanese Society for Esophageal Diseases (JSED), the annual incidence of esophageal adenocarcioma, mainly BCa, among total esophageal carcinomas (mainly squamous cell carcinoma) was low and unchanged at 0.8%–2.2% over the 10 years from 1988 to 1997 [2, 3]. Even if cases are limited to tumors of the abdominal esophagus where most esophageal adenocarcinomas develop, the incidence of adenocarcinoma is around 4%. In this chapter, we report the clinicopathologic characteristics of BCa patients and lesions we have treated in two institutions in Tokyo, Japan, an area with a low incidence of the tumor, and then discuss the histologic changes with high risk for adenocarcinoma development in Barrett esophagus (BE), i.e., the columnar-lined mucosa of the lower esophagus.

Definition of BCa

We followed the classic definition: BCa is an adenocarcinoma located above the esophagogastric junction (EGJ), which should be diagnosed by stepwise sectioning of specimens containing the EGJ (Fig. 1) and by confirmation of remnant esophageal cardiac glands, multilayered glands, squamous islands, etc. (Figs. 2 and 3) in columnar-lined mucosa. If possible, the beginning of what is called the "sling fiber" (internal oblique muscle of the stomach) should be confirmed. The tumor location is determined based on the epicenter or predominant part of the tumor.

Departments of [1]Pathology and [2]Digestive Surgery, Cancer Institute, Japanese Foundation for Cancer Research, 1-37-1 Kami-Ikebukuro, Toshima-ku, Tokyo 170-8455, Japan
[3]Department of Pathology, Toranomon Hospital, Tokyo 105-0001, Japan

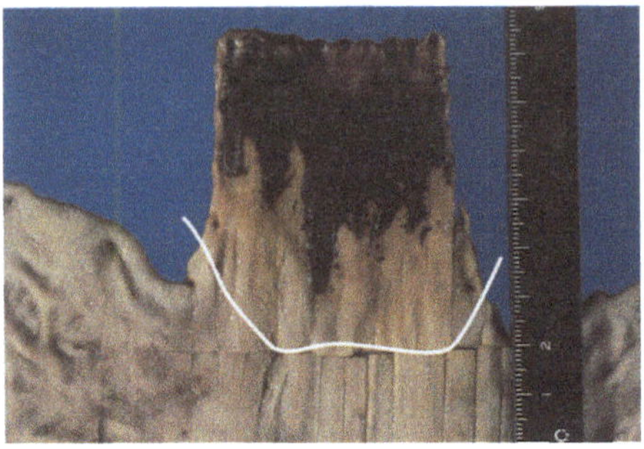

Fig. 1

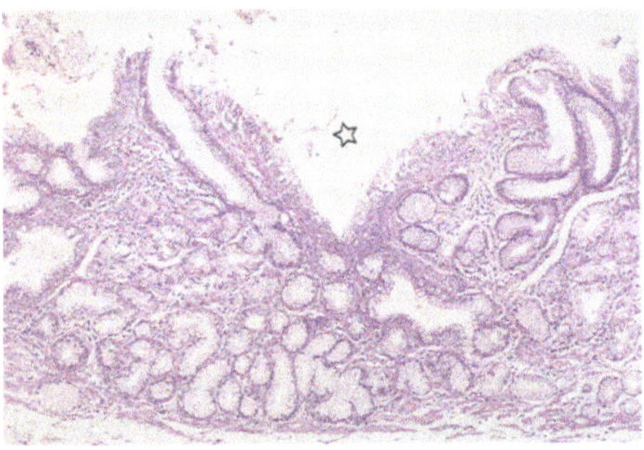

Fig. 2

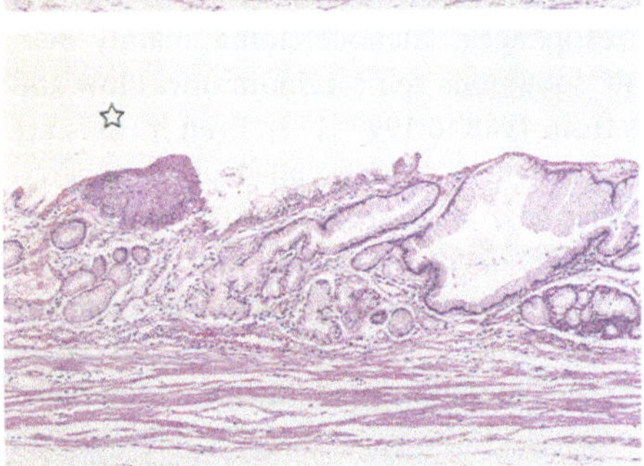

Fig. 3

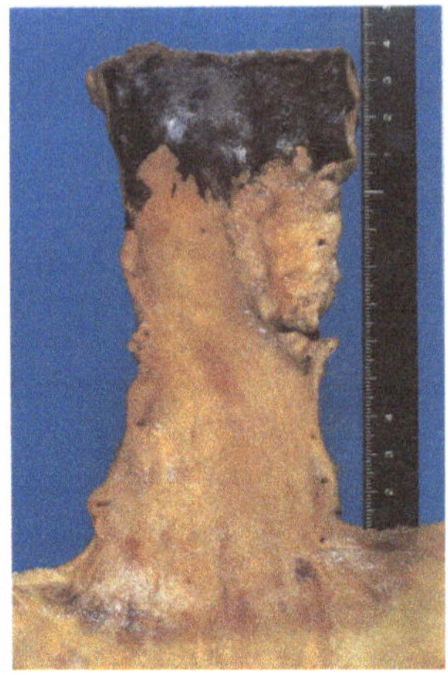

Fig. 4

Fig. 1. Esophagogastric junction (EGJ) should be determined by stepwise sectioning of the specimen. *White line*, EGJ (Lugol-stained specimen)

Fig. 2. "Multilayered gland," a gland with multilayered epithelium, suggesting a remnant of the proper esophageal gland, particularly of its duct (asterisk). ×10

Fig. 3. "Squamous island" in columnar-lined esophagus, i.e., Barrett esophagus (BE); a remnant of the esophageal squamous epithelium (asterisk). ×10

Fig. 4. A typical case of Barrett carcinoma (BCa) located orally to BE. Lugol-stained specimen

Clinicopathologic Characteristics of BCa

According to the above criteria, seven patients with nine BCas (including two cases of double cancer) were listed in the series of surgical cases in two institutions, the Cancer Institute Hospital (CIH) and Toranomon Hospital (TH), up to 1996 (Table 1). The incidence of BCa in the total number of esophageal carcinomas operated on in the CIH was around 0.4% [T. Matsubara, personal communication, 1999], slightly lower than the incidence of cases registered with the JSED. The rate of cases of multiple carcinomas was 29% (two of seven patients). The average age of the patients was 58 years and all were men. Most tumors were located in the abdominal esophagus, that is, in short-segment BE, and only one in long-segment BE. Six of nine lesions were superficial carcinomas, including five intramucosal lesions. Seven of the nine tumors were the well-differentiated type, and only two were moderately to poorly differentiated advanced lesions. All superficial carcinomas were the well-differentiated type, and all

TABLE 1. Clinicopathological data on seven cases of Barrett carcinoma (BCa)

Case	Age	Sex	Location	Gross	Grade of adenocarcinoma	Depth of invasion	Size (mm)
1	69	M	Ut	2	Moderately-poorly	a3	50 × 47
			Mt	0 (IIb)	Well[a]	m[a]	5 × 4
2	51	M	Lt-Ae	0 (I + IIa + IIb)	Well	sm2	30 × 28
			Ae	0 (IIc)	Well[a]	m[a]	16 × 15
3	63	M	Ae	0 (IIc)	Well	mp	21 × 15
4	51	M	Ae	0 (IIc)	Well[a]	m[a]	17 × 7
5	54	M	Ae-Lt	2	Moderately-poorly	a2	70 × 68
6	59	M	Ae	0 (IIc)	Well[a]	m[a]	10 × 8
7	58	M	Lt	0 (IIa)	Well*	m[a]	19 × 15

Ut, upper thoracic; Mt, middle thoracic; Lt, lower thoracic; Ae, abdominal esophagus; m, mucosa; sm2, middle 1/3 of submucosa; mp, muscularis propria; a2, deeper than shallow adventitia; a3, invading adjacent organ(s)

[a] These lesions correspond to "high-grade neoplasia" in the Vienna classification

TABLE 2. Circularity and length of BE and tumor location relative to BE

Case	Circularity	Length (mm)		Tumor location relative to BE
		Max.	Min.	
1	Total	58	40	In the middle of
2	Total	18	2	Oral to
3	4/5	10	2	Oral to
4	Total	22	6	Oral to
5	1/3	9	4	Oral to
6	2/3	13	3	Oral to
7	4/5	30	4	Oral to

the intramucosal carcinomas diagnosed by our criteria corresponded to "high-grade neoplasia" in the Vienna classification [4] (Table 1).

The circularity and length of BE were as shown in Table 2. Totally circular BE was found in three out of seven cases and the circularity of 4/5–2/3 in three of seven. Thus, in most of these cases, the BE involvement nearly surrounded the esophageal tube. However, the length of BE from the EGJ was estimated to be less than 30 mm in six of seven cases. Thus, most cases corresponded to short-segment BE and only one was compatible with long-segment BE. In general, the tumors were located orally to the BE (Fig. 4).

Mucin Phenotype of Tumors and Surrounding Mucosa

The mucin status of the Barrett tumors, surrounding mucosa, and tiny dysplastic lesions found incidentally was examined by conventional mucin staining (periodic acid-Schiff [PAS], Alcian blue, pH 2.5) and by immunohistochemistry for 45M1 (gastric mucin), Muc 2 (goblet cell mucin), and CD10 (absorptive cell brush border).

TABLE 3. Mucin typing

	Conventional staining		Immunohistochmistry		
Mucin type	PAS	AB (pH 2.5)	45M1[a]	MUC2[b]	CD10[c]
Gastric	+	–	+	–	–
Intestinal, incomplete	+	+	+	+/–	–/+
Intestinal, complete	+	+	–	+	+

[a] positive for foveolar neutral mucin
[b] positive for goblet mucin
[c] positive for brush border

TABLE 4. Mucin phenotype of carcinoma, surrounding mucosa, and dysplasia

	Mucin phenotype (CS)			Mucin phenotype (IHC)		
Case	Carcinoma	Surrounding mucosa	Dysplasia	Carcinoma	Surrounding mucosa	Dysplasia
1	I	I	I	I	I	I
2	I	G		G	G	
3	G = I	I		G	G	
4	I	I		I > G	I	
5	I	G	G	G	G	G
6	I	I	I,I	I	G	G > I,G > I
7	I	I		I	G	

CS, conventional staining such as HE, periodic acid-schiff, and antibody (pH 2.5); IHC, immunohistochemistry for 45M1, Muc2, and CD10; I, intestinal; G, gastric

The mucin phenotypes of the lesion and mucosa were determined by the staining patterns (Table 3) [5] and predominant mucin type.

As shown in Table 4, using conventional staining, most carcinomas were the intestinal type and many were surrounded by mucosa of the intestinal type, i.e., mucosa with intestinal metaplasia, particularly of the incomplete type. Only two lesions were surrounded by gastric-type mucosa. However, by immunohistochemistry three of the seven carcinomas were classified as the gastric type and many were surrounded by gastric-type mucosa. Only two lesions were surrounded by intestinal-type mucosa. A similar tendency was shown for the four incidentally discovered dysplastic lesions. The discrepancy in the results between conventional staining and immunohistochemistry may be because tumors or lesions of the incomplete intestinal type in BE contain more gastric mucin than expected, yielding strong positivity for gastric mucin on immunohistochemical staining (Fig. 5a–d).

p53 Immunostaining of Tumors and Surrounding Mucosa

p53 Immunostaining was performed using the monoclonal antibody DO-7 and streptavidin-biotinylated antibody (SAB) method. When the nuclei of tumor cells were continuously and diffusely positive, the tumor was considered positive, and the

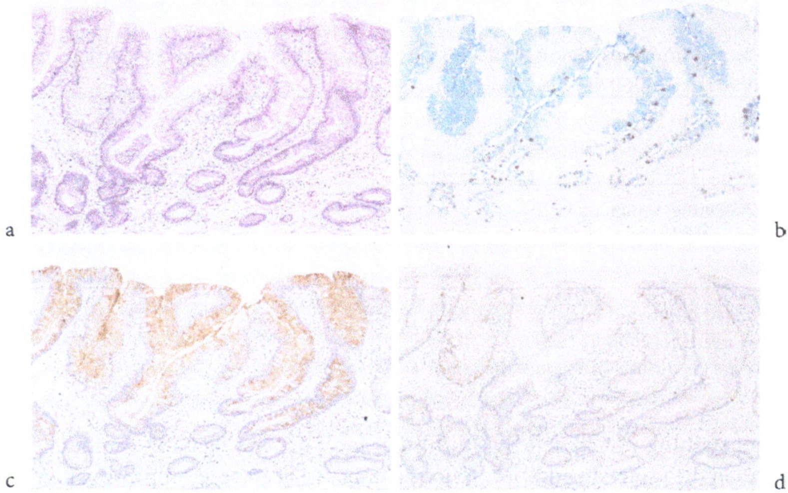

FIG. 5. Mucin status of surrounding mucosa, i.e., the mucosa surrounding BCa. **a** Typical "specialized columnar epithelium" with many goblet cells. HE stain. **b** Alcian blue staining at pH 2.5 is strongly positive. The incomplete intestinal type is suggested by mucin status. **c** Immunohistochemistry (IHC) for 45M1 (gastric mucin) is strongly positive. **d** IHC for MUC2 (goblet cell mucin) is negative. Thus, the mucosa has the gastirc-type mucin status based on mucin IHC

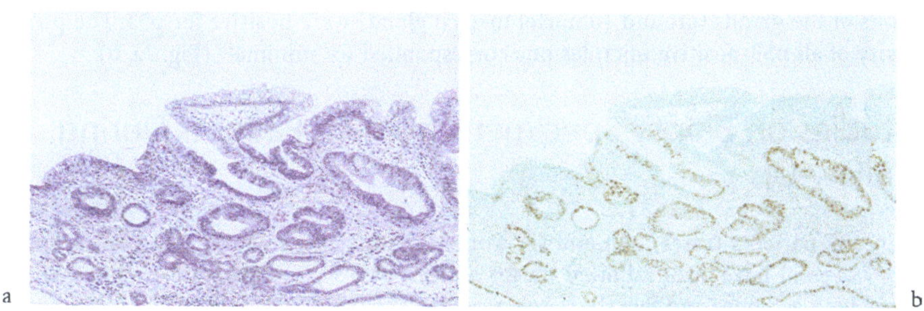

FIG. 6. p53 immunostaining for mucosal carcinoma, very well-differentiated carcinoma (case 6). (from [6]) **a** HE staining. **b** p53 immunostaining. Nuclei are continuously and diffusely positive throughout the lesion

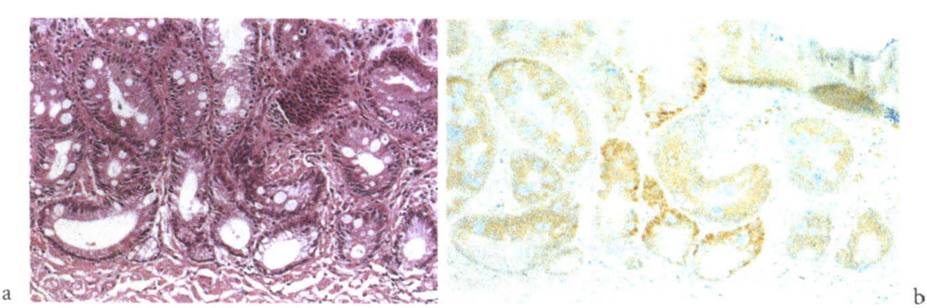

FIG. 7. A p53-positive microlesion found in BE (case 1). (From [6]) **a** HE staining. Glands correspond to the incomplete intestinal type. **b** p53 immunostaining. Four glands are positive

TABLE 5. p53 Immunostaining results for carcinoma, dysplasia, and p53-positive microlesions found in BE (7 surgical cases)

Rate of p53 (+) lesion	Carcinoma ($n = 7$) 57.1% (4/7)	Dysplasia ($n = 4$) 75.0% (3/4)	p53-Positive microlesions ($n = 5$)
Grade of staining: minimal[a]	0	1	5
focal[b]	0	2	0
diffuse[c]	4	0	0

[a] Only limited number of nuclei are positive in glands
[b] Positive area is focal in the tumor
[c] Positive area is diffuse throughout the tumor

grade of staining was classified as diffuse or focal depending on the amount of positive area in the tumor. In addition, lesions composed of 10 or fewer p53-positive glands in the Barrett mucosa were classified as "p53-positive microlesions." Glands with sporadically positive nuclei were not considered positive. As a result, five microlesions were detected in four of the seven cases.

As shown in Table 5, four (57.1%) of seven carcinomas, and three (75%) of four dysplasias were positive for p53 staining. All p53-positive carcinomas showed diffuse positivity throughout the tumor (Fig. 6a, b). However, of three p53-positive dysplasias, two presented focal positivity and one minimal positivity in which only limited portions of the glands (around 10 nuclei in each gland) were positive for p53. The positivity of all p53-positive microlesions corresponded to "minimal" (Fig. 7a, b).

Studies on Biopsy Specimens from BE Patients During Follow-Up

Nine BE patients (three men and six women) with a mean age of 64.4 years (range 45–78 years) have been followed up for a mean of 2.5 years (range 1–6 years). Four have long-segment and five short-segment BE. The length of the BE has not changed during the follow-up period. Forty-three biopsy specimens, consisting of 23 gastric- and 20 intestinal-type mucosa, have been examined. Neither dysplasia nor a p53-positive lesion has so far been detected.

Discussion

According to Nishi et al., who reviewed 81 Japanese cases of BCa from the literature published over 13 years (1973–1985), the average patient age was 60.3 years, the male/female ratio was 3/1, most lesions were the superficial type (the depth of tumor invasion is limited to the submucosa), the average tumor size was 3.6 cm, and the histological type was mostly well-differentiated [7]. Our data are comparable with the report of Nishi et al., except that all patients in our series are men. Reports from Western countries list the following as characteristic of adenocarcinoma of the esophagus: a high preponderance of male patients; a higher incidence among Caucasians; and an average age at the time of diagnosis of approximately 65 years [8]. It appears that typical esophageal squamous cell carcinoma in Japan has at least the first and third characteristics.

Most of our BE patients have short-segment disease. In Western countries, short-segment BE also predominates, but the risk of developing adenocarcinoma is reported to be higher in long-segment than in short-segment BE [9]. There does not appear to be a major difference between Japanese and Western patients in terms of tumor location, that is, most tumors develop in the proximal verge of BE [10]. It is interesting that the advancing area of reflux esophagitis is at higher risk for the development of dysplasia or carcinoma, and this finding is referred to as the "seashore phenomenon."

The mucin phenotype of most of tumors and surrounding mucosa was the intestinal type, particularly the incomplete type, in our patient series. These findings are consistent with those previously reported [11]. However, it is interesting that the gastric phenotype is more frequently seen using immunohistochemistry than with conventional staining. Two of seven cases using conventional staining, and five of seven cases with immunohistochemistry were surrounded by gastric-type mucosa. This is understandable when a tumor or lesion of the incomplete intestinal type contains more gastric mucin than expected. Therefore, it is unreasonable to designate only the metaplastic mucosa as Barrett mucosa or epithelium.

p53 Mutation is the best characterized somatic alteration found in human tumors, and it is reported that 60% of BCa cases exhibit this mutation [12]. By immunohistochemistry, nearly 60% of our cases showed p53 overexpression, and the data were comparable with the results of genetic analysis. Five p53-positive microlesions occurred in seven cases, for a rate of 0.7/case. The rate is lower than 3.7/case in the stomach with severe intestinal metaplasia [K. Aizu and Y. Kato, unpublished data, 2000]. However, considering the number of specimens examined, the rate could be four or five times higher, that is, 2.8 or 3.5/case, or almost the same as in the stomach with severe intestinal metaplasia.

In our follow-up study of BE aptients, no histologically atypical changes, including p53-positive microlesions, have been noted in biopsy specimens. Most cases of BCa are associated with intestinal metaplasia, including specialized columnar epithelium, and nonmetaplastic columnar epithelium should not be called BE. However, since at least 30% of carcinomas in our series were surrounded by nonmetaplastic mucosa and 20% of cases in the West are associated with nonmetaplastic mucosa [8], our practice is to follow up patients irrespective of the presence or absence of intestinal metaplasia. The significance of the presence of p53-positive glands in the columnar-lined mucosa during follow-up remains to be clarified.

Conclusion

Seven cases of BCa developing in Japan, an area with a low incidence of the disease, were compared with cases in Western countries. No significant difference was found in terms of clinicopathologic characteristics. Since most of the carcinomas developed in the proximal verge of BE, the advancing area of reflux esophagitis can be at high risk for the development of dysplasia or adenocarcinoma due to the seashore phenomenon. At least 30% of the tumors in our series were surrounded by nonmetaplastic mucosa, and 20% of cases in Western countries are associated with nonmetaplastic mucosa. Therefore our practice is to follow up BE patients irrespective of the presence or absence of intestinal metaplasia. The significance of p53-positive glands in the columnar-lined mucosa on follow-up remains to be clarified.

Acknowledgment. We thank Miss Junko Okazaki for typing the manuscript.

References

1. Blot WJ, Devesa SS, Kneller RW, et al (1991) Rising incidence of adenocarcinoma of the esophagus and gastric cardia. JAMA 265:1287–1289
2. Japanese Society for Esophageal Diseases (1998) Annual statistics of Esophageal Cancer Registered (cases of 1988–1994) (in Japanese). Japanese Society for Esophageal Diseases
3. Japanese Society for Esophageal Diseases (2001) Annual statistics of esophageal cancer registered (cases of 1995–1997) (in English). Japanese Society for Esophageal Diseases
4. Schlemper RJ, Riddel RH, Kato Y, et al (2000) The Vienna classification of gastrointestinal epithelial neoplasia. Gut 47:251–255
5. Koseki K, Takizawa T, Koike M, et al (1999) Subclassification of well-differentiated gastric cancer with reference of biological behavior and malignancy, gastric type vs intestinal type, and papillary carcinoma vs tubular carcinoma. Stomach Intestine 34: 507–512 (Japanese with English abstract)
6. Tomimatsu H, Kato Y, Sakai Y, et al (1999) Clinicopathological study on Bavretl's cancer with analysis of its precancerous state. Gastroenterology 28:42–50 (Japanese)
7. Nishi T, Makuuchi H, Machimura T, et al (1995) A small adenocarcinoma arising in Barrett esophagus—A case report. Endoscopia Digestiva 7:557–563 (Japanese with English abstract)
8. Siewert JR, Stein HJ (1998) Classification of adenocarcinoma of the esophagogastric junction. Br J Surg 85:1457–1459
9. Sharma P, Morales T, Bhattacharrya A, et al (1997) Dysplasia in short segment Barrett's esophagus: a prospective 3-year follow up. Am J Gastroenterol 92:2012–2016
10. Werner M, Flejou JF, Hainaut P, et al (2000) Adenocarcinoma of the esophagus. In: Hamilton SR and Aaltonen LA (eds) WHO classification. Tumours of the digestive systems. IARC, Lyon, pp 20–26
11. Rogers EL, Goldkind SF, Iseri OA, et al (1986) Adenocarcinoma of the lower esophagus. A disease primarily of white men with Barrett's esophagus. J Clin Gastroenterol 8:613–618
12. Ireland AP, Clark GW, Demeester TR (1997) Barrett's esophagus. The significance of p53 in clinical practice. Ann Surg 225:17–30

Q & A after Dr. Kato's presentation

Dr. Jass (University of Queensland, Australia): I was interested that your illustration was similar to mine. You showed *p*53 in nondysplastic glands exclusively from patients who had dysplasia or cancer elsewhere. Hence the change in a nondysplastic gland seems to be a some kind of marker of increased risk of neoplasia. Can you comment on that?

Dr. Kato: I have the same suspicions. We saw it in some definite neoplastic lesions and a *p*53 overexpression focus here and there in the Barrett mucosa with Barrett carcinoma; but in the follow-up case, unfortunately, we saw no such lesions.

Barrett's Esophagus and Adenocarcinoma: Surgical Results of Superficial Adenocarcinoma of the Esophagus

Arnulf H. Hölscher, Elfriede Bollschweiler, Futoshe Myazono, Christian Gutschow, Hartmut Schäfer, and Wolfgang Schröder

Introduction

Adenocarcinoma of the esophagus is of topical importance as a strong increase in the incidence of this entity has been observed in North America and Europe [1]. Most adenocarcinomas develop in a columnar cell-lined lower esophagus that is due to chronic gastroesophageal reflux. Early detection of Barrett's adenocarcinoma is difficult because the symptoms of patients with superficial carcinoma are uncharacteristic and rare [2]. Early detection is possible by endoscopic surveillance programs of patients with Barrett's esophagus [3, 4], although the histological criteria, especially for mucosal esophageal or gastric adenocarcinoma, are controversial between Western and Japanese pathologists [5].

Early esophageal cancer is defined as a tumor limited to the mucosa or submucosa and consequently offers favorable prerequisites for complete healing after surgical resection [6]. Most previous series of esophageal pathological tumor stage pT1 adenocarcinoma included carcinoma of the cardia or were too small for a representative analysis of clinicopathological characteristics and long-term outcome [7–11]. We report a larger series of patients who had undergone resection of early esophageal adenocarcinoma [2]. The purpose of this study was to analyze the rate of multicentricity and lymph node involvement and to evaluate the prognosis according to the depth of tumor infiltration and the presence of lymphatic metastasis.

Clinical Results

Adenocarcinoma of the esophagus was defined as a tumor centered more than 1 cm above the anatomical cardia according to preoperative endoscopy and radiography and postoperative examination of the resected specimen [12, 13]. Patients whose lesions were staged as pT1 after preoperative radiotherapy or chemotherapy (or both) were excluded [6]. Routine preoperative staging included endoscopy, percutaneous ultrasonography, computed tomography, and endoscopic ultrasonography.

Department of Visceral and Vascular Surgery, University of Cologne, Joseph-Stelzmann-Strasse 9, 50931 Köln, Germany

Histopathological examination of all resected specimens consisted of a thorough evaluation of tumor stage, residual tumor (R category), grading, and the number of resected and involved lymph nodes. The ratio of the number of infiltrated to resected lymph nodes was termed the lymph node ratio [13]. The pT1 tumors were further subclassified as pT1a (limited to the mucosa) or pT1b (limited to the submucosa) [14]. The median duration of follow-up of the whole series was 5.5 years (range 0.7–12.9 years). The median age of the patients was 60 years (range 28–82 years). The male/female ratio was 8:1.

The treatment of choice for early adenocarcinoma of the distal esophagus was transhiatal radical subtotal esophagectomy and partial gastrectomy [13, 15–17], which included widely incising the diaphragm from in front of the esophageal hiatus and exposing the lower mediastinum by inserting two long hooks. The periesophageal tissue of the lower mediastinum between the pericardium and aorta was resected in continuity with the esophagus. The proximal two-thirds of the lesser curvature of the stomach was removed by linear stapler up to the uppermost point of the fundus. In addition to this partial lymphadenectomy of compartment I, complete lymphadenectomy of compartment II was added [15, 18, 19]. Three patients with proximal extension of Barrett's epithelium and adenocarcinoma in the mid or upper thoracic portion of the esophagus underwent transthoracic en bloc esophagectomy with extended mediastinal lymphadenectomy [15]. After both types of resection the reconstruction was made with a 4–5 cm wide gastric tube fashioned along the greater curvature [13]. The stomach interposition was placed in the posterior mediastinum, and all anastomoses were performed in the neck.

Some 28 of 41 patients were symptomatic, whereas 13 were asymptomatic (Table 1). Of the 13 asymptomatic patients, 8 underwent endoscopy during the course of a regular surveillance program for Barrett's esophagus. The adenocarcinomas detected by this program included six mucosal and two submucosal tumors.

Postoperative surgical and general complications occurred in 18 of the 41 patients; one patient died within 30 days of operation and another within 90 days (4.8% mortality). In all cases complete resection (R0) of the tumor was achieved. On average, 23 (range 10–48) lymph nodes were removed. Some 36 early adenocarcinomas had developed in a columnar cell-lined lower esophagus, as proven by endoscopy and histology, with a minimum length of 3 cm. The mean length of Barrett's esophagus in these 36 patients was 6.3 cm (range 3–15 cm). The mean maximum extent of all pT1 carci-

TABLE 1. Symptoms of 41 patients with superficial adenocarcinoma of the esophagus

Symptoms	No.
Symptomatic (68%)	28
Dysphagia	10
Epigastric pain	10
Retrosternal pressure	4
Other symptoms	4
Asymptomatic (32%)	13
Endoscopic surveillance program of Barrett's esophagus	8
Endoscopy for other reasons	5

nomas was 2.5 cm (0.1–8.0 cm). In 10 of the 41 patients the carcinoma was limited to the mucosa (pT1a) including three patients with slight encroachment of the muscularis mucosae (m3 according to the Japanese classification) (Table 2). Altogether, 31 patients had infiltration of the submucosa (pT1b). In 6 cases there was multicentric tumor development in Barrett's esophagus on histology; 28 cases showed high-grade dysplasia within the specialized epithelium, and 13 had low-grade dysplasia. Histological grading identified 5 G1, 26 G2, and 9 G3 tumors; there was 1 G4 tumor.

No patient with mucosal adenocarcinoma had lymph node metastasis; all patients with lymphatic spread had submucosal infiltration (Table 2). The localization and infiltrated/removed lymph node ratio for the five pN1 cases is shown in Table 3. On average, 19% of the removed lymph nodes were infiltrated for the pN1 carcinomas. Regional lymph nodes were involved in four cases (paraesophageal, paracardial, or lesser curvature), and in one patient a cervical lymph node was also infiltrated (pT1N1M1). Two patients had second primary cancers: One underwent thyroidectomy for papillary thyroid carcinoma 18 months before esophagectomy, and the other developed squamous cell cancer of the lung 11 years after esophagectomy.

The causes of death during long-term follow-up were postoperative mortality in two patients and distant metastases in four. Some 83% [95% confidence interval (CI) 80%–85%] of the group of 41 patients with esophageal adenocarcinomas survived for 5 years (Fig. 1). There was a limited number of cases in the subgroups, and no significant differences were found between the survival curves of patients with mucosal or submucosal infiltration (5-year survival: 100% versus 79%) (Fig. 2). Patients in the pN0 and pN1 categories had survival rates of 81% and 50%, the difference was also not significant (Fig. 3). All patients with carcinoma detected during the course of endoscopic surveillance have survived disease-free for 1.2, 1.3, 1.7, 4.1, 4.3, 5.9, 8.1, and 12.2 years after esophagectomy. For patients without a diagnosis by endoscopic surveillance, the 5-year survival rate was 79%.

TABLE 2. Lymph node metastases in patients with mucosal or submucosal infiltration with esophageal adenocarcinoma ($n = 41$)

Site of adenocarcinoma	No.	pN1 (%)
Mucosa	10	0
Submucosa	31	16

TABLE 3. Lymph node metastases from five adenocarcinomas

Lymph node ratio (infiltrated LNs/ removed LNs)	Site of infiltrated LN	Site of adenocarcinoma
2/12	Paracardial	Lower esophagus
1/10	Paraesophageal	Mid-esophagus
3/13	Paraesophageal (2), paracardial (1)	Lower esophagus
1/41	Left gastric artery	Lower esophagus
7/17	Left gastric artery (5), paracardial (1), cervical (1)	Lower esophagus

LN, lymph nodes

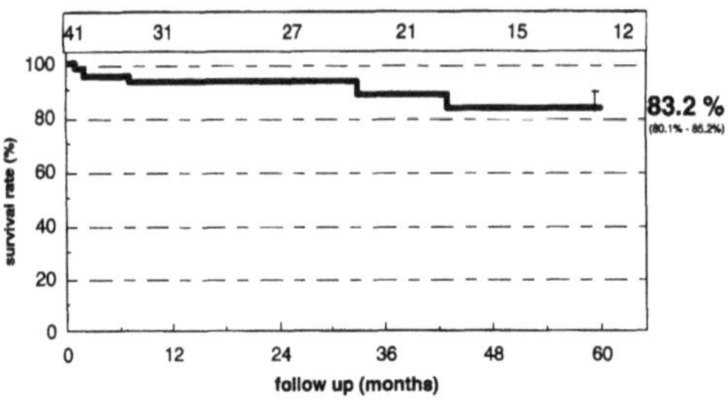

FIG. 1. Survival of 41 patients with resected pT1 adenocarcinoma of the esophagus. (From [2], with permission)

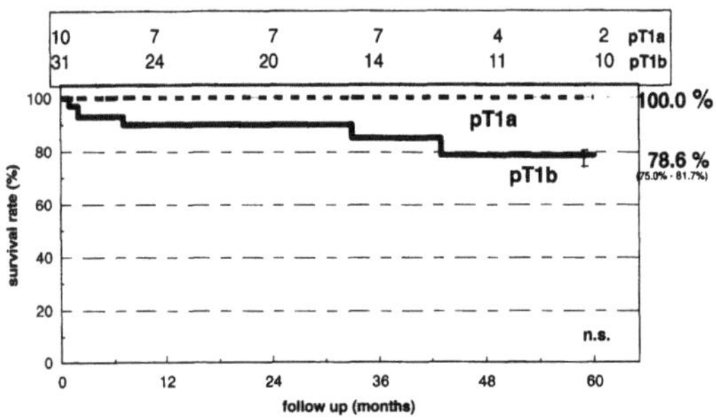

FIG. 2. Survival of 41 patients with resected pT1 adenocarcinoma of the esophagus, comparing infiltration of the mucosa (pT1a) and submucosa (pT1b). (From [2], with permission)

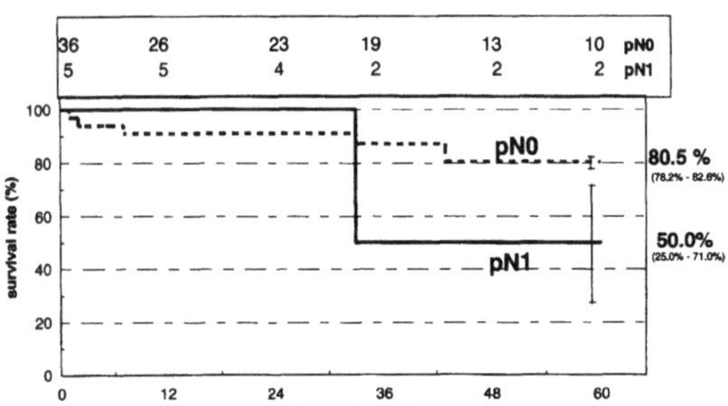

FIG. 3. Survival of 41 patients with resected pT1 adenocarcinoma of the esophagus, comparing pN0 and pN1 categories. (From [2], with permission)

Discussion

It is desirable to detect esophageal adenocarcinoma in the pT1 stage because prognosis is significantly correlated with the pT1 category [13]. The most significant variation in long-term survival is found between pT1 and pT2 tumors owing to an increase in lymph node metastasis [13, 14]. As the columnar cell-lined lower esophagus is premalignant, endoscopic surveillance programs have been initiated to detect malignant degeneration of Barrett's epithelium as early as possible. However, the impact of this surveillance on long-term results of esophagectomy for carcinoma has been demonstrated in only one study and several reports [3, 4, 8, 20–26]. The present analysis supports the development of endoscopic surveillance programs for Barrett's esophagus, as eight early adenocarcinomas (mostly mucosal tumors) were found as a result of the regular review. These eight patients also had a potentially more favorable outcome than the group diagnosed without surveillance. Early detection of adenocarcinoma is difficult because one-third of the patients are asymptomatic, and the others often have uncharacteristic symptoms.

An important finding is the frequency of multicentricity of early Barrett's carcinoma and the rate of concomitant high-grade dysplasia in Barrett's epithelium. The multifocal development of this lesion with additional foci of high-grade dysplasia or carcinoma in situ has been described by others [3, 4, 8, 27]. It is generally accepted that the entire columnar cell-lined lower esophagus must be resected together with the adenocarcinoma. The multifocal nature of this carcinoma is an argument against local endoscopic mucosectomy for early lesions. One alternative treatment is resection of the distal esophagus and interposition of a jejunal loop according to the operation of Merendino [28] (Fig. 4). The management plan for high-grade dysplasia in Barrett's esophagus is suggested in Fig. 5.

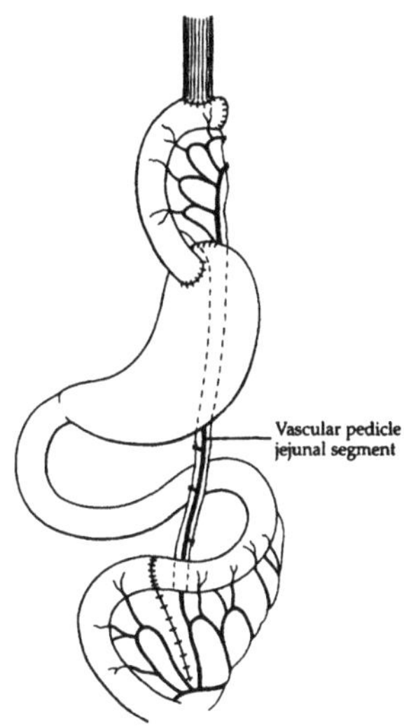

FIG. 4. Final position of the jejunum after replacing the distal esophagus by jejunal interposition and esophagojejunostomy plus jejunogastrostomy (Merendino operation). (From [28], with permission)

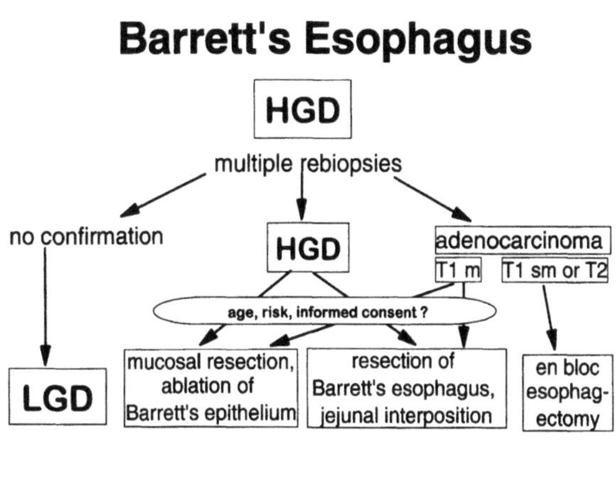

FIG. 5. Strategy for management of Barrett's esophagus with high-grade dysplasia (*HGD*). *LGD*, low grade dysplasia

TABLE 4. Survey of the literature on survival according to infiltration of mucosa or submucosa after resection of early adenocarcinoma of the esophagus

Study	Year	No.	Mucosa	Submucosa	Total
Streitz et al. [21]	1991	14	100	86 (3 years)	—
Menke-Pluymers et al. [22]	1992	12	100	63	—
Lerut et al. [26]	1993	24	100	100	100
Siewert & Hölscher [28]	1997	41	100	78.6	83.2

Important issues are the rate and localization of lymph node metastasis of early adenocarcinoma of the esophagus. Lymphatic involvement should not be expected with mucosal adenocarcinoma. However, preoperative distinction between mucosal and submucosal infiltration by endoscopy or endoscopic ultrasonography is difficult. It can only be differentiated by endoscopic mucosal resection [11, 29]. Even if complete removal of the carcinoma is possible by endoscopic mucosal resection, the danger of malignant degeneration of the remaining esophageal Barrett's epithelium persists. For most cases of early esophageal adenocarcinoma, therefore, the treatment of choice is still radical subtotal esophagectomy and lymphadenectomy. This can be performed by en bloc esophagectomy but also by means of a transhiatal approach because lymphatic metastasis of adenocarcinoma usually involves the lower thoracic paraesophageal and paracardial nodes [2, 30]. As most patients with pN1 lesions have involvement only of regional lymph nodes and the infiltration rate is less than 30% of the removed nodes, lymphadenectomy should be worthwhile for early adenocarcinoma and may improve the prognosis [2, 13]. The long-term results for pT1a carcinoma suggest that esophageal adenocarcinoma limited to the mucosa may be cured by surgical resection, a finding confirmed by other series [20, 22, 26, 31, 32] (Table 4). Although the difference in survival between patients with mucosal and submucosal infiltration was not significant in various studies owing to the small numbers of these subgroups, the overall trend seems obvious (Table 4). Early detection of esophageal adenocarcinoma is worthwhile because the risks of esophagectomy are low and the long-term prognosis is favorable.

References

1. Bollschweiler E, Hölscher AH (2000) Rising incidence of esophageal adenocarinoma. Dtsch Ärzteblatt 97(27):1896–1900
2. Hölscher AH, Bollschweiler E, Schneider PM, Siewert JR (1997) Early adenocarcinoma in Barrett's esophagus. Br J Surg 84:1470–1473
3. Reid BJ, Weinstein WM, Lewin KJ, et al (1988) Endoscopic biopsy can detect high-grade dysplasia or early adenocarcinoma in Barrett's oesophagus without grossly recognizable neoplastic lesions. Gastroenterology 94:81–90
4. Altorki NK, Sunagawa M, Little AG, Skinner DB (1991) High-grade dysplasia in the columnar-lined esophagus. Am J Surg 161:99–100
5. Schlemper RJ, Itabashi M, Kato Y, Lewin J, Riddell RH, Shimoda T, Sipponen P, Stolte M, Watanabe H, Takahashi H, Fujita R (1997) Differences in diagnostic criteria for gastric carcinoma between Japanese and Western pathologists. Lancet 349:1725–1729
6. Union International Contra la Cancrum (UICC) (1992) In: Hermanek P, Sobin LH (eds) TNM classification of malignant tumors, 4th edn. Springer, Berlin

7. Hamilton SR, Smith RRL, Cameron JL (1988) Prevalence and characteristics of Barrett's esophagus in patients with adenocarcinoma of the esophagus or esophagogastric junction. Hum Pathol 19:942–948
8. Hameeteman W, Tytgat GNJ, Houthoff HJ, van den Tweel JG (1989) Barrett's esophagus: development of dysplasia and adenocarcinoma. Gastroenterology 96:1249–1256
9. Kuster GGR, Foroozan P (1989) Early diagnosis of adenocarcinoma developing in Barrett's esophagus. Arch Surg 124:925–928
10. Geisinger KR, Teot LA, Richter JE (1992) A comparative cytopathologic and histologic study of atypia, dysplasia and adenocarcinoma in Barrett's esophagus. Cancer 69:8–16
11. Moghissi K (1992) Surgical resection for stage I cancer of the esophagus and cardia. Br J Surg 79:935–337
12. Hölscher AH, Bumm R, Siewert JR (1994) Oesophagogastrectomy for adenocarcinoma of the oesophagus and cardia. In: Jamieson GG, Debas HT (eds) Rob and Smith's operative surgery. surgery of the upper gastrointestinal tract. Chapman & Hall, London, pp 280–291
13. Hölscher AH, Bollschweiler E, Bumm R, Bartels H, Höfler H, Siewert JR (1995) Prognostic factors of resected adenocarcinoma of the esophagus. Surgery 118:845–855
14. Union International Contra la Cancrum (UICC) (1993) In: Hermanek P, Henson E, Hutter RVP, Sobin LH (eds) TNM supplement. Springer, Berlin
15. Siewert JR, Hölscher AH (1989) Eingriffe beim Oesophaguscarcinom. In: Siewert JR (ed) Breitner Chirurgische Operationslehre, vol. IV. Chirurgie des Abdomens 2. Oesophagus, Magen und Duodenum. Urban & Schwarzenberg, Munich, pp 17–54
16. Bumm R, Hölscher AH, Feussner H, Tachibana M, Bartels H, Siewert JR (1993) Endodissection of the esophagus: technique and clinicial results in transhiatal esophagectomy. Ann Surg 218:97–104
17. Alderson D, Courtney SP, Kennedy RH (1994) Radical transhiatal esophagectomy under direct vision. Br J Surg 81:404–407
18. Kajitani T (1981) Japanese Research Society for Gastric Cancer: the general rules for the gastric cancer study in surgery and pathology. Part 1. Clinical classification. Jpn J Surg 11:127–139
19. Maruyama K, Okabayashi K, Kinoshita T (1987) Progress in gastric cancer surgery in Japan and its limits of radicality. World J Surg 11:418–425
20. Streitz JM Jr, Ellis FH Jr, Gibb SP, Balogh K, Watkins E Jr (1991) Adenocarcinoma in Barrett's esophagus: a clinocopathologic study of 65 cases. Ann Surg 213:122–125
21. Streitz JM, Ellis FH Jr, Andrews C (1993) The impact of close surveillance of Barrett's esophagus patients on the results of esophagogastrectomy for carcinoma. In: Nabeya K, Hanaoka T, Nogami H (eds) Recent advances in diseases of the esophagus. Springer, Tokyo, pp 760–765
22. Menke-Pluymers MBE, Schoute NM, Mulder AH, Hop WCJ, van Blankenstein M, Tilanus HW (1992) Outcome of surgical treatment of adenocarcinoma in Barrett's esophagus. Gut 33:1456–1458
23. Pera M, Cameron AJ, Trastek VF, Carpenter HA, Zinsmeister AR (1993) Increasing incidence of adenocarcinoma of the esophagus and esophagogastric junction. Gastroenterology 104:510–513
24. Provenzale D, Kemp JA, Arora S, Wong JB (1994) A guide for surveillance of patients with Barrett's esophagus. Am J Gastroenterol 89:670–680
25. DeMeester TR, Attwood SEA, Smyrk TC, Therkildsen DH, Hinder RA (1990) Surgical therapy in Barrett's esophagus. Ann Surg 212:528–542
26. Lerut T, Coosemans W, Dillemans B, et al (1993) Surgical treatment of Barrett's carcinoma: correlation between morphologic findings and prognosis. In: Nabeya K, Hanoka T, Nogami H (eds) Recent advances in diseases of the esophagus. Springer, Tokyo, pp 162–168

27. Nishimaki T, Hölscher AH, Schüler M, Bollschweiler E, Becker K, Siewert JR (1991) Histopathologic characteristics of early adenocarcinoma in Barrett's esophagus. Cancer 68:1731–1736
28. Siewert JR, Hölscher AH (1997) Jejunal interposition in esophageal replacement. In: Nyhus LM, Baker RJ, Fischer JE (eds) Mastery of surgery, 3rd edn, vol I. Little, Brown, Boston, pp 802–812
29. Ell C, May A, Gossner L, Pech O, Gunter E, Mayer G, et al (2000) Endoscopic mucosal resection of early cancer and high-grade dysplasia in Barrett's esophagus. Gastroenterology 118:670–677
30. Clark GWB, Peters JH, Ireland AP, et al (1994) Nodal metastasis and sites of recurrence after en bloc esophagectomy for adenocarcinoma. Ann Thorac Surg 58:646–654
31. Pera M, Trastek VF, Carpenter HA, Allen MS, Deschamps C, Pairolero PC (1992) Barrett's esophagus with high-grade dysplasia: an indication for esophagectomy? Ann Thorac Surg 54:199–204
32. Levine DS, Haggitt RC, Blount PL, Rabinovitch PS, Rusch VW, Reid BJ (1993) An endoscopic biopsy protocol can differentiate high-grade dysplasia from early adenocarcinoma in Barrett's esophagus. Gastroenterology 105:40–50

Q & A after Dr. Hölscher's presentation

Dr. Aikou (Kagoshima University, Japan): Do you change strategies according to the cell type—superficial adenocarcinoma and superficial squamous cell carcinoma? As you showed the distribution of the lymph node metastasis is a bit different for these two cancers.

Dr. Hölscher: The series was not large, as we reported on 41 adenocarcinomas and 60 squamous cell carcinomas, so it is clearly difficult to detect significant differences. If you want to treat adenocarcinomas definitively, you must remove the whole Barrett's esophagus because it is an area of malignant potential. Therefore, mucosal resection alone is not a good solution because you can expect high-grade dysplasia or adenocarcinoma at another area of Barrett's esophagus within the next few years. The situation is somewhat different for squamous cell carcinoma, but of course there are some cases of high-grade dysplasia or superficial adenocarcinoma in Barrett's esophagus that you cannot resect because, for instance, the patients are old or have heart problems. You can attempt mucosal resection and ablation of Barrett's esophagus, but there are no long-term results of mucosal ablation with photodynamic therapy up to now, and carcinoma development is still possible after these treatments.

Dr. Ando (Keio University, Japan): I want to ask about the lymph node metastasis of T1 adenocarcinoma of Barrett's esophagus. Based on your data of 41 patients the 5-year survival for patients with pT1b is 78% with submucosal infiltration. If we compare those data with results of pT1b squamous cell carcinoma, they are good. Did all the patients undergo transthoracic esophagectomy with en bloc resection?

Dr. Hölscher: Patients with adenocarcinoma mostly underwent transhiatal resection, but we also performed extensive lymphadenectomy through the hiatus. We open the distal diaphragm and operate through the hiatus into the lower mediastinum, performing lymphadenectomy quite high up. Lymph node metastases were detected in all these cases.

Dr. Ando: You mean below the carina?

Dr. Hölscher: Yes, below the carina. Up to now we have not found lymph node metastasis above the carina with the advanced adenocarcinomas. We also have analyzed advanced adenocarcinomas and performed en bloc esophagectomy. Concerning the difference in 5-year survivals between squamous cell carcinoma and adenocarcinoma, there is of course the epidemiological background. As you know, most patients with squamous cell carcinoma, especially in our country, have high alcohol intake and they smoke. They are considerably different from patients with adenocarcinoma. The latter have more heart problems and are slightly obese; but patients who have squamous cell crcinoma have other risks and they may die for other reasons.

Dr. Ando: In your policy for the patients with pT1b adenocarcinoma of Barrett's esophagus, is it not necessary to dissect above the carina?

Dr. Hölscher: In patients whose adenocarcinoma or squamous cell carcinoma is below the carina, we always perform transthoracic en bloc esophagectomy now, with complete lymphadenectomy of the mediastinum. So there is no difference.

Dr. Ando: No difference? Even in cases of pT1b with submucosal invasions?

Dr. Hölscher: That's right.

Dr. Imamura (Kyoto University, Japan): I was surprised to hear about the poor results of antireflux surgery to reflux esophagitis related adenocarcinoma. Please comment on antireflux surgery with endoscopic mucosectomy of the diseased esophagus. Also, I agree with you that vagus nerve-preserving partial esophageal resection is useful; we also use it. What do you think about the extent of the resection of the stomach, and have you ever performed 24-h pH monitoring after the operation and examined the reflux state of the gastric acid to the jejunum?

Dr. Hölscher: Concerning the first question, this operation has already been reported, especially from Finland, by Salo, who examined the antireflux operation and ablation of Barrett's esophagus with the argon beam. He has had good results, with complete regression in these patients. This is something we should look at intensively during the next few years, although there are no long-term results yet. The results I showed are all without mucosal ablation. They are observations of Barrett's esophagus after antireflux surgery, and we selected only those with *effective* antireflux surgery. If antireflux surgery fails, it is the same as without surgery. Concerning the second question, about acid exposure of the distal esophagus in these patients, we did not find pathological acid or bile reflux into the esophagus by postoperative 24-h pH monitoring or bilimetry.

Selective Surgical Approach to Superficial Barrett's-Associated Adenocarcinoma

Jeffrey A. Hagen

Introduction

Over the past two decades a dramatic change has occurred in the epidemiology of esophageal cancer [1]. Adenocarcinoma has replaced squamous cell carcinoma as the most common esophageal malignancy in most centers, as the incidence of adenocarcinoma has risen faster than any other malignancy in the United States [2]. Description of the relation between Barrett's esophagus (a known complication of gastroesophageal reflux disease) and adenocarcinoma of the distal esophagus and gastroesophageal junction has linked one of the most deadly malignancies known to humans to the most common upper gastrointestinal disorder in Western civilization. Recognition of this relation has resulted in increased detection of early esophageal cancers through early endoscopy in patients with reflux symptoms and the performance of surveillance endoscopy in those with Barrett's esophagus.

As the epidemiology of esophageal cancer has changed, management strategies have also evolved. Historically, therapy was based on lessons learned during treatment of patients with squamous cell carcinoma, most of whom presented with advanced disease [3–5]. These strategies emphasized the classical principles of surgical oncology, including complete resection of the primary tumor and systematic removal of all potentially involved lymph nodes. As increasing numbers of patients are detected with early-stage tumors, the need for such extensive surgical procedures has been questioned. In addition, a variety of nonsurgical therapeutic techniques have been described including photodynamic therapy (PDT) and endoscopic mucosal resection. Before reductions in the extent of surgery or these alternative therapies are accepted, it is imperative that the extent of disease in patients with early tumors be known so as not to compromise the benefits of early detection by incomplete removal.

Section of Thoracic/Foregut Surgery, Keck School of Medicine, University of Southern California, LAC-USC Medical Center, 1441 Eastlake Avenue, Suite 7418, Los Angeles, CA 90033, USA

Definition of Superficial Esophageal Adenocarcinoma

For the purposes of this chapter, superficial esophageal adenocarcinoma is defined as a tumor limited to the mucosal or submucosal layers of the esophagus. This classification is consistent with the present TNM classification of esophageal cancer [6], which classifies both of these lesions as T1 tumors. More importantly, this classification recognizes the clinical difficulty of differentiating between T1 mucosal (T1m) and T1 submucosal (T1sm) disease (see below). Because it is also often difficult to differentiate clinically between T1 and T2 disease, it is wise from a practical standpoint to consider all patients with tumors confined to the esophageal wall as a group when defining the management approach to patients with early or superficial esophageal adenocarcinoma.

Historical Approach to Esophageal Cancer Surgery

To understand the changes that are occurring in the management of esophageal cancer today, it is important that we keep them in the perspective of the lessons we have learned in the past. Historically, the treatment approach to esophageal cancer was based on the Halstead theory of cancer progression, which posits that cancer progresses in an orderly fashion from local disease, to locoregional disease with lymph node metastases, to systemic disease. According to this concept, radical operations can be developed that can effectively treat patients with local or locoregional disease. Such an operation must ensure complete removal of the primary tumor and all potentially involved lymph nodes. For esophageal cancer, this has included a total thoracic esophagectomy with so-called en bloc resection of the mediastinal and upper abdominal lymph nodes. This approach was based largely on observations made when treating squamous cell cancers at a time when most patients presented with advanced disease. In the process, impressions regarding the patterns of lymphatic spread were biased by these relatively advanced tumors, in comparison to those seen today.

In the early reports [7, 8] lymph node spread was said to be extremely common in patients with esophageal cancer, and the nodes involved were widespread. These observations encouraged performance of a wide en bloc resection with systematic lymphadenectomy to encompass all potentially involved nodes. In many centers this evolved into adding neck dissection or three-field lymph node dissection to the treatment of esophageal cancer [9–11]. It was concluded that more surgery was better, and it was routine to perform a radical operation in all patients who could tolerate the procedure.

Because the epidemiology of esophageal cancer has changed, and the number of patients with early tumors has increased, this aggressive surgical approach to esophageal cancer must be revisited. Careful analysis of the literature reporting on the use of systematic node dissection can form the basis for determining whether there are circumstances in which it might be safe to perform a more limited resection and maintain the possibility of cure. This analysis must focus on the importance of lymph node involvement as a determinant of outcome and on the prevalence and location of lymph node metastases with early esophageal cancer. The extent of resection necessary to achieve a complete (R0) resection can then be defined.

Importance of Lymph Node Metastases

The importance of lymph node spread, from a prognostic standpoint, is well recognized. What is debated, however, is whether removal of these potentially involved nodes is of benefit to the patient. Because there is little effective therapy for patients with recurrent esophageal cancer, it makes sense that any procedure that decreases the likelihood of local recurrence should result in improved survival. This would be expected to be true only if it could be shown that there are significant numbers of patients with locoregional lymph node involvement in the absence of systemic metastases. It is in these patients in whom the difference between complete surgical eradication of cancer rests on the completeness of locoregional control. Proponents of a systematic lymph node dissection maintain that this is in fact the case, although prospective studies documenting the benefit of formal node dissection are lacking.

The alternative view, advocated more recently, is that esophageal cancer is a systemic disease in virtually all patients at the time of diagnosis. This hypothesis has led to the conclusion that lymph node dissection is of no benefit, as it is the presence of occult systemic metastases that is responsible for the poor survival in esophageal cancer. As a result, neoadjuvant therapy has been widely adopted in conjunction with simple or transhiatal esophagectomy, despite the fact that most recent studies have shown no benefit in survival [12–15].

Several recent studies have reemphasized the importance of lymph node metastases in esophageal cancer in terms of prognosis and the risk of locoregional recurrence. Many of these same series, summarized in the sections that follow, have also shown that the number of patients with locoregional lymph node involvement without systemic metastases appears to be relatively large. This conclusion is based on the observation that surgical resection alone can result in cure in many of these patients. This indicates that they did not, in fact, have systemic disease at the time of diagnosis, despite of the presence of locally advanced disease.

Number of Involved Nodes

Several series have documented that the presence of node metastases is an independent predictor of survival, including a report by Killinger and associates [16], which suggests that it is the presence of N1 disease that is the primary determinant of survival, exceeding tumor depth for predicting ultimate recurrence or cancer death. As such, the status of the locoregional nodes is included in all staging classification systems of esophageal cancer proposed to date. Recent data, however, suggest that the mere presence or absence of node metastases does not adequately stratify patients from a prognostic standpoint, and the absolute number of involved lymph nodes has been proposed as a better means of staging patients with esophageal cancer [4, 17, 18]. Most of these series have used a threshold of more than four involved lymph nodes as identifying patients at high risk for cancer death.

In 1994 we reported a series of 43 patients with Barrett's-associated adenocarcinoma in whom en bloc resection was performed [19]. This was the first series to demonstrate the importance of the number of lymph nodes for determining prognosis in a group of patients with esophageal adenocarcinoma, with significantly better survival demonstrated in patients with limited nodal disease (four or fewer nodes). Long-term survival was achieved in nearly 50% of the patients with limited lymph node involvement following en bloc resection alone. Even in the presence of more than four involved nodes, approximately 30% were alive 5 years after en bloc resection. These data indicate that long-term survival is still possible in a number of patients with esophageal cancer in the presence of node metastases, provided adequate resection has been performed. That is, there are a number of patients with locoregional disease in the absence of systemic metastases in whom the magnitude of the operation performed may make a difference.

Lymph Node Ratio

A clinically more useful way to approach this same concept has been promoted by a number of centers around the world [20–22]. According to this concept a ratio is calculated by dividing the number of involved nodes by the total number of lymph nodes removed. This concept is based on the hypothesis that a single positive node among only one or two nodes that might have been removed by a limited resection seems likely to be more ominous than when 30–40 or more nodes are removed, with tumor present in only one node. The precise cutoff value for the involved/removed lymph node ratio associated with poor survival remains to be determined, but reported values range from 10% to 30%. Based on these observations, it seems that a group of patients can be defined, with one to four positive nodes or fewer than 10%–30% of their nodes involved, who have locoregional disease as defined by Halstead that is potentially amenable to cure if an adequate operation is performed.

Lymph Node Micrometastases

The study of node metastases has been taken one step further recently using immunohistochemical (IHC) staining techniques. Izbicki et al. [23] published one of the first reports using these techniques, adding significantly to our understanding of the patterns of spread of esophageal cancer. They performed anti-epithelial antibody staining on lymph nodes removed from patients with esophageal cancer. They found evidence of micrometastases in 17% of the nodes that were negative for metastases by conventional histology. More importantly, they documented evidence of lymph node involvement in 15 of 30 patients (50%) who had no evidence of lymph node involvement in any of their nodes detected by routine histology. These data suggest that there are large numbers of patients thought to have only local disease with no evidence of lymph node metastases who in fact have locoregional disease with limited lymph node involvement when the specimen is subjected to a more sensitive analysis. It thus appears that the number of patients with locoregional disease who require systematic node dissection is larger than what we have historically thought. It also emphasizes the importance of a detailed assessment of all potentially involved nodes as we study the patterns of lymph node spread in patients with early esophageal cancer.

Importance of Tumor Depth

The depth of invasion of the primary tumor is the second most important determinant of outcome in most series reporting survival after esophageal cancer. The major importance of the depth of tumor invasion, from the standpoint of surgical treatment, lies in the need to ensure complete removal of the primary tumor. When comparing

TABLE 1. Lymph node prevalence and number in patients undergoing en bloc esophagectomy

Tumor depth	Prevalence of involved nodes	No. of involved nodes (median, range)
Intramucosal	1/15 (7%)*	0 (0–1)
Submucosal	6/12 (50%)*	0.5 (0–9)**
Intramuscular	8/10 (80%)*	1.0 (0-6)**

* $\chi^2 = 14.05$, $P = 0.00089$
** $P < 0.01$ vs. intramucosal group

the various operations for esophageal cancer, this is of little importance in terms of the treatment of superficial cancer. Essentially, all operations described for esophageal cancer remove the entire esophageal wall. However, accurate assessment of the tumor depth is critical when considering such techniques as mucosal ablation or endoscopic mucosal resection, where the extent of tumor invasion relative to the depth of treatment takes on considerable importance.

Studies have shown that the depth of tumor invasion is also of importance as a predictor of the likelihood of lymph node spread. Rice and colleagues [24] were the first to document this association for esophageal adenocarcinoma. They studied 295 patients who underwent esophagectomy with lymph node dissection for adenocarcinoma. They found a progressive increase in the frequency of lymph node metastases with increasing tumor depth. Fewer than 3% of patient with T1(m) tumors had involved nodes, compared to 21% of those with T1(sm) tumors, and rising to 83% for patients with T3 disease. We have found a similar relation between tumor depth and the prevalence of lymph node metastases in a series of 37 patients who underwent en bloc resection for Barrett's-associated adenocarcinoma [25] (Table 1). In only one case was lymph node spread found in a patient with a tumor confined to the mucosa. These observations have led to the concept that a formal lymph node dissection might be safely eliminated in patients with tumors that are known to be limited to the mucosal layer if they can be identified with precision.

Endoscopic Ultrasonography Staging Study

Endoscopic ultrasonography (EUS) is at present the preferred means for assessing the locoregional extent of disease for esophageal cancer. It was initially hoped that this technology would allow us to identify accurately patients with superficial esophageal cancer (tumors that are confined to the mucosa) who may be candidates for a more limited resection. Unfortunately, experience has shown that EUS is not accurate enough overall to allow clear definition of the extent of disease present in patients with early cancers.

The overall accuracy of EUS for staging esophageal cancer is reported to be about 70% [26, 27]. A more detailed analysis has shown that differentiating tumors confined to the mucosal layer from those that are more deeply invasive remains difficult unless extremely high frequency ultrasound is used [28, 29]. Reported accuracy rates for the diagnosis of disease limited to the mucosa and submucosa range from a low as 14%

to, at best, 59%. As a result, our ability to determine safely when a tumor is confined to the mucosa, and thus potentially amenable to limited resection, is restricted. The accuracy of EUS seems to improve, however, when differentiating between tumors that are confined to the wall of the esophagus and those in which there is transmural invasion. In our experience and that reported by Salminen, this is possible in 80%–90% of cases, which has led us to use this factor as a major determinant of the optimal treatment approach.

Management of Cancers Confined to the Esophageal Wall

In January 1999 we reported a series of patients treated for Barrett's-associated adenocarcinoma with tumors confined to the esophageal wall [25]. The goal of this study was to determine whether these patients with early tumors required an extensive operation including lymph node dissection or a lesser operation. To make this determination, a clear understanding of the prevalence and location of lymph node involvement was required. A total of 65 patients were studied: 37 following en bloc resection and 28 following transhiatal esophagectomy. As mentioned previously, there was a clear relation between tumor depth and the presence of node metastases; 80% of the patients who had tumors that invaded beyond the submucosa had involved nodes. In most cases, however, the total number of involved nodes was small; in all but three cases there were four or fewer positive nodes (Table 1). These data indicate that lymph node dissection is necessary for patients with tumors confined to the esophageal wall (seen on EUS), as most have positive locoregional node disease.

We then sought to determine the extent of the lymphadenectomy needed to ensure a curative (R0) resection. To do so required that the location of the potentially involved nodes be defined. Figure 1 shows the results of this analysis. As the tumor invades deeper into the esophageal wall, nodes can be found in virtually all locations in the lower mediastinum and upper abdomen, especially when the muscle layer is involved. This wide distribution of node metastases emphasizes the need for a systematic lymph node dissection to include all of these potentially involved node groups if an R0 resection is to be accomplished. As a result, we recommend en bloc resection with mediastinal and upper abdominal lymph node dissection in patients whose tumors are confined to the esophageal wall.

Management of "Occult" Esophageal Cancer

Data that demonstrate frequent, widespread lymph node involvement of early esophageal adenocarcinoma has led many to conclude that lymph node dissection is required in all patients with esophageal cancer. In fact, that was our approach until recently. However, as Barrett's endoscopic surveillance programs have become more widespread, increasing numbers of patients have been identified with high-grade dysplasia or microscopic invasive cancer in the absence of a grossly detectable tumor mass. The need for such an extensive resection and lymph node dissection, particularly when only high-grade dysplasia is found, has been questioned; and a

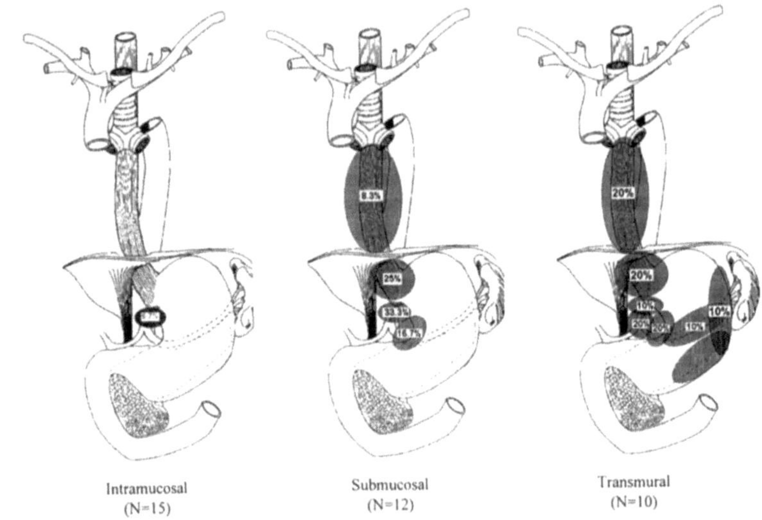

FIG. 1. Prevalence of lymph node involvement for tumors of various depths, by lymph node group

number of less invasive treatment options have been proposed for treating these patients. They include nonoperative treatments, such as photodynamic therapy and endoscopic mucosal resection, and less extensive surgical procedures, such as the vagal-sparing esophagectomy [5]. Before these lesser treatments are accepted, however, the likelihood of lymph node spread must be determined, so the benefits of early detection are not compromised by incomplete tumor removal. This led us to review our experience with these early cancers in an attempt to identify patients in whom the operation might be safely tailored back, with an emphasis on improved long-term function.

The patients on whom we focused were those whose cancers were detected during the course of surveillance endoscopy for Barrett's esophagus [30]. This is an important group of patients to study because it not only represents the group with the earliest tumors, it is also the group being proposed for more limited treatment, such as endoscopic resection and mucosal ablation. A total of 27 patients with extremely early Barrett's-associated adenocarcinoma were identified whose cancers were detected on biopsies performed for Barrett's surveillance. In all cases, the patients were asymptomatic, with no visible tumor in the esophagus.

Reviewing the endoscopy notes on these patients, a number were identified who had tiny areas of nodularity in Barrett's mucosa or areas of ulceration. We found that the presence or absence of such an area of ulceration or nodularity noted on endoscopy predicted the likelihood of a more locally advanced tumor at the time of resection. In the absence of a visible lesion, more than 85% of the tumors were limited to the mucosa (Fig. 2), with the remainder of the tumors confined to the submucosa. In contrast, when a nodule or area of ulceration was seen at endoscopy, 75% of the patients had tumors that invaded the submucosa or beyond, with muscular or trans-

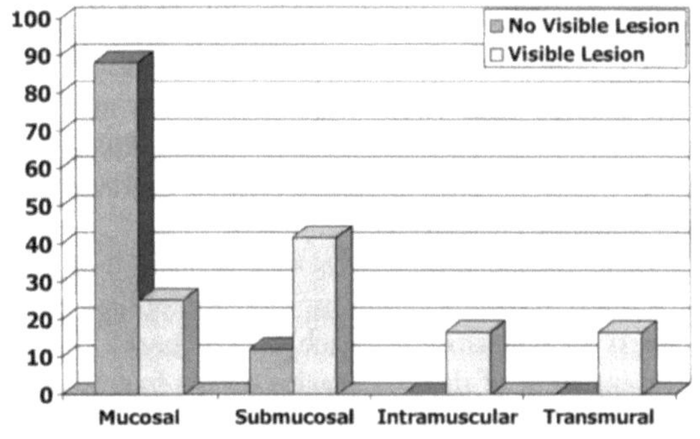

FIG. 2. Depth of tumor invasion for patients with and without an endoscopically visible lesion on surveillance endoscopy

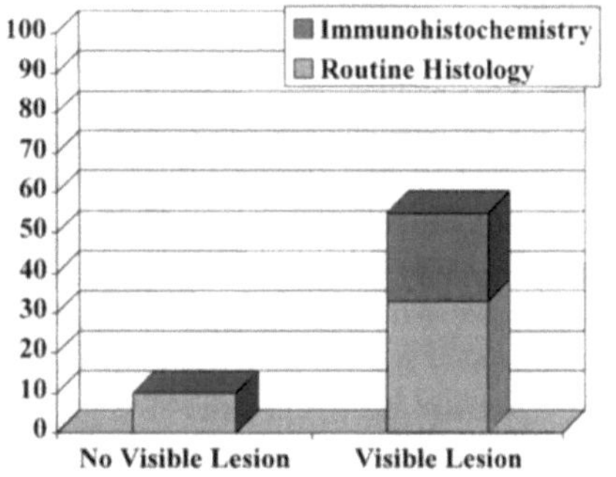

FIG. 3. Frequency of lymph node metastases in patients with and without an endoscopically visible lesion on surveillance endoscopy

mural invasion in about one-third. This factor, the presence or absence of an endoscopically visible lesion, far exceeds the reported accuracy of EUS under these circumstances for predicting disease limited to the mucosa.

Patients with endoscopically visible lesions were also significantly more likely to have lymph node metastases (Fig. 3). More than half of the patients with endoscopically visible ulcers or nodules had evidence of lymph node involvement compared to a single patient with a single involved node in the group without a visible lesion. These data suggest that no formal lymph node dissection is required in patients with a biopsy showing adenocarcinoma in the absence of a visible lesion. As a result, we recommend resection without formal lymph node dissection, preferably by vagal-sparing techniques that maximize the long-term functional outcome. Because a number of these patients have tumors that invade deeply into the mucosa or even into the submucosa, we continue to recommend resection until techniques of mucosal ablation or endoscopic mucosal resection can reliably be shown to remove the full thickness of the esophageal mucosa.

In patients with visible lesions, the presence of involved nodes in half of the patients suggests that some form of lymph node dissection should be performed. However, analysis of the number and locations of the involved nodes suggest that transthoracic en bloc resection is more surgery than is necessary. We found that in all but two patients there was only one involved lymph node. More importantly, in all cases the involved nodes were in the left gastric or distal paraesophageal location, areas that are readily accessible without the need for thoracotomy. We perform an extended transhiatal resection in these patients, an operation that removes all of the upper abdominal retroperitoneal nodes, with a lower mediastinal node dissection performed through an enlarged esophageal hiatus. This approach should encompass all potentially involved nodes in patients with an endoscopically visible lesion detected during surveillance for Barrett's esophagus.

Based on the results of several series reported in the recent literature, a tailored approach to patients with superficial esophageal adenocarcinoma can be defined that selects an operation for each patient based on the clinical scenarios in which they present. Each of these scenarios differs from the others in subtle yet important ways, which affects how they should be managed. When surveillance endoscopy for Barrett's esophagus shows high-grade dysplasia or intramucosal cancer in the absence of a visible lesion, the goal of surgery should be to remove the full thickness of the esophageal wall that contains the early tumor, with a focus on long-term alimentary function by vagal-sparing esophagectomy using colon interposition. When a lesion is visible on surveillance endoscopy, it is likely that the tumor invades the submucosa or beyond, and local nodes are involved in half of the patients. In this setting we recommend extended transhiatal esophagectomy with upper abdominal and lower mediastinal lymph node dissection to maximize the chances of complete resection.

Patients who present with symptomatic tumors require a different approach. We recommend EUS in these patients to determine whether the tumor extends beyond the muscular layer. When the tumor is confined to the esophageal wall, we recommend en bloc esophagectomy, knowing that as many as 80% have involved nodes, which in almost all cases are limited in number. The management of patients with a transmural tumor remains less well defined. Although en bloc resection results in cure of a number of these patients [3], particularly when there is limited node involvement [21], in most cases the presence of multiple and widespread node metastases precludes cure by surgery alone, and consideration should be given to administration of neoadjuvant or adjuvant chemotherapy.

Conclusions

The approach to patients with esophageal cancer has changed dramatically over the past several decades as the epidemiology of the disease has changed and new treatment modalities have been described. Through a number of recent observations, it has become clear that institutions dedicated to the management of this disease must have a variety of tools in their armamentarium to select the proper operation for the extent of disease present in a given patient. This chapter focused on the selective surgical approach that we use in the management of patients with Barrett's-associated adenocarcinoma and the rationale behind the algorithm described. This approach emphasizes several important changes in the management of patients with early Barrett's-associated cancers.

References

1. Wang HH, Antonioli DA, Goldman H (1986) Comparative features of esophageal and gastric adenocarcinomas: recent changes in type and frequency. Hum Pathol 17: 482–487

2. Hesketh PJ, Clapp RW, Doos WG, Spechler SJ (1989) The increasing frequence of adenocarcinoma of the esophagus. Cancer 64:526–530
3. Altorki NK, Girardi L, Skinner DB (1997) En bloc esophagectomy improves survival for stage III esophageal cancer. J Thorac Cardiovasc Surg 114:948–956
4. Hagen JA, Peters JH, DeMeester TR (1993) Superiority of extended en bloc esophagogastrectomy for carcinoma of the lower esophagus and cardia. J Thorac Cardiovasc Surg 106:850–859
5. Akiyama H, Tsurumaru M, Ono Y, Udagawa H, Kajiyama Y (1994) Esophagectomy without thoracotomy with vagal preservation. J Am Coll Surg 178:83–85
6. Anonymous (1997) AJCC Cancer staging manual, 5th edn. Lippincott-Raven, Philadelphia, pp 65–69
7. Akiyama H, Tsurumaru M, Udagawa H, Kajiyama Y (1981) Principles of surgical treatment for carcinoma of the esophagus: analysis of lymph node involvement. Ann Surg 194:438–446
8. Skinner DB (1983) En bloc resection for neoplasms of the esophagus and cardia. J Thorac Cardiovasc Surg 85:59–71
9. Akiyama H, Tsurumaru M, Udagawa H, Kajiyama Y (1994) Radical lymph node dissection for cancer of the thoracic esophagus. Ann Surg 220:364–373
10. Altorki NK, Skinner DB (1997) Occult cervical nodal metastasis in esophageal cancer: preliminary results of three-field lymphadenectomy. J Thorac Cardiovasc Surg 113: 540–544
11. Fujita H, Kakegawa T, Yamana H, et al (1995) Mortality and morbidity rates, postoperative course, quality of life, and prognosis after extended radical lymphadenectomy for esophageal cancer: comparison of three-field lymphadenectomy with two-field lymphadenectomy. Ann Surg 222:654–662
12. Bhansali MS, Patil PK, Badwe RA, Havaldar R, Desai PB (1997) Historical control bias: adjuvant chemotherapy in esophageal cancer. Dis Esophagus 10:51–54
13. Law S, Fok M, Chow S, Chu KM, Wong J (1997) Preoperative chemotherapy versus surgical therapy alone for squamous cell carcinoma of the esophagus: a prospective randomized trial. J Thorac Cardiovasc Surg 114:210–217
14. Kelsen DP, Ginsberg R, Pajak TF, et al (1998) Chemotherapy followed by surgery compared with surgery alone for localized esophageal cancer. N Engl J Med 339:1979–1984
15. Urba SG, Orringer MB, Turrisi A, Iannettoni M, Forastiere A, Strawderman M (2001) Randomized trial of preoperative chemoradiation versus surgery alone in patients with locoregional esophageal carcinoma. J Clin Oncol 19:305–331
16. Killinger WA Jr, Rice TW, Adelstein DJ, et al (1996) Stage II esophageal carcinoma: the significance of T and N. J Thorac Cardiovasc Surg 111:935–940
17. Ellis FH, Watkins E, Krasna MJ, et al (1993) Staging of carcinoma of the esophagus and cardia: a comparison of different staging criteria. J Surg Oncol 52:231–235
18. Korst RJ, Rusch VW, Venkatraman E, et al (1998) Proposed revision of the staging classification for esophageal cancer. J Thorac Cardiovasc Surg 115:660–669
19. Clark GW, Peters JH, Ireland AP, et al (1994) Nodal metastases and sites of recurrence after en bloc esophagectomy for adenocarcinoma. Ann Thorac Surg 58:646–654
20. Roder JD, Busch R, Stein HJ, Fink U, Siewert JR (1994) Ratio of invaded to removed lymph nodes as a predictor of survival in squamous cell carcinoma of the oesophagus. Br J Surg 81:410–413
21. Nigro JJ, DeMeester SR, Hagen JA, et al (1999) Node status in transmural esophageal adenocarcinoma and outcome after en bloc esophagectomy. J Thorac Cardiovasc Surg 117:960–968
22. Holscher AH, Bollschweiler E, Bumm R, Bartels H, Hofler H, Siewert JR (1995) Prognostic factors of resected adenocarcinoma of the esophagus. Surg 118:845–855
23. Izbicki JR, Hosch SB, Pichlmeier U, et al (1997) Prognostic value of immunohistochemically identifiable tumor cells in lymph nodes of patients with completely resected esophageal cancer. N Engl J Med 337:1188–1194

24. Rice TW, Zuccaro G Jr, Adelstein DJ, Rybicki LA, Blackstone EH, Goldblum JR (1998) Esophageal carcinoma: depth of tumor invasion is predictive of regional lymph node status. Ann Thorac Surg 65:787–792
25. Nigro JJ, Hagen JA, DeMeester TR, et al (1999) Prevalence and location of nodal metastases in distal esophageal adenocarcinoma confined to the wall: implications for therapy. J Thorac Cardiovasc Surg 117:16–25
26. Peters JH, Hoeft SF, Heimbucher J, et al (1994) Selection of patients for curative or palliative resection of esophageal cancer based on preoperative endoscopic ultrasonography. Arch Surg 129:534–539
27. Salminen JT, Farkkila MA, Ramo OJ, et al (1999) Endoscopic ultrasonography in the preoperative staging of adenocarcinoma of the distal oesophagus and oesophagogastric junction. Scand J Gastroenterol 34:1178–1182
28. Rice TW, Boyce GA, Sivak MV, Adelstein DJ, Kirby TJ (1992) Esophageal carcinoma: esophageal ultrasound assessment of preoperative chemotherapy. Ann Thorac Surg 53: 972–977
29. Fukuda M, Hirata K, Natori H (2000) Endoscopic ultrasonography of the esophagus. World J Surg 24:216–226
30. Nigro JJ, Hagen JA, DeMeester TR, et al (1999) Occult esophageal adenocarcinoma: extent of disease and implications for effective therapy. Ann Surg 230:433–440

Q & A after Dr. Hagen's presentation

Dr. Imamura (Kyoto University, Japan): You said that you use endoscopic ultrasonography (EUS) before operations. Do you also use computed tomography (CT) scans for estimating the lymph nodes preoperatively? What is your opinion of lymph node dissection around the celiac axis or paraaortic region?

Dr. Hagen: Yes, we do use EUS in all these patients, and practically speaking they all undergo CT scans before operation as well. The only exceptions are patients who have Barrett's esophagus with high-grade dysplasia or intramucosal cancer: We decided that it is not likely to be cost-effective to study these patients with a CT scan. Having said that, I think it affects treatment very little. Occasionally you find patients with unsuspected metastases to the liver, but for most of these early cases it is not helpful, particularly with lymph node involvement. As to the second question: for us, abdominal lymph node dissection includes dissection from the porta hepatis down to the celiac artery and then across to remove the spleen and splenic artery and all retroperitoneal tissues above that. We have not been dissecting inferior to the celiac axis along the aorta; but from the celiac axis upward it is a complete lymphadenectomy.

Dr. Jankowski (Birmingham University, UK): What do you find when you look at these mucosal abnormalities—the irregular legions you see when you examine patients endoscopically for these dysplastic inflamed lesions? What does the phenotype look like?

Dr. Hagen: It's a bit all over the map. Sometimes when we biopsy these nodules we see a focus of intramucosal cancer but this is no means universal. Many times the nodules do not show cancer, but there is high-grade dysplasia and cancer elsewhere in the esophagus. Sometimes the lesions have just dysplastic changes; it's rare when they are completely normal, but by no means is there a diagnosis of cancer in all of these nodules.

Dr. Udagawa (Toranomon Hospital, Japan): You say that mostly you used the data of Dr. Izabesky for your radical operation, but he himself said there is no use for radical operation for that kind of systemic disease patient. I completely agree with you. I noted that you didn't include the height level of the tumor in your strategy. You must have experienced, for instance, neck lymph node metastases or superior mediastinal lymph node metastases in patients with mid-esophageal tumors, but you limited your operation to the lower mediastinum. What is your opinion about paratracheal or neck dissection?

Dr. Hagen: First, the demographics of our patient population is such that most of these tumors are located in the distal esophagus or GE junction area. It's rare that we see patients with mid-esophageal Barrett's cancers. It does happen; but because of the heightened awareness of reflux disease, the long segments of Barrett's esophagus in our experience seem to be much less common than they once were. Most of these cancers are confined to the distal esophagus. With respect to the value of lymph node dissection, I am not sure what to make of the data on that. It's conflicting in many ways. I think that most of the patients who have lymph nodes involved in the neck would have to have extensive lymph node involvement elsewhere, with more than 10%–20% of their nodes involved. Curable surgery is not likely in those patients. It's the rare patient with limited lymph node disease who has cervical metastases—certainly those with lower esophageal cancers and arguably middle esophageal lesions. Clearly high thoracic cancers require cervical lymph node dissection because there are local lymph nodes in those tumors.

Dr. Baba (Kagoshima University, Japan): You questioned that patients with transmural cancer had extensive lymph node metastases, but you are dealing with these patients perhaps daily. If patients coming to your institution are diagnosed preoperatively to have four or more lymph node metastases and transmural tumor, how do you deal with them?

Dr. Hagen: That's a good question. There are basically two ways the patient is assigned to that category. The first is on the basis of preoperative endoscopic ultrasonography showing transmural tumor with many lymph nodes involved. In that circumstance, we recommend that the patient undergo neoadjuvant chemoradiotherapy followed by resection. Without going into details, this approach to advanced disease is purely our own; its efficacy has not been proved. What we are doing presently is treating these patients with neoadjuvant therapy; if they show a good response objectively, we use it as a marker of favorable prognosis and then treat the patient with lymph node dissection and en bloc esophagectomy. If they don't respond to therapy or if the disease progresses while on therapy, a simple transhiatal esophagectomy is usually performed. Just as commonly, though, we operate on patients who we think have more limited disease but are proven on histologic analysis to have a lot of positive nodes. Those patients are subjected to chemotherapy postoperatively on the basis of some molecular biology studies that seem to be a predictor of sensitivity to chemotherapy.

Dr. Baba: Who judges the status of patients who respond to the preoperative therapy?

Dr. Hagen: We perform all of our endoscopies, so our definition of response to therapy is a comparison. They are all done with video, so when there is any question we can go back and look thoroughly and carefully to what extent the disease was present before and then after. We have that luxury because we do the endoscopies ourselves before and after therapy on all of these patients. If you don't do that it's difficult because it can be highly subjective at times regarding whether there has been partial response. I think that by using such prospective, repeated studies done by the surgeons who are doing the operations, our characterization of response is pretty good.

Clinical Strategies for Adenocarcinoma of the Esophagus at the National Cancer Center, Japan

Yuji Tachimori

Introduction

The incidence of adenocarcinoma of the esophagus has been increasing in most Western countries over the past 25 years. In the United States adenocarcinoma has replaced squamous cell carcinoma as the most common esophageal cancer. In Japan, however, squamous cell carcinoma is still the most common histological type of esophageal carcinoma. In this study the incidence of adenocarcinoma of the esophagus in Japan over the past three decades was assessed based on the data from the nationwide registry.

The frequency of the association of Barrett's esophagus with adenocarcinoma of the esophagus was studied in another nationwide registry. Surgical strategies for adenocarcinoma of the esophagus are discussed based on the experience of our institution.

Incidence of Adenocarcinoma of the Esophagus in Japan

The patient data in the registry of esophageal carcinoma in Japan [1–15], conducted by the Japanese Society for Esophageal Diseases (JSED), provided an opportunity for estimating the incidence trend for adenocarcinoma. Registration of esophageal carcinoma was started as a task force of the JSED in 1976. Patients as far back as 1966 were registered retrospectively, and the registry data were submitted by more than 200 institutions across the nation. The association of Barrett's esophagus was not studied for these registrations.

The numbers of registered patients with tumor of the esophagus are shown in Fig. 1. During 1966 and 1994 a total of 37060 patients with esophageal tumor were registered, with 526 (1.4%) patients having adenocarcinoma. The incidence of adenocarcinoma did not increase during these 29 years. During the 1980s, among 17439

Department of Surgery, National Cancer Center Hospital, Tsukiji 5-1-1, Chuo-ku, Tokyo 104-0045, Japan

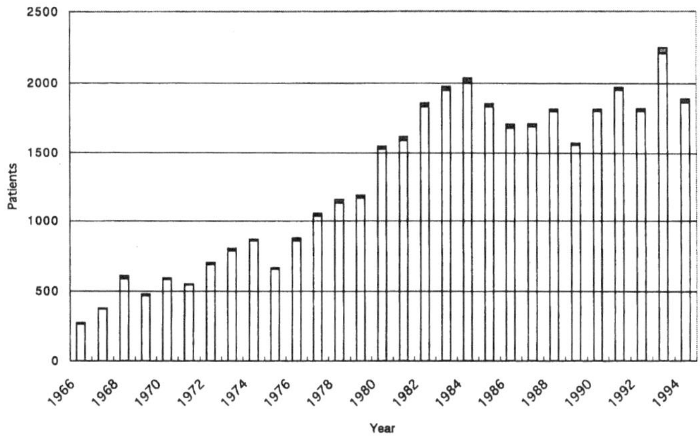

FIG. 1. Incidence trend for adenocarcinoma of the esophagus on the nationwide registration in Japan. *Black area*, adenocarcinoma; *open area*, other histological types

resected esophageal tumors, adenocarcinoma accounted for only 1.4%. During the next 4 years adenocarcinoma was still less than 2% among 9611 resected esophageal tumors.

During the last 30 years the Japanese diet has changed to Western-style food. The incidence of gastric cancer has decreased, and that of colorectal cancer has increased. The incidence of adenocarcinoma of the esophagus has not yet increased.

In the follow-up report [16] of registered patients, the survival curve of patients with adenocarcinoma was no different from that for patients with squamous cell carcinoma (Fig. 2). The 5-year survival rate was almost 40% for both histological types.

Adenocarcinoma of the Esophagogastric Junction and Barrett's Mucosa

The histology of carcinoma of the esophagogastric junction and the association of Barrett's esophagus was studied in another registry of carcinoma of the esophagogastric junction conducted by the JSED. Hiroko Ide, chief of the Registration Committee for Esophageal Cancer, conducted the registration of carcinoma of the esophagogastric junction, and the data were presented at the annual meeting of the Society in June 2000 [17]. The registry collected 2013 cases of carcinoma of the esophagogastric junction among 11 317 esophagectomy cases and 49 887 gastrectomy cases seen in 97 institutions throughout Japan between 1990 and 1999. Tumors of the esophagogastric junction had their centers within 5 cm proximal to the anatomical esophagogastric junction. Squamous cell carcinoma without involvement of the esophagogastric junction was excluded. In this registry carcinoma of the esophagogastric junction was differentiated according to the classification proposed by Siewert et al. and Hölscher et al. [18, 19]. Type I tumor has its center in the tubular

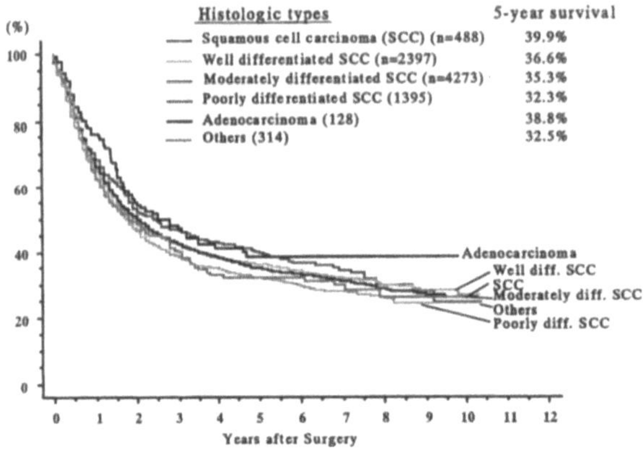

FIG. 2. Survival curves of patients who underwent esophagectomy for esophageal carcinoma. (From [16], with permission)

TABLE 1. Histology of carcinoma of the esophagogastric junction (1990–1999, 97 institutions)

Cancer	Type I	Type II
Adenocarcinoma	116 (17.3%)	1004 (76.2%)
Squamous cell	529 (79.1%)	285 (21.8%)
Others	24	20
Total	669	1309

From [17], with permission

esophagus, and type II tumor has its center in the junction. Type III tumor, with its center in the stomach, was excluded as a gastric carcinoma in this registry.

Almost half of the tumors were adenocarcinoma. Most of the type I tumors were squamous cell carcinoma. In contrast, most of the adenocarcinomas were type II tumors, located not in the tubular esophagus but in the junction (Table 1).

About 30% of type I adenocarcinomas were associated with Barrett's esophagus (Table 2), although Barrett's esophagus was associated with only 4% of type II adenocarcinomas. This means that in Japan most type II adenocarcinomas of the esophagogastric junction originated from gastric mucosa as gastric cancer. The incidence of Barrett's esophagus was low among patients with squamous cell carcinoma of the esophagogastric junction. This result supports the low incidence of Barrett's esophagus in the general population in Japan.

The frequency of mediastinal lymph node involvement was lower than that of squamous cell carcinoma (Table 3). However, the upper mediastinum was dissected in only 30% for type I tumors and less than 10% for type II tumors. Postoperative survival was better for patients with adenocarcinoma than for those with squamous cell carcinoma (Fig. 3). This result was due to the more advanced disease in patients with squamous cell carcinoma. Based on these reports from nationwide registries adenocarcinoma of the esophagus still holds quite a minor position among esophageal carcinomas in Japan.

TABLE 2. Incidence of Barrett's mucosa in patients with carcinoma of the esophagogastric junction (1990–1999, 97 institutions)

Cancer	Type I	Type II
Adenocarcinoma	34/116 (29.3%)	40/1004 (4.0%)
Squamous cell	6/529 (1.1%)	3/285 (1.1%)
Others	4/24 (16.7%)	0/20

From [17], with permission

TABLE 3. Frequency of lymph node involvement from adenocarcinoma of the esophagogastric junction (1990–1999, 97 institutions)

Node area	Type I (%)	Type II (%)
Upper mediastinum	4	0.5
Middle mediastinum	3	2
Lower mediastinum	9	7
Abdominal	31	36

From [17], with permission

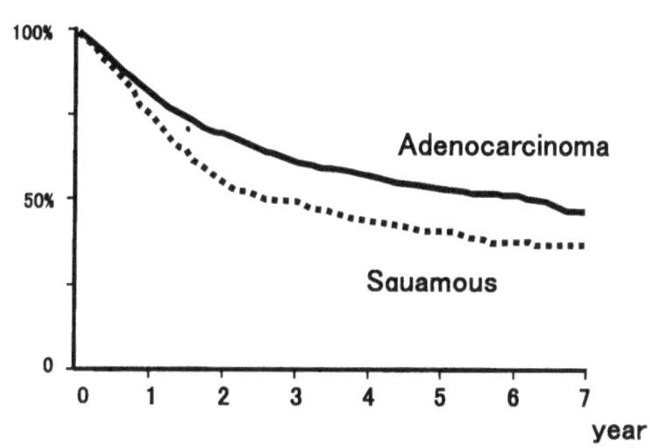

FIG. 3. Survival curves of patients who underwent surgery for carcinoma of the esophagogastric junction. (From [17], with permission)

Experience at National Cancer Center Hospital

At the National Cancer Center Hospital we have seen only 30 patients with adenocarcinoma of the esophagus and esophagogastric junction during a recent 20-year period (Table 4). The incidence of adenocarcinoma was about 2.2% among 1387 esophagectomies, almost the same as reported in the nationwide registry. Barrett's esophagus was associated with adenocarcinoma in only nine patients.

When the center of the tumor was located in the lower tubular esophagus, three of nine patients had lymph node involvement in the upper mediastinum (Table 5). When the center of the tumor was located in the esophagogastric junction, the frequency of lymph node involvement in the upper mediastinum was low, but there was lymph node involvement in the middle mediastinum in more than 10% of patients.

TABLE 4. Histology of carcinoma of the esophagus (1980–1999, National Cancer Center Hospital)

	Tumor location (no.)					
Cancer	Cervical	Upper	Middle	Lower	Junction	Total
Adenocarcinoma	1	0	1	9 (5)	19 (4)	30 (9)
Squamous	122	136	664	315	32	1269
Others	4	3	48	28	5	88
	127	139	713	352	56	1387

Numbers in parentheses are patients with Barrett's mucosa

TABLE 5. Area of lymph node involvement from adenocarcinoma of the esophagogastric junction (1980–1999, National Cancer Center Hospital)

	Tumor location (no.)	
Node area	Lower ($n = 9$)	Junction ($n = 19$)
Upper mediastinum	3	1
Middle mediastinum	2	3
Lower mediastinum	3	6
Abdominal	6	13

TABLE 6. Area of lymph node involvement from Barrett's carcinoma of the esophagogastric junction (1980–1999, National Cancer Center Hospital)

	Tumor location	
Node area	Lower ($n = 5$)	Junction ($n = 4$)
Upper mediastinum	2	
Middle mediastinum	2	
Lower mediastinum	2	
Abdominal	4	1

In patients with adenocarcinoma associated with Barrett's esophagus, the areas of lymph node involvement were related to the tumor location (Table 6). In four patients with superficial Barrett's-associated adenocarcinoma, no lymph node metastasis was detected.

Discussion

When the tumor involves the esophagogastric junction, middle and lower mediastinal dissection through a left thoracotomy is recommended for adenocarcinoma of the esophagus. When the adenocarcinoma is located in the lower tubular esophagus, the upper mediastinum including the area along the recurrent laryngeal nerves should be dissected through a right thoracotomy. Because of the limited experience with adenocarcinoma of the esophagus, the indication of three-field dissection is not proposed owing to a lack of exact data. The surgical approach for adenocarcinoma is indicated based on the anatomical location of the tumor, similar to that for squamous cell carcinoma of the esophagus.

The incidence of adenocarcinoma of the esophagus has not increased. However, among the nine cases of Barrett's-associated adenocarcinoma, eight were seen in the most recent 10 years. This year we have already experienced three cases of Barrett's-associated adenocarcinoma, and no doubt we will see more of this lesion in the near future.

References

1. Japanese Society for Esophageal Diseases (1982) The report of treatment results of esophageal carcinoma in Japan (1969, 1970, 1971, 1972, 1973)
2. Japanese Society for Esophageal Diseases (1985) The report of treatment results of esophageal carcinoma in Japan (1974, 1975, 1976, 1977, 1978)
3. Japanese Society for Esophageal Diseases (1979) The report of the registration of esophageal carcinoma in Japan (1976)
4. Japanese Society for Esophageal Diseases (1980) The report of the registration of esophageal carcinoma in Japan (1977)
5. Japanese Society for Esophageal Diseases (1983) The report of the registration of esophageal carcinoma in Japan (1978)
6. Japanese Society for Esophageal Diseases (1984) The report of the registration of esophageal carcinoma in Japan (1979)
7. Japanese Society for Esophageal Diseases (1986) The report of the registration of esophageal carcinoma in Japan (1980)
8. Japanese Society for Esophageal Diseases (1987) The report of the registration of esophageal carcinoma in Japan (1981)
9. Japanese Society for Esophageal Diseases (1988) The report of the registration of esophageal carcinoma in Japan (1982)
10. Japanese Society for Esophageal Diseases (1992) The report of the registration of esophageal carcinoma in Japan (1983)
11. Japanese Society for Esophageal Diseases (1992) The report of the registration of esophageal carcinoma in Japan (1984)
12. Japanese Society for Esophageal Diseases (1994) The report of the registration of esophageal carcinoma in Japan (1985)
13. Japanese Society for Esophageal Diseases (1994) The report of the registration of esophageal carcinoma in Japan (1986)
14. Japanese Society for Esophageal Diseases (1995) The report of the registration of esophageal carcinoma in Japan (1987)
15. Japanese Society for Esophageal Diseases (1998) The report of the registration of esophageal carcinoma in Japan (1988–1994)
16. Japanese Society for Esophageal Diseases (2000) Comprehensive registry of esophageal cancer in Japan (1988–1994)
17. Ide H. Resected cases with carcinoma of the esophago-gastric junction in Japan. Presented at the 54th annual meeting of the Japanese Society for Esophageal Diseases, Tokyo, June 2000
18. Siewert JR, Hölscher AH, Becker K, Gössner W (1987) Kardiacarcinom: Versuch einer therapeutisch relevanten Klassifikation. Chirurg 58:25–32
19. Hölscher AH, Siewert JR, Böttcher K, et al (1987) Surgical classification for adenocarcinomas of the gastroesophageal junction. In: Siewert JR, Hölscher AH (eds) Diseases of the esophagus. Springer, Berlin, pp 571–578

Q & A after Dr. Tachimori's presentation

Dr. Jankowski (Birmingham University, UK): The most important conclusion you have come to is the fact that Barrett's esophagus is rare in Japan. What could be the explanation? Could it be missed diagnoses? How do you endoscopically classify the lower gastroesophageal junction—is that a possible explanation? Is there something different about the cancers themselves? In the West we often say that if you have the cancer it may overgrow a small segment of Barrett's esophagus that was originally there. Has there been any attempt to look for that? Is there truly a difference in this disease in Japan? Is it possible that the disease in Japan is different from that in the West? For example, is protein pump inhibitor usage less common here than in the West?

Dr. Tachimori: As I noted in my presentation, Barrett's esophagus in the general population in Japan is quite low. Only 1.1% of the patients with squamous cell carcinoma have Barrett's esophagus not associated with carcinoma. A Japanese commission also check for the presence of Barrett's esophagus in resected specimens, but the incidence of Barrett's esophagus was still low. Adenocarcinoma of the esophagus in Japan is still quite different than the Barrett's esophagus-associated adenocarcinoma in Western countries. In Japan, in recent years, many have adopted a Western life style and Western food, and we are now experiencing more obese persons with reflux disease. We anticipate having the same experience as in Western countries in the near future.

Dr. Jass (University of Queensland, Australia): I want to make just one point: that we have contrasting pathology and surgical approaches to adenocarcinoma of Barrett's esophagus. It occurs to me that surgeons proceed regardless of whether we as pathologists diagnose high-grade dysplasia adenocarcinoma in situ or superficial carcinoma that affects the mucosa. As far as I can tell, the management and prognosis are the same, regardless of whether we categorize these entities together or separately. As a pathologist I can often "split" biopsies in that way, and it seems not to matter. The important thing I think is the difficulty of interpreting biopsies and, in particular, distinguishing reactive change from genuine neoplasia. Surgeons want to have confidence in the pathologists' judgments about whether it is neoplastic, high-grade dysplasia, or early cancer. They really want to know if it is neoplastic; then they can proceed with management.

Part 3
Dysplasia and Superficial Squamous Cell Carcinoma

International Consensus Classification of Gastrointestinal Epithelial Neoplasia: Usefulness for Esophageal Squamous Epithelium

RONALD J. SCHLEMPER

Introduction

In 1998 a review of 21 esophageal squamous biopsy and resection specimens by 31 pathologists from 12 countries showed that definite carcinoma was the diagnosis in fewer than 20% of assessments by the Western pathologists but in more than 80% by the 9 Japanese specialists in gastrointestinal pathology [1]. There was agreement between the Western and Japanese viewpoints for only 14% of the specimens [2, 3]. In many cases Western pathologists diagnosed high-grade dysplasia when the Japanese diagnosed carcinoma. Western pathologists considered invasion into the lamina propria of the mucosa mandatory for the diagnosis of carcinoma, whereas nuclear and structural features were more important for the Japanese. Most Western pathologists made a discrepant diagnosis of dysplasia in the biopsy specimen and carcinoma in the resected specimen in some of the cases where they assessed both biopsy and resection specimens from the same esophageal lesion [1]. Similar differences were found between the Western and Japanese pathologists in the diagnosis of adenoma/dysplasia versus carcinoma in 35 gastric and 20 colorectal glandular lesions [1–3].

Among the 31 pathologists, 27 met in Vienna in 1998 and reached a consensus on the terminology for esophageal and gastrointestinal epithelial neoplasia; the "Vienna classification" thus emerged, as shown in Table 1 [2]. With this classification, the diagnoses high-grade dysplasia, carcinoma in situ, and suspicious for invasive carcinoma, which cannot be reproducibly distinguished, are clustered into one category, as the treatment recommendation would be the same for any of these three diagnoses. This classification is meant to be used for diagnosis of both biopsy and resected specimens [2]. When the original assessments of the 21 esophageal specimens were regrouped into the five categories of the Vienna classification, the agreement between the Western and Japanese pathologists increased from 14% to 62% [2, 3].

In the present study, I examined whether the use of the Vienna classification could also lead to a decreased number of discrepant diagnoses between biopsy specimens and corresponding resected specimens.

Department of Internal Medicine, Fukuoka University School of Medicine, 7-45-1 Nanakuma, Jonan-ku, Fukuoka 814-0180, Japan

TABLE 1. Vienna classification of esophageal and gastrointestinal epithelial neoplasia and clinical implications

Category	Clinical consideration
C1: Negative for neoplasia	Optional follow-up
C2: Indefinite for neoplasia	Follow-up
C3: Noninvasive low-grade neoplasia (low-grade adenoma/dysplasia)	Endoscopic treatment or follow-up[a]
C4: Noninvasive high-grade neoplasia	Endoscopic or surgical local treatment[a]
C4.1: High-grade adenoma/dysplasia	
C4.2: Noninvasive carcinoma (carcinoma in situ)[b]	
C4.3: Suspicious for invasive carcinoma	
C5: Invasive neoplasia	
C5.1: Intramucosal carcinoma[c]	Endoscopic or surgical local treatment[a]
C5.2: Submucosal carcinoma or beyond	Surgical treatment[a]

[a] The treatment modality depends on the size of the lesion, the endoscopic/radiographic/ultrasonographic assessment of the depth of invasion, and factors such as the patient's age and morbidity. Additional surgery after "complete" endoscopic resection may or may not be required depending on tumor differentiation and lymphatic vessel invasion
[b] Noninvasive: absence of evident invasion
[c] Intramucosal: invasion of the lamina propria or muscularis mucosae

Methods

Additional analyses were performed using data collected for a study reported in 1999 and 2000 [1–3]. In the previous study, 31 pathologists from 12 countries (listed in the Acknowledgments) individually reviewed a circulating slide set in 1998. There were 20 pathologists from Western countries and 11 from Japan (two general pathologists and nine specialists in gastrointestinal pathology).

The slide set consisted of glass slides plus photomicrographs of 21 esophageal specimens obtained from Japanese patients who underwent endoscopic mucosal resection for early squamous neoplastic lesions. Details of this material have been reported elsewhere [4]. Both biopsy and resected specimens were assessed for five lesions. The pathologists were not told the relation of the biopsy and resected specimens.

The pathologists were asked to diagnose each histologic specimen by choosing from the following categories: (1a) negative for neoplasia/dysplasia (normal, reactive, or regenerative epithelium); (1b) indefinite for neoplasia/dysplasia; (2) low-grade dysplasia; (3) high-grade dysplasia; (4) suspicious for carcinoma; or (5) definite carcinoma, subclassified by the depth of invasion: (5a) no invasion (Japanese viewpoint), (5b) intramucosal invasion (into the lamina propria or muscularis mucosae), (5c) submucosal invasion.

In the statistical analysis, 95% confidence intervals (CI) for proportions were based on binomial distributions. The two Japanese general pathologists were included in the group of Western pathologists, as they had (and also considered themselves as having) a Western viewpoint. Conventional Western and Japanese diagnoses were classified into the five categories mentioned above. Regrouping of diagnoses was done according to the five categories in Table 1. If there were two or more biopsies (or two or more resection specimens) from the same lesion, the severest diagnosis (i.e., highest category) was taken as the pathologist's biopsy diagnosis (or resection diagnosis) for that lesion.

Results

In the five cases for which there were both biopsy specimens and corresponding resected specimens, the 22 pathologists with a Western viewpoint made 37 of 110 assessments (34%; 95% CI 25%–43%) of reactive epithelium or dysplasia in the biopsy specimen and suspected or definite carcinoma in the resected specimen (Table 2, A). In 18 of these discrepant assessments the biopsy diagnosis was high-grade dysplasia, and the resection diagnosis was invasive carcinoma. There were 21 consistent assessments of high-grade dysplasia from both biopsy and resection specimens. Moreover, the Western pathologists made 30 of 110 assessments (27%; 95% CI 19%–36%) of reactive epithelium or low-grade dysplasia in the biopsy specimen and high-grade dysplasia or suspected/definite carcinoma in the corresponding resected specimen (Table 2, B). In 8 of these 30 assessments the resection diagnosis was suspected carcinoma; in 6 it was invasive carcinoma. The nine Japanese specialists in gastrointestinal pathology did not make such discrepant diagnoses, as all their biopsy and resection diagnoses were suspected or definite carcinoma.

When high-grade dysplasia, carcinoma in situ, and suspicious for invasive carcinoma were grouped into one category of noninvasive high-grade neoplasia according to the Vienna classification (Table 1), the 22 pathologists with a Western viewpoint made 30 of 110 assessments (27%; 95% CI 19%–36%) of noninvasive neoplasia in the biopsy specimen and invasive neoplasia in the resected specimen (Table 3, A). The nine Japanese specialists in gastrointestinal pathology made such discrepant diagnoses in 12 of 45 assessments (27%; 95% CI 15%–42%) (Table 3, B).

TABLE 2. Discrepant assessments by 22 pathologists with a Western viewpoint for five esophageal squamous lesions

(A) Benign vs. malignant diagnoses[a]				(B) Low-grade vs. high-grade diagnoses[a]			
	EMR diagnosis				EMR diagnosis		
Diagnosis	R + L + H	S + D	Total	Diagnosis	R + L	H + S + D	Total
Biopsy				Biopsy			
R + L + H	45 (41%)	37 (34%)	82	R + L	8 (7%)	30 (27%)	38
S + D	4 (4%)	24 (22%)	28	H + S + D	3 (3%)	69 (63%)	72
Total	49	61	110	Total	11	99	110

R, reactive or regenerative epithelium; L, low-grade dysplasia; H, high-grade dysplasia; S, suspected carcinoma; D, definite carcinoma; EMR, endoscopic mucosal resection

[a]Data are for conventional diagnoses divided into benign versus malignant (A) or into low-grade versus high-grade neoplasia (B) diagnoses

TABLE 3. Discrepant assessments by 22 pathologists with a Western viewpoint and by 9 Japanese specialists in gastrointestinal pathology for five esophageal squamous lesions

(A) Western viewpoint				(B) Japanese viewpoint			
	EMR diagnosis				EMR diagnosis		
Diagnosis	C1–C4	C5	Total	Diagnosis	C1–C4	C5	Total
Biopsy				Biopsy			
C1–C4	62 (56%)	30 (27%)	92	C1–C4	20 (44%)	12 (27%)	32
C5	4 (4%)	14 (13%)	18	C5	2 (4%)	11 (24%)	13
Total	66	44	110	Total	22	23	45

C1–C4, negative for neoplasia (C1), indefinite for neoplasia (C2), noninvasive low-grade neoplasia (C3), or noninvasive high-grade neoplasia (C4); C5, invasive neoplasia; EMR, endoscopic mucosal resection

Diagnoses were based on the Vienna classification

Discussion

This study confirms that Western pathologists often make a discrepant diagnosis of high-grade dysplasia from the biopsy specimen and invasive carcinoma from the resected specimen of the same esophageal lesion. Moreover, they sometimes diagnose low-grade dysplasia from the biopsy and invasive carcinoma from the corresponding resected specimen. The Japanese pathologists did not make such discrepant assessments in this material. However, when the carcinoma diagnoses were classified by invasion status according to the Vienna classification, there was a discrepant diagnosis of noninvasive neoplasia (category ≤ 4) from the biopsy and invasive neoplasia (category 5) from the corresponding resected specimen in about one-quarter of all assessments by both Japanese and Western pathologists.

These results have important implications for the clinical management of patients with superficial esophageal neoplastic lesions. Because in Western countries low-grade dysplasia usually is dealt with by endoscopic follow-up, the current Western diagnostic practice may lead to underdiagnosis of carcinoma and delayed treatment. On the other hand, esophagectomy is usually recommended for high-grade dysplasia, as endoscopic local resection is not performed in most Western countries; this can lead to overtreatment of lesions with no evident invasion. In comparison, the Japanese approach of diagnosing carcinoma in patients with noninvasive lesions may lead to overdiagnosis and unnecessary treatment, but this problem is mitigated by the availability of endoscopic mucosal resection, which has a low rate of complications [5–7].

To resolve many of the diagnostic and therapeutic differences between Western and Japanese pathologists, it was agreed that the Vienna classification should include categories based on invasion status, and clinical considerations were suggested (Table 1) [2]. However, the findings of this study show that the use of the Vienna classification would not diminish the discrepancies between biopsy and resection diagnoses, particularly with regard to the diagnosis of category 4 versus 5. This problem is due to the sampling error of endoscopic biopsies, which may miss the presence of nearby invasion [4]. Therefore, one should always keep in mind that the histologic diagnosis of biopsy specimens should be supplemented by available endoscopic [8], ultrasonographic [7], and radiographic assessments of the depth of invasion before a choice between endoscopic and surgical treatment is made [5]. To stress this point, pathologists could add the note "at least" to the category number when using the Vienna classification for biopsy diagnoses.

Three additional problems remain with the use of the Vienna classification. First, many lesions that Western pathologists would interpret as category 3, low-grade neoplasia, would be regarded as category 4, high-grade neoplasia, by Japanese pathologists. Second, there are lesions that Western pathologists would interpret as category 4 lesions without evident invasion but that the Japanese would diagnose as category 5.1, carcinoma with intramucosal invasion [2]. Invasion into the lamina propria is difficult to define, not only for glandular epithelium [1, 9] but also for squamous epithelium [4]. Third, the categories do not properly match the therapeutic implications. For example, categories 4 and 5.1 have the same clinical implication (i.e., local resection whenever possible) [6]. Conversely, within category 5, subcategories 5.1 and 5.2 should be treated differently (i.e., endoscopic treatment versus esophagectomy plus lymph node dissection for most mucosal versus submucosal lesions).

A previous study has shown that there are some nuclear features that Japanese pathologists judge to be clues for the diagnosis of carcinoma but that most Western pathologists either do not take into consideration (e.g., irregular shape) or to which they do not attach similar importance (e.g., marked hyperchromatism and variable size or enlargement) [4]. Furthermore, there are structural features Japanese pathologists consider more weighty (e.g., a sharp lateral border between normal and atypical epithelium for the diagnosis of carcinoma) and structural features the Western pathologists find more important (e.g., whether there are increased undifferentiated cells only in the lower half or also in the upper half of the epithelium for the diagnosis of low-grade versus high-grade dysplasia) [4]. The different interpretation of such nuclear and structural features accounts for lesions being diagnosed as category 3 by Western pathologists and as category 4 by Japanese pathologists. This difference in histologic interpretation is probably due to a difference in experience with early neoplastic lesions, a problem that could be reduced by an increased East-West exchange through histologic slide seminars [2, 4, 9, 10], training of Western pathologists and endoscopists in Japan, and an increased endoscopic detection rate of early neoplastic lesions in Western countries.

The problem of different diagnoses of category 4 versus 5.1 between Western and Japanese pathologists and the problem that categories 4 and 5 do not properly match the therapeutic implications could both be resolved by changing 5.1 of the Vienna classification to 4.4, thus including intramucosal carcinoma into a new category 4, named "mucosal high-grade neoplasia" [1]. Using this modification the definitional problem of intramucosal invasion is avoided, and a clear, clinically relevant distinction is made between mucosal neoplasia (categories 3 and 4) and submucosal invasion of neoplasia (category 5). The lymph node metastasis rate of esophageal carcinoma invading the submucosa is about 40%, but that of mucosal neoplasia is negligible [5, 6, 11, 12]; it is not significantly higher than the mortality rate of esophagectomy with three-field lymph node dissection, which is 3% in the best surgeon's hands [13]. Thus even for m3 carcinomas that have reached the muscularis mucosae, for which the lymph node metastasis rate is about 5% [5, 6, 11, 12], endoscopic resection is preferable when technically possible [6]. If a locally resected specimen shows only slight invasion into the submucosa, additional surgical treatment is not required when the tumor is well differentiated and there is no lymphatic vessel invasion [11, 14].

As there will always be discrepancies between biopsy and resection diagnoses, the Vienna classification with or without modification should be used for biopsy specimens only in combination with a clinical assessment of the depth of invasion. Only then can the recommendation for local treatment of category 4 be an important advantage. The classification is particularly useful for endoscopically resected specimens to determine whether additional surgery with lymph node dissection is required [15].

Conclusions

In summary, esophageal, gastric, and colorectal lesions considered dysplasia by Western pathologists are often diagnosed as carcinoma by Japanese pathologists. In 1998 a group of 31 pathologists from 12 countries proposed common worldwide terminology, which became known as the Vienna classification of gastrointestinal epithelial neoplasia. This classification consists of five categories: (1) negative for neoplasia; (2) indefinite for neoplasia; (3) noninvasive low-grade neoplasia; (4) noninvasive high-grade neoplasia; (5) invasive neoplasia, subdivided into (5.1) intramucosal carcinoma and (5.2) submucosal carcinoma or beyond. The clinical usefulness of this consensus classification for esophageal lesions requires evaluation.

Data from an individual review of 21 esophageal histologic specimens by 31 pathologists were analyzed with regard to the number of discrepant diagnoses for five squamous epithelial lesions of which there were both biopsy and resected specimens. Diagnoses were classified conventionally and according to the Vienna classification. In 34% of cases the 22 pathologists with a Western viewpoint diagnosed dysplasia from the biopsy but suspected or definite carcinoma from the resected specimen of the same lesion. In 27% of cases they assessed the biopsy as low-grade neoplasia but the corresponding resected specimen as high-grade neoplasia. Such discrepancies were not observed for the nine Japanese specialists in gastrointestinal pathology, as they diagnosed suspected or definite carcinoma in all specimens. However, in 27% of cases both Western and Japanese pathologists diagnosed noninvasive neoplasia from the biopsy but invasive neoplasia from the resected specimen of the same lesion.

With the use of the Vienna classification, the problem of frequent discrepant diagnoses between biopsy and resected specimens thus remained. Because of sampling error, one should not rely on a biopsy diagnosis of noninvasive or intramucosally invasive neoplasia for the choice between endoscopic and surgical treatment but, rather, on the depth of invasion estimated by endoscopy and ultrasonography or radiography. The classification is useful for endoscopically resected specimens to determine whether additional esophagectomy with lymph node dissection is necessary.

Acknowledgments. I thank F. Borchard, H.S. Cooper, S.M. Dawsey, M.F. Dixon, C.M. Fenoglio-Preiser, J-F. Fléjou, K. Geboes, T. Hattori, T. Hirota, M. Itabashi, M. Iwafuchi, A. Iwashita, Y. Kato, Y.I. Kim, T. Kirchner, M. Klimpfinger, M. Koike, G.Y. Lauwers, K. J. Lewin, G. Oberhuber, A.B. Price, R.H. Riddell, C.A. Rubio, M. Rugge, M. Shimizu, T.

Shimoda, P. Sipponen, E. Solcia, M. Stolte, H. Watanabe, and H. Yamabe for their histopathologic assessments.

References

1. Schlemper RJ, Kato Y, Stolte M (2000) Diagnostic criteria for gastrointestinal carcinomas in Japan and Western countries: proposal for a new classification system of gastrointestinal epithelial neoplasia. J Gastroenterol Hepatol 15:G49–G57
2. Schlemper RJ, Riddell RH, Kato Y, et al (2000) The Vienna classification of gastrointestinal epithelial neoplasia. Gut 47:251–255
3. Schlemper RJ, Kato Y, Riddell RH, et al (1999) New international consensus classification of gastrointestinal epithelial neoplasia (Vienna classification). Stomach Intestine 34:1043–1049
4. Schlemper RJ, Dawsey SM, Itabashi M, et al (2000) Differences in diagnostic criteria for esophageal squamous cell carcinoma between Japanese and Western pathologists. Cancer 88:996–1006
5. Momma K, Yoshida M, Nakamura J, et al (1997) Endoscopic mucosal resection for mucosal cancer of the esophagus. Clin Gastroenterol 12:1733–1740
6. Makuuchi H (1996) Endoscopic mucosal resection for early esophageal cancer: indications and techniques. Dig Endosc 8:175–179
7. Takeshita K, Tani M, Inoue H, et al (1997) Endoscopic treatment of early oesophageal or gastric cancer. Gut 40:123–127
8. Makuuchi H, Shimoda H, Mizutani K, et al (1997) Endoscopic criteria for invasive depth of superficial esophageal cancer. Dig Endosc 9:110–115
9. Schlemper RJ, Itabashi M, Kato Y, et al (1997) Differences in diagnostic criteria for gastric carcinoma between Japanese and Western pathologists. Lancet 349:1725–1729
10. Schlemper RJ, Borchard F, Dixon MF, et al (2000) International comparability of the pathological diagnosis for early cancer of the digestive tract: Munich meeting. J Gastroenterol 35(suppl XII):102–110
11. Tajima Y, Nakanishi Y, Ochiai A, et al (2000) Histopathologic findings predicting lymph node metastasis and prognosis of patients with superficial esophageal carcinoma: analysis of 240 surgically resected tumors. Cancer 88:1285–1293
12. Watanabe H, Komukai S, Ajioka Y, et al (1998) Histopathology of m3 and sm1 invasive squamous cell carcinoma of the esophagus with special reference to endoscopic resection. Stomach Intestine 33:985–992
13. Isono K, Sato H, Nakayama K (1991) Results of a nationwide study on the three-field lymph node dissection of esophageal cancer. Oncology 48:411–420
14. Makuuchi H, Shimada H, Chino O, et al (1998) Possibility of endoscopic mucosal resection in patients with m3 and sm1 esophageal cancer. Stomach Intestine 33:993–1002
15 Schlemper RJ, Kato Y, Stolte M (2001) Review of histological classifications of gastrointestinal epithelial neoplasia: differences in diagnosis of early carcinomas between Japanese and Western pathologists. J Gastroenterol 36:445–456

Q & A after Dr. Schlemper's presentation

Dr. Jankowski (Birmingham University, UK): It seems that the final arbiter of whether this is useful is long-term follow-up data. Do you have any evidence on that? It would be good to know whether the Japanese view that the intraepithelial structural abnormality and nuclei are important is correct or the Western view that invasion is more important.

Dr. Schlemper: There are still no data on the use of the Vienna classification, but I am advising all Japanese pathologists to start using it in addition to the current terminology, also in their biopsy reports. If they later obtain follow-up data such as from resected specimens, it can be seen whether or not biopsy diagnoses based on this classification are helpful for predicting patient outcomes. However, such data are not yet available.

Dr. Jankowski: Could it be one of the recommendations of this conference to pick a handful of pathologists who are willing to use this classification in addition to their own? Then, maybe after a year or so you could see what the long-term follow-up of some of the high-grade dysplasia cases would be.

Dr. Schlemper: I know they are using it at the National Cancer Center and in Hiroshima as well. Hopefully, after a couple of years, we will see some results.

Dr. Itabashi (Ibaragi Prefectural Central Hospital, Tomobe, Japan): Dr. Schlemper, will you please introduce and explain Dawsey's papers concerning the Chinese people's follow-up data?

Dr. Schlemper: My main conclusion regarding Dr. Dawsey's papers of 1994 and 1998 published in the journal "Cancer" (which is his conclusion as well) is that conventional classifications cause misunderstandings about prognosis and about the value of iodine staining. Diagnoses should be stratified by invasion status, otherwise it is impossible to compare Wastern and Japanese studies. Moreover, the distinction between high-grade dysplasia and carcinoma in situ is clinically irrelevant and should be abandoned.

Dr. Chandrasoma (Los Angeles County-USC Medical Center, USA): Do you make the distinction between intramucosal carcinoma and submucosal invasive carcinoma? Is it based on the biopsy or the resected specimen?

Dr. Schlemper: It should not be based on the biopsy because of the possibility of sampling error. After complete local resection, you can do a proper assessment, because there are no longer any sampling errors. For intramucosal lesions endoscopic resection is sufficient, but for submucosal lesions additional surgical resection is often required because of the high rate of lymph node metastases. So, for the therapeutic implications of this classification, information gained from the complete local resection should be used to avoid sampling error. Dr. Nakanishi's paper will show the histopathologic findings that can be used as markers to identify patients who require additional surgical lymph node dissection after endoscopic local resection.

Histopathologic Findings Predicting Lymph Node Metastasis and Prognosis of Patients with Superficial Esophageal Carcinoma

Yukihiro Nakanishi

Introduction

Studies on patients with superficial squamous cell carcinoma of the esophagus (SSCCE) revealed that 0%–8.7% of mucosal carcinomas had lymph node metastases, whereas the incidence of lymph node metastasis in those with submucosal carcinomas was 43.6%–53.3% [1, 2]. In recent years, endoscopic mucosal resection (EMR), a minimally invasive surgical procedure, has been performed with excellent results [3]. It has been proposed that EMR be indicated as a radical resection procedure for mucosal carcinomas [4]. EMR is associated with a low incidence of postoperative complications, and so far no patients have died as a result of this surgical technique [1]. Therefore, the indications for EMR may be able to be extended. To do so, it is important to establish the histopathologic findings that affect lymph node metastasis, so patients without lymph node metastasis can be excluded. However, as far as we are aware, there have been no studies involving a large number of patients with SSCCE in which the relation between the histopathologic findings and lymph node metastasis has been evaluated by multivariate analysis.

In this study, histopathologic findings in SSCCE were evaluated to abstract the factors strongly related to lymph node metastasis and prognosis. Afterward the cases in which tumors had invaded the lamina muscularis mucosa or slightly invaded the submucosa were reviewed to abstract those for which additional surgical resection is not required after EMR.

Materials and Methods

Patients

Our series consisted of 240 consecutive patients who had undergone esophagectomy for SSCCE at the National Cancer Center Hospital, Tokyo, Japan, between February 1968 and December 1996 (Table 1). The group comprised 219 men and 21 women age

Pathology Division, National Cancer Center Research Institute, 1-1 Tsukiji 5 chome, Chuo-ku, Tokyo 104-0045, Japan

TABLE 1. Characteristics of tumors

Characteristic	No. of cases (%)
Depth of invasion	
m	54 (22.5)
mm	20 (8.3)
sm	166 (69.2)
Multicentric esophageal lesions	
1	174 (72.5)
2	41 (17.1)
3	12 (5.0)
4	6 (2.5)
5+	7 (2.9)
Mean no. of dissected lymph nodes	52.3 ± 27.2
Location	
Cervical	15 (6.3)
Thoracic	
Upper	34 (14.2)
Middle	118 (49.2)
Lower	73 (30.4)
Multiple tumors of other organs	
Pharynx	25 (10.4)
Colon	6 (2.5)
Oral cavity	4 (1.7)
Larynx	4 (1.7)
Prostate	2 (0.8)
Stomach	23 (9.6)
Thyroid	5 (2.1)
Tongue	4 (1.7)
Lung	2 (0.8)
Others	5 (2.1)
Total	80 Tumors in 71 patients

Numbers in parentheses are percents
(CANCER 2000;88:1285–93.)

60.9 ± 9.5 years (mean ± SD). Each patient underwent thoracoabdominal (two-field) or cervicothoracoabdominal (three-field) lymphadenectomy. Altogether, 66 patients (27.5%) had multicentric esophageal lesions, and 71 (29.6%) had synchronous or metachronous multiple carcinomas in other organs. No preoperative radiotherapy or chemotherapy was performed. When a patient had multicentric lesions, the histopathologic factors of the lesion showing the greatest invasion depth were evaluated.

Histopathologic Review

Serial 5mm thick tissue sections of the entire lesion were cut from resected specimens fixed with 10% buffered formalin, embedded in paraffin, and stained with hematoxylin and eosin (H&E) using routine methods. The tumor size, depth of invasion (vertical tumor invasion depth in the submucosal layer; VTIDsm), lymphatic invasion, blood vessel invasion, lymph node metastasis, tumor differentiation, degree of nuclear atypia, growth pattern, and histologic grade were examined histopathologically. The depth of invasion was subclassified as m (intraepithelial carcinomas and tumors invading the lamina propria mucosa), mm (invasive tumors in contact with or invading the lamina muscularis mucosa), or sm (tumors invading the submucosa). The distance from the lower edge of the lamina muscularis mucosa to the deepest portion of the invading tumor was measured by microscopy with an ocular lens scale and defined as VTIDsm. In specimens in which the lamina muscularis mucosa was disrupted by ulceration or tumor invasion, a tentative lamina muscularis mucosal level was drawn by connecting the two ends of the remaining lamina muscularis mucosa. Tumor differentiation was assessed using the World Health Organization classification [5]. The degree of nuclear atypia was classified as low (nuclei of uniform size and shape with homogeneous chromatin: 1 point) or high (polymorphic nuclei with vesicular or dot-like chromatin: 2 points) (Fig. 1a,b). The growth pattern was classified as expansive (large solid nests with a clear tumor margin: 1 point) or infiltrative (small nests and dissociated cells with an unclear tumor margin: 2 points) (Fig. 1c,d). The degree of nuclear atypia and the growth pattern were evaluated in the deepest area of the invading tumor. The histologic grade of each tumor was calculated by adding the nuclear atypia and growth pattern scores to obtain grade 1 (2 points), grade 2 (3 points), or grade 3 (4 points).

Statistical Analysis

Survival rates were calculated as described by Kaplan and Meier, and prognostic factors were analyzed using the proportional hazards model of Cox. Patients who died of operative complications or other diseases were excluded. The effects of histopathologic factors on lymph node metastasis were examined using logistic regression analysis. The level of significance was set at $P < 0.05$.

Results

Incidence of Lymph Node Metastasis and 5-Year Survival Rates in 240 Patients with Superficial Esophageal Carcinomas of Varying Invasion Depths

None of the 54 patients with m carcinomas and just one of the 20 (5.0%) with mm carcinomas had lymph node metastasis; the 5-year survival rates for both groups were 100%. Altogether, 79 of the 166 (47.6%) patients with sm carcinomas had lymph node metastasis, and the 5-year survival rate of this group was 78.4%. Accordingly, we analyzed the relations between the histopathologic findings and lymph node metastasis and prognosis of the 186 patients with mm and sm carcinomas.

Relations Between Histopathologic Findings and Lymph Node Metastasis in Patients with mm and sm Carcinomas

The relations between the histopathologic findings and lymph node metastasis in 186 patients with mm and sm carcinomas determined by univariate and multivariate

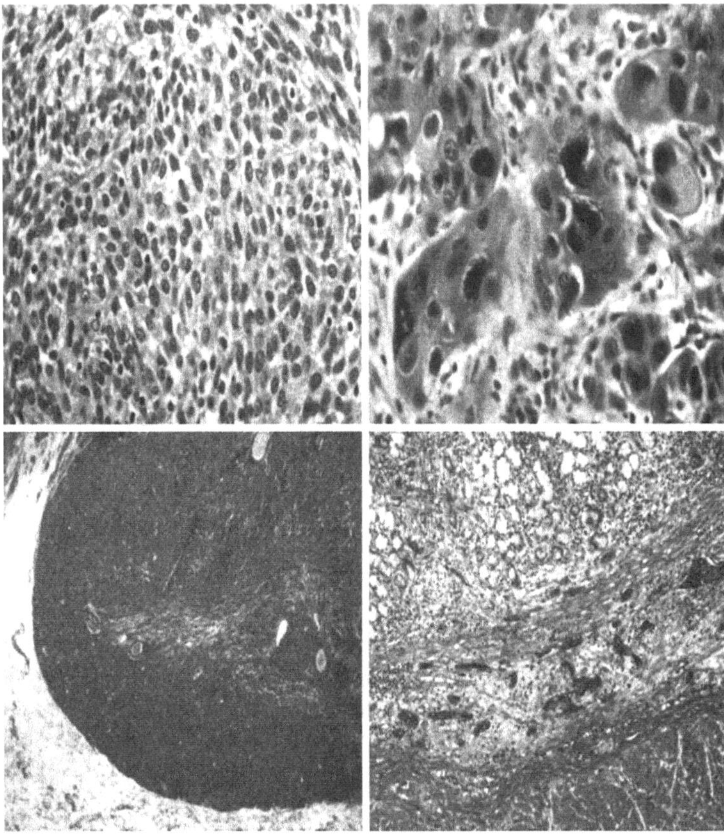

FIG. 1. **a,b** Photomicrographs of superficial esophageal carcinomas showing different degrees of nuclear atypia. **a** Nuclei of uniform sizes and shapes with homogeneous chromatin are considered to indicate a low degree of nuclear atypia. (H&E, ×200). **b** Polymorphic nuclei with vesicular or dot-like chromatin are considered to indicate a high degree of nuclear atypia. (H&E, ×400) **c,d** Photomicrographs of superficial esophageal cancers showing different growth patterns. **c** Large solid nests and a clear tumor margin are considered to indicate an expansive growth pattern. (H&E, ×40). **d** Small nests, dissociated cells, and an unclear tumor margin are considered to indicate an infiltrative growth pattern. (H&E, ×100). (CANCER 2000;88:1285–93.)

analysis are shown in Table 2. Univariate analysis showed that each of the following histopathologic factors had a significant influence on lymph node metastasis: VTIDsm, lymphatic permeation, blood vessel permeation, degree of nuclear atypia, and histologic grade (P = 0.0090, 0.0001, 0.0011, 0.074, and 0.0080, respectively), whereas multivariate analysis showed that only lymphatic permeation correlated with lymph node metastasis ($P < 0.0001$). When the data for the same patients were analyzed using both the degree of nuclear atypia and the growth pattern instead of the histologic grade, similar results were obtained (data not shown).

TABLE 2. Relations between histopathologic findings and lymph node metastasis in mm and sm carcinomas (186 cases)

Histopathologic factor	Lymph node metastasis positive ($n = 80$)	Lymph node metastasis negative ($n = 106$)	Univariate analysis *P*	Multivariate analysis OR	Multivariate analysis CI	Multivariate analysis *P*
Tumor size						
<30 mm	36 (45.0)	52 (49.1)	0.58			NS
≥30 mm	44 (55.0)	54 (50.9)				
VTIDsm						
<500 μm	15 (18.8)	38 (35.8)	0.0090			NS
<1000 μm	24 (30.0)	30 (28.3)				
1000 μm	41 (51.3)	38 (35.8)				
Ly						
Negative	18 (22.5)	74 (69.8)	<0.0001	7.00	3.30–14.9	<0.0001
Positive	62 (77.5)	32 (30.2)				
V						
Negative	54 (67.5)	93 (87.7)	0.0011			NS
Positive	26 (32.5)	13 (12.3)				
Differentiation						
Well, moderately	37 (46.3)	59 (55.7)	0.20			NS
Poorly	43 (53.8)	47 (44.3)				
Degree of nuclear atypia						
Low	43 (53.7)	74 (69.8)	0.026		Not analyzed	
High	37 (46.3)	32 (30.2)				
Growth pattern						
Expansive	23 (28.8)	44 (41.5)	0.074		Not analyzed	
Infiltrative	57 (71.3)	62 (58.5)				
Histologic grade						
1	12 (15.0)	36 (34.0)	0.0080			NS
2	42 (52.5)	46 (43.4)				
3	26 (32.5)	24 (22.5)				

Numbers in parentheses are percents
OR, odds ratio; CI, 95% confidence interval; Ly, lymphatic permeation; V, blood vessel permeation
(CANCER 2000;88:1285–93.)

Relations Between Histopathologic Findings and Prognosis in Patients with mm and sm Carcinomas

The relations between the histopathologic findings and prognosis in 186 patients with mm and sm carcinomas determined by univariate and multivariate analysis are shown in Table 3. The former showed that each of the following histopathologic factors had a significant deleterious influence on prognosis: presence of lymphatic permeation, presence of lymph node metastasis, high-degree nuclear atypia, an infiltrative growth pattern, and a high histologic grade ($P = 0.021, 0.001, 0.025, 0.024$, and 0.0028, respectively). Multivariate analysis showed that the presence of lymph node metastasis and a high histologic grade were independent factors predictive of a poor prognosis ($P =$ 0.0061 and 0.023, respectively). When the data for the same patients were analyzed using the degree of nuclear atypia and the growth pattern scores instead of the histologic grade, their effect on prognosis was reduced, and only lymph node metastasis was a significant prognostic factor ($P = 0.0052$).

Relations Between Histopathologic Findings and Lymph Node Metastasis in Patients with Carcinomas with a VTIDsm less than 500 μm

The relations among VTIDsm, lymphatic permeation, blood vessel permeation, and the histologic grade and lymph node metastasis in 53 patients in whom VTIDsm was less than 500 μm (17 and 36 with mm and sm carcinomas, respectively) were analyzed. As described above, lymphatic permeation had a significant influence on lymph node metastasis ($P = 0.0003$) in this group. The incidence of lymph node metastasis in the 17 patients with lymphatic permeation was high (64.7%; 11/17) irrespective of VTIDsm, blood vessel permeation, or the histologic grade (Table 4), whereas only 4 (11.1%) of those without lymphatic permeation had lymph node metastasis (Table 5). The respective VTIDsm values and histologic grades of these four were 200 μm and 3300 μm and 2 (2 patients), and 320 μm and 2. One patient with an mm carcinoma of histologic grade 3 had blood vessel permeation. No lymph node metastases were found in the lymphatic permeation-negative and blood vessel permeation-negative patients whose VTIDsm values were less than 200 μm and histologic grades were 1 or 2 (Table 5).

Discussion

As far as we are aware, there are no reported studies involving a large number of patients with SSCCE in which the relations between the histopathologic findings and lymph node metastasis have been evaluated by multivariate analysis. In our study, univariate analysis of 186 patients with mm and sm carcinomas showed that VTIDsm, lymphatic permeation, blood vessel permeation, degree of nuclear atypia, and histologic grade correlated with lymph node metastasis, whereas multivariate analysis showed a correlation between lymphatic permeation and lymph node metastasis. Therefore, lymphatic permeation is the most important histopathologic factor that predicts lymph node metastasis in patients with mm and sm carcinomas.

TABLE 3. Relations between histopathologic findings and prognosis using univariate and multivariate analysis in mm and sm carcinomas (186 cases)

	Univariate analysis	Multivariate analysis A			Multivariate analysis B[a]		
Histopathologic factor	*P*	HR	CI	*P*	HR	CI	*P*
Tumor size							
<30 mm	0.58			NS			NS
≥30 mm							
VTIDsm							
<500 μm	0.24			NS			NS
<1000 μm							
≥1000 μm							
Multicentric lesions							
Negative	0.64			NS			NS
Positive							
Ly							
Negative	0.021			NS			NS
Positive							
V							
Negative	0.53			NS			NS
Positive							
Lymph node metastasis							
Negative	0.001	6.21	2.83–16.34	0.0052	6.08	2.77–16.06	0.0061
Positive							
Differentiation							
Well, moderately	0.34			NS			NS
Poorly							
Degree of nuclear atypia							
Low	0.025			NS		Not analyzed	
High							
Growth pattern							
Expansive	0.024			NS		Not analyzed	
Infiltrative							
Histologic grade							
1	0.0028		Not analyzed		2.77	1.27–6.02	0.023
2							
3							

HR, hazards ratio; CI, 95% confidence intervals; Ly, lymphatic permeation; V, blood vessel permeation
[a] The material was analyzed for the same cases using the two components (degree of nuclear atypia and growth pattern, respectively) instead of histologic grade in multivariate analysis B
(CANCER 2000;88:1285–93.)

TABLE 4. Lymphatic permeation-positive tumors with VTIDsm <500 μm (17 cases)

VTIDsm (μm)	Histologic grade	Blood vessel permeation	Lymph node metastasis
mm Invasion			
0	2	−	Negative
0	2	−	Negative
0	3	−	Positive
sm Invasion			
50	1	−	Positive
80	1	−	Positive
100	1	+	Negative
100	1	−	Positive
100	3	+	Positive
130	1	−	Negative
200	2	+	Positive
300	3	−	Positive
350	2	−	Negative
400	1	+	Negative
400	2	−	Positive
400	2	−	Positive
450	2	−	Positive
480	3	−	Positive

(CANCER 2000;88:1285–93.)

Previous studies showed that the 5-year survival rates of patients with mucosal and submucosal carcinomas were 83.5%–87.6% and 54.9%–63.6%, respectively. In particular, the 5-year survival rate of patients with submucosal carcinomas with lymph node metastasis was reported to be much poorer, 27.0%–43.6% [2, 6, 7]. Endo and Kawano performed univariate analysis of 230 patients with SSCCE and showed that the prognosis of those with mucosal carcinomas was superior to that of those with submucosal carcinomas, and that vessel (lymphatic and blood vessel) permeation and lymph node metastasis correlated with prognosis [8]. However, to the best of our knowledge, there have been no studies involving multivariate analysis of the relations between the histopathologic factors and prognosis of a large number of patients with SSCCE. Our multivariate analysis showed that the presence of lymph node metastasis and a high histologic grade were independent factors predictive of a poor prognosis. Therefore, careful postoperative follow-up is required for patients with lymph node metastasis, high histologic grade or both. In patients with breast cancer, multivariate analysis indicated that the histologic grade based on the degree of architectural atypia, degree of nuclear atypia, and number of mitotic figures was an independent prognostic factor, as was the number of positive lymph nodes [9]. Hitherto, the prognostic significance of the degree of nuclear atypia and growth pattern in combination had not been investigated in patients with SSCCE. In this study we found that the histologic grade, determined by combining the degree of nuclear atypia and the growth pattern, was a useful prognostic factor.

Further study should be advocated to establish the most appropriate treatment strategy for patients with carcinomas invading the lamina muscularis mucosa or

TABLE 5. Lymphatic permeation-negative tumors with VTIDsm <500 μm (36 cases)

VTIDsm (μm)	Histologic grade	Blood vessel permeation	Lymph node metastasis
mm Invasion			
0	1	–	Negative
0	1	–	Negative
0	1	–	Negative
0	1	–	Negative
0	1	–	Negative
0	1	–	Negative
0	1	–	Negative
0	1	–	Negative
0	1	–	Negative
0	1	–	Negative
0	1	–	Negative
0	1	–	Negative
0	2	–	Negative
0	2	–	Negative
0	2	–	Negative
0	2	–	Negative
0	3	+	Negative
sm Invasion			
100	1	–	Negative
150	1	–	Negative
150	1	–	Negative
200	2	–	Negative
200	2	–	Negative
200	3	–	Positive
230	2	–	Negative
230	2	–	Negative
250	1	–	Negative
250	2	–	Negative
300	1	–	Negative
300	2	–	Positive
300	2	–	Positive
320	2	–	Positive
350	2	–	Negative
350	1	–	Negative
400	2	–	Negative
400	2	–	Negative
450	2	–	Negative

(CANCER 2000;88:1285–93.)

slightly invading the submucosa with a relatively low incidence of lymph node metastasis.

The indications for EMR treatment should be extended because EMR is a safe, feasible procedure. Therefore, it is important to establish which histopathologic factors predict lymph node metastasis of carcinomas that invade the lamina muscularis mucosa or slightly invade the submucosa.

Our multivariate analysis showed that lymphatic permeation was the most important histopathologic factor that predicted lymph node metastasis in patients with mm and sm carcinomas. In addition to lymphatic permeation, other histopathologic factors shown by univariate analysis to correlate with lymph node metastasis (i.e., blood vessel permeation, VTIDsm, histologic grade) in 53 patients in whom the VTIDsm values were less than 500 μm were analyzed to predict lymph node metastasis as accurately and comprehensively as possible. A cutoff value of 500 μm was chosen for these patients because about one-third of those with submucosal invasion had VTIDsm values below 500 μm. Of the 17 patients with lymphatic permeation, 11 (64.7%) had lymph node metastasis irrespective of blood vessel permeation, VTIDsm, or histologic grade. Therefore, in this group it is difficult to separate patients with and without lymph node metastasis. However, only 4 (11.1%) of the 36 patients without lymphatic permeation had lymph node metastasis. No lymph node metastasis occurred in lymphatic permeation-negative and blood vessel permeation-negative patients whose VTIDsm values were less than 200 μm with histologic grades of 1 or 2. These results indicate that the presence of vessel permeation (lymphatic permeation and blood vessel permeation), VTIDsm, and histologic grade should be considered to identify patients who do not require additional surgical resection after EMR. If vessel permeation is present, additional surgical resection after EMR is required for all patients with invasion depths greater than mm. If vessel permeation is not present, additional surgical resection after EMR is not required for patients with histologic grades 1 or 2 and VTIDsm values below 200 μm.

Acknowledgment. The author is grateful to Drs. Tadakazu Shimoda (Clinical Laboratory Division, National Cancer Center Hospital); Atsushi Ochiai (Pathology Division, National Cancer Center Research Institute East); Yusuke Tajima (Second Department of Surgery, Faculty of Medicine, Showa University); Kimio Yoshimura (Cancer Information and Epidemiology Division, National Cancer Center Research Institute); Yuji Tachimori, Hoichi Kato, Hiroshi Watanabe (Department of Surgery, National Cancer Center Hospital); and Hajime Yamaguchi (Department of Internal Medicine, National Cancer Center Hospital) for valuable advice.

References

1. Nabeya K, Nakata Y (1997) Extent of resection and lymphadenectomy in early squamous cell esophageal cancer. Dis Esophagus 10:159–161
2. Tachibana M, Yoshimura H, Kinugasa S, Hashimoto N, Dipok Kumar Dhar, Abe S, et al (1997) Clinicopathological features of superficial squamous cell carcinoma of the esophagus. Am J Surg 174:49–53
3. Makuuchi H, Machimura T, Mizutani K (1993) Endoscopic mucosal resection for early carcinoma of the esophagus. In: Takanishi T (ed) Recent advances in management of digestive cancer. Springer, Tokyo, pp 94–97
4. Sugawara K, Sayama J, Nishihira T, Hirayama K, Akaishi T, Shineha R, et al (1993) How should therapies for superficial cancer of the esophagus be performed? In: Nabeya K, Hanaoka T, Nogami H (eds) Recent advances in diseases of the esophagus. Springer, New York, pp 780–785
5. World Health Organization (1990) Histological typing of oesophageal and gastric tumors, 2nd edn. Springer, Berlin, p 2

6. Kato H, Tachimori Y, Watanabe H, Yamaguchi H, Ishikawa T, Itabashi M (1990) Superficial esophageal carcinoma: surgical treatment and the results. Cancer 66:2319–2323
7. Bonavina L, Ruol A, Ancona E, Peracchia A (1997) Prognosis of early squamous cell carcinoma of the esophagus after surgical therapy. Dis Esophagus 10:162–164
8. Endo M, Kawano T (1997) Detection and classification of early squamous cell esophageal cancer. Dis Esophagus 10:155–158
9. Tsuda H, Hirohashi S, Shimosato Y, Hirota T, Tsugane S, Watanabe S, et al (1990) Correlation between histologic grade of malignancy and copy number of c-erbB2 gene in breast carcinoma. Cancer 65:1794–1800

Q & A after Dr. Nakanishi's presentation

Dr. Jankowski (Birmingham University, UK): From my way of thinking tumorigenesis in any organ, is progressive, from abnormal cells, clonal expansion through the gland, and a stage of commitment to invasion. There is invasion directly into the tissue or into the lymphatic structure.

Dr. Nakanishi: We classify tumors into two types: expansive pattern or infiltrative growth pattern. Is that sufficient?

Dr. Jankowski: That's fine. But you said that the pattern of invasion was not analyzed for independent prognostic significance.

Dr. Nakanishi: Yes, growth pattern was not found to be an independent prognostic factor. Multivariate analysis showed that the presence of lymph node (LN) metastasis and high histologic grades were independent factors predictive of a poor prognosis. When the data for the same patient were analyzed using both nuclear atypia and growth pattern scores instead of histologic grades, their effect on prognosis was reduced, and only LN metastasis was a significant factor.

Dr. Jankowski: I just want to make sure it is quite clear because it seems that you must have a degree of invasion whether it is expansive or infiltrative to get to the LN in the first place. I am unclear about whether you actually analyzed the pattern of invasion. To get to the LN, by definition, you must first have an invasion, and you said you didn't independently assess invasion. Have I misunderstood? Oh, I understand now. You clearly had invasion in all these cases, but you did not analyze the *pattern* of invasion. That is quite significant. I think it is important for you to analyze the pattern of invasion. Does that make sense?

Dr. Nakanishi: Univariate analysis showed that an invasive growth pattern in a significant factor.

Dr. Itabashi (Ibaragi Prefectural Central Hospital, Tomobe, Japan): But in multivariate analysis, it was not significant.

Dr. Chanvitan (Khaengkoi Medical Center, Thailand): I was interested in your presentation about the chance of dysplasia progressing to cancer. How many cases in your report did you have to change from dysplasia to cancer, and what was the timing for the change? What factors were involved in the change?

Dr. Nakanishi: Dr. Ishiguro examined 25 cases, and only 2 cases of dysplasia progressed to cancer. The longest follow-up period was 6 years.

Dr. Chanvitan: What was the method of diagnosis for dysplasia in the biopsied specimens?

Dr. Nakanishi: We first examined the biopsy specimen and later examined the corresponding resected specimen.

Dr. Itabashi: Dr. Rubio may have some comments on these pathologic presentations. He attended the meeting about the Vienna classification, and he understands the Japanese, American, and European histological criteria for GI tract neoplasias.

Dr. Rubio (Karolinska Institute, Sweden): Here in Japan, because of your searching for small lesions, you have many more cases of very early lesions, especially squamous epithelial lesions such as severe dysplasia and carcinoma in situ. In the West, we don't see such lesions. Mostly we see invasive carcinoma. There is not much discrepancy except among particularly difficult cases, such as those being presented here. Despite the differences, when we make the second review of these cases there is rather good agreement between the classification used in the West and that used in Japan. As a matter of fact, we have learned from the Japanese how to classify these lesions. Therefore, thanks to the meetings, to the work of Dr. Schalemper, and the work of all the pathologists here in Japan trying to arrive at some agreement with the West we are diminishing the differences and are coming to some agreement. These meetings are very important to this goal.

Esophageal Superficial Neoplasms: Results of Surgery: Primary Early-Stage Squamous Cell Carcinomas versus Tumors Down-Staged to an Early Stage by Neoadjuvant Chemoradiotherapy

Stefano Merigliano, Alberto Ruol, Matteo Cagol, Sabrina Scappin, Rita Alfieri, Magdalena Epifani, and Ermanno Ancona

Introduction

Early squamous cell carcinoma of the esophagus has been defined as a tumor limited to the mucosa or submucosa without nodal metastasis in the resected specimen [1]. This corresponds to pTis-T1N0M0 or stage 0-I according to the TNM classification. Superficial esophageal cancer has been defined by endoscopic evidence of a tumor that does not extend beyond the submucosa regardless of the presence of lymph node metastasis.

The reported incidence of superficial esophageal cancer has steadily increased in Japan and other Far East countries as a result of the widespread use of endoscopy and the effectiveness of mass screening programs. In contrast, in Western countries, where the incidence of the disease is low, esophageal cancer is rarely diagnosed until dysphagia occurs; therefore, only few patients with superficial esophageal cancer (i.e., fewer than 5%) are seen [2].

Neoadjuvant chemoradiotherapy possibly followed by surgery has been acknowledged as the treatment of choice for locally advanced esophageal cancer (T4anyNM0), because it guarantees tumor down-staging in a significant percentage of patients and improves long-term survival. On the other hand, neoadjuvant chemoradiotherapy is still investigational for potentially resectable esophageal cancer (T1-T3anyNM0) and should be used only in prospective controlled studies. After neoadjuvant chemotherapy or chemoradiotherapy, it is not unusual to find in the operative specimen an esophageal tumor that has been down-staged to complete response (pT0N0M0) or an early-stage tumor (pTis-T1) [3, 4].

The aim of this study was to compare the early and long-term results after primary surgery in patients with superficial squamous cell carcinoma of the esophagus and in patients with tumors down-staged to superficial cancer by neoadjuvant chemotherapy or chemoradiotherapy (CRT-surgery).

Clinica Chirurgica 4°, University of Padova School of Medicine, Via Giustiniani 2, 35128 Padova, Italy

Materials and Methods

The computerized hospital records of patients with squamous cell carcinoma of the esophagus who were observed from 1980 to 1999 were reviewed using a dedicated software program.

The preferred approach for esophageal resection was transthoracic esophagectomy. Transhiatal esophagectomy was used only when thoracotomy was contraindicated, when the tumor was intraepithelial or intramucosal, or when tumor location was limited to the cervical esophagus. Esophagectomy plus two-field or three-field lymph node dissection, depending on tumor location, was the standard operative procedure. The stomach was the most commonly used esophageal substitute. The anastomosis was performed with a circular stapler in the chest and manually in the neck.

Postoperative morbidity was defined as any type of major or minor postoperative complication. Postoperative mortality was defined as any deaths occurring before hospital discharge or occurring even later if possibly related to the surgical procedure. Survival was measured from the date of surgery in the primary surgery group or from the date of chemotherapy in the CRT-surgery group to death or last date of follow-up. Survival rates were calculated by the Kaplan-Meier method, including deaths from all causes except postoperative mortality. All the patients had at least 24 months of follow-up.

In patients with locally advanced esophageal cancer (T4anyNM0) the first-line chemotherapy possibly followed by surgery was the combined-modality treatment of choice from 1983 to 1992; since then, first-line chemoradiotherapy possibly followed by surgery became the treatment of choice in these patients. The standard regimen included four cycles of concomitant chemotherapy (cisplatin/5-fluorocuracil, or DDP/5FU) and radiotherapy (45 Gy) followed by surgery when adequate tumor downstaging was documented.

Patients with a potentially resectable esophageal cancer (T1-T3anyNM0) entered a randomized trial of surgery alone versus neoadjuvant chemotherapy (DDP/5FU) from 1992 to 1997.

From 1980 to 1998 a series of 1225 (53%) of 2300 patients with squamous cell carcinoma of the esophagus underwent resection of their tumors: 943 (41%) patients underwent primary surgery, and 282 (12%) underwent surgery after neoadjuvant chemotherapy or chemoradiotherapy (CRT-surgery).

Of the 943 patients in the primary surgery group, 118 (12.5%) had a superficial tumor documented by pathological examination of the surgical specimen. There were 21 pTisN0M0 tumors, and 97 pT1 tumors (8 with mucosal and 89 with submucosal involvement). Of 89 submucosal pT1 tumors, 16 (19%) had lymph node metastasis (pN^+). The preoperative clinical staging of the above 118 patients was as follows: 14 with Tis, 61 with T1, 28 with T2, and 15 with T3; all patients were node-negative.

Altogether, 88 (74%) patients were male and 30 (26%) female; the mean age was 61 years. The tumor was located in the cervical esophagus in 5 (4%) cases, in the upper thoracic esophagus in 34 (29%), in the mid-thoracic esophagus in 44 (37%), and in the lower thoracic esophagus in 35 (30%).

Of 282 patients in the CRT-surgery group, 65 (5.1%) had a superficial tumor documented by pathological examination of the surgical specimen. There were 38 complete-response tumors (pT0), 6 pTis tumors, and 21 pT1 tumors (3 with mucosal and 18 with submucosal involvement). Altogether, 6 (16%) of 38 pT0 tumors, 1 (17%) of 6 pTis tumors, 2 (67%) of 3 mucosal pT1 tumors, and 9 (50%) of 18 submucosal pT1 tumors had lymph node metastasis (pN^+). The initial pretreatment clinical staging of the above 65 patients was as follows: 15 with T2, 25 with T3, and 25 with T4; 38 node-negative and 27 node-positive tumors. Altogether, 53 (81%) patients were male, and 12 (19%) were female. The mean age was 61 years. The tumor was located in the cervical esophagus in 11 (17%), in the upper thoracic esophagus in 21 (32%), in the mid-thoracic esophagus in 18 (28%), and in the lower thoracic esophagus in 15 (23%).

On average, lymph node dissection included 13 lymph nodes per patient (range 5–45). Most patients with nodal metastasis (78%) had only one or two metastatic lymph nodes.

Results

The overall incidence of postoperative complications was 57% (68/118) in the primary surgery group and 61% (40/65) in the CRT-surgery group. The incidence of anastomotic leaks or ischemic necrosis of the esophageal substitute was 17% (20/118; 11 were asymptomatic and were demonstrated only radiologically) in the primary surgery group and 18% (12/65; 5 were asymptomatic and were demonstrated only radiologically) in the CRT-surgery group; other "surgical" complications (e.g., chylothorax, bleeding) occurred in 4.2% (5/118) and 1.5% (1/65) of the cases, respectively; other "medical" complications (infectious, respiratory, cardiovascular, metabolic, and miscellaneous complications) occurred in 36.4% (43/118) and 41.5% (27/65) of the cases, respectively.

Postoperative mortality was 4.2% (5/118) in the primary surgery group (one due to anastomotic leak, one due to necrosis of the esophageal substitute, three due to "medical" complications) and 7.7% (5/65) in the CRT-surgery group (one due to anastomotic leak, one due to necrosis of the esophageal substitute, three due to "medical" complications).

Table 1 shows the survival rates according to patient group (primary surgery versus CRT-surgery) and pathologic tumor stage. In both groups the prognosis was sig-

TABLE 1. Survival rates in relation to patient group and pathologic tumor stage

	Survival (%)				
Condition No.	1 Year	2 Years	3 Years	4 Years	5 Years
Primary surgery					
pTisN0M0 20	95	95	95	95	89*
pT1N0M0 77	95	81	63	58	54**
pT1N1M0 16	87	47	47	40	32***
CRT surgery					
pT0-TisN0M0 34	94	91	76	72	67*
pT1N0M0 10	90	80	60	48	48**
pT0-TisN1M0 7	82	41	41	20	20
pT1N1M0 9	78	33	33	33	33***

Log-rank test: * $P = 0.2$; ** $P = 0.98$; *** $P = 0.46$

nificantly better for pTis tumors than for pT1 tumors ($P < 0.05$). In both groups the prognosis was significantly worse in the presence of lymph node metastasis ($P < 0.05$). The long-term survival was comparable in patients who underwent primary surgery and those who underwent CRT-surgery when they were stratified by pathologic tumor stage, with the 5-year survivals as follows: pT0-TisN0M0, 89% vs. 67% ($P = 0.2$); pT1N0M0, 54% vs. 48% ($P = 0.98$); and pT1N^{+}M0, 32% vs. 33% ($P = 0.8$). It is worth noting that patients in the CRT-surgery group whose tumor showed a complete pathologic response (pT0) in the presence of nodal metastasis (pN^{+}) had a grim prognosis (5-year survival 20%).

Discussion

Esophagectomy represents the standard of care for patients with clinically resectable esophageal cancer who are medically fit for an operation [3–5]. Resection is our treatment of choice also for T1 tumors of the esophagus, especially for submucosal tumors, because of the high prevalence of metastatic lymph nodes.

In patients with more advanced tumors (especially with a locally advanced T4 tumor), surgery is increasingly being combined with preoperative chemotherapy or chemoradiotherapy with the aim of increasing the resection rate and improving the long-term prognosis [3, 4]. The available results of phase II and randomized phase III studies show that patients who respond to preoperative chemotherapy or chemoradiotherapy and subsequently undergo a complete R0 resection have a significantly better long-term prognosis than nonresponders or patients who undergo an R0 resection without preoperative chemotherapy. A significant survival advantage is particularly evident for patients who show a complete response to preoperative treatments and subsequently undergo a curative resection [6, 9]. Because in the literature it is reported that 21%–62% of clinically complete responders actually do not have a pathologically complete response [6, 8], surgical resection should be considered an indispensable component of multimodality treatment for esophageal cancer.

Our study shows that the long-term prognosis of patients with squamous cell carcinoma of the esophagus who undergo chemotherapy or chemoradiotherapy plus resection and obtain a complete or nearly complete pathologic response is comparable to that of patients who present with an early-stage carcinoma of the esophagus and are treated with surgery alone. In both groups of patients the lymph node status is a significant determinant of survival.

Endoscopic mucosectomy may be a valid alternative to surgery in patients with intraepithelial or intramucosal esophageal cancer; on the other hand, surgery is preferred for submucosal cancers because of the high prevalence of lymph node metastasis [10]. In our opinion, surgery should always be the treatment of choice in patients with a good response to neoadjuvant chemotherapy or chemoradiotherapy.

References

1. Japanese Society for Esophageal Diseases (1976) Guidelines for the clinical and pathological studies on carcinoma of the esophagus. Jpn J Surg 6:69–78
2. Bonavina L, Group European pour l'Etude des Maladies de l'Oesophage (1995) Early oesophageal cancer: results of a European multicentre study. Br J Surg 82:98–101

3. Ruol A, Panel of Experts (1996) Multimodality treatment for non-metastatic cancer of the thoracic esophagus: results of a consensus conference held at the 6th world Congress of the International Society for Diseases of the Esophagus. Dis Esophagus 9:39–55
4. Lehnert T (1999) Multimodal therapy for squamous carcinoma of the oesophagus. Br J Surg 86:727–739
5. Kelsen DP, Ginsberg R, Pajak TF, et al (1998) Chemotherapy followed by surgery compared with surgery alone for localized esophageal cancer. N Engl J Med 339:1979–1984
6. Vogel SB, Mendenhall WM, Sombeck MD, et al (1995) Downstaging of esophageal cancer after preoperative radiation and chemotherapy. Ann Surg 221:685–695
7. Forastiere AA, Orriger MB, Perez-Tamayo C, et al (1993) Preoperative chemoradiation followed by transhiatal esophagectomy for carcinoma of the esophagus: final report. J Clin Oncol 11:1118–1123
8. Triboulet JP, Amrouni H, Guillem P, et al (1998) Devenir des cancers epidermoides de l'oesophage en response complete apres chimio-radiotherapie preoperatoire. Ann Chir 52:503–508
9. Kitamura K, Kuwano H, Arari K, et al (1998) Clinicopathologic features of patients with oesophageal cancer obtaining a histological complete response for preoperative hyperthermo-chemoradiotherapy. Int J Hyperthermia 14:233–243
10. Lambert R (2000) Endoscopic mucosectomy: an alternative treatment for superficial esophageal cancer. Recent Results Cancer Res 155:183–192

Q & A after Dr. Merigliano's presentation

Dr. Jankowski (Birmingham University, UK): You showed slides of no cancer in the esophagus but with a tumor underneath. We now recognize familial cancer syndromes of diffuse esophageal cancer that have been reported particularly with E-cadherin gene mutations for gastroesophageal cancer. Do some of your esophageal cancers represent this familial cancer syndrome? Do you routinely take a family history of esophageal cancer? Some of your slides of diffuse esophageal cancer would fit very well with the familial syndrome.

Dr. Merigliano: It's a good question. I don't know. We often observe these diffuse tumors. That is the reason there is an attitude suggesting extensive resection of the esophagus up to the upper mediastinal level or to the cervical level. I learned from Professor Perracchia that esophageal diffusion is very important, and so you need to remove tissue at least 10 cm from the tumor to be safe. There are cases that even after chemoradiation therapy can be identified in these situation. We don't know much about this problem, but that is why we perform extensive resection of the esophagus.

Dr. Bumm (Technishe University, München, Germany): You recommended transthoracic esophagectomy, but we have seen that you treated many patients with transhiatal esophagectomy as well. In Munich, we perform about 90% transthoracic esophagectomies on esophagus squamous cell carcinoma. What is your decision-making process? When the patient comes to you, how do you decide when to use the transhiatal approach and when to use the transthoracic approach? Second, do you perform a two-stage operation after neoadjuvant treatment or do you use one-step resection and reconstruction?

Dr. Merigliano: The problem with this series of data is time; you can see that the data are from 1980 to 1995, with corresponding different experiences and different attitudes. Up to now, we have decided in this way: If the patient is not yet 75 years old or does not have severe, compromising biorespiratory problems, we recommend the transthoracic approach. If there is a minor general complication or the patient is older, we prefer the transhiatal approach which is less invasive. What we recommend today, especially after chemoradiotherapy, is the transthoracic approach. The answer to the second question is that for 95% of the patients treated we preferred the one-step surgical approach. The approach with two steps—resection and later reconstruction (about 30 days afterward)—is not recommended even if you don't have special patients. I think that maybe 2%–3% of our patients might have undergone the two-step approach.

Dr. Rubio (Karolinska Institute, Sweden): Many years ago I was working in Ling Xian County in Heng Nang Province in China. There were many cases of cancer of the esophagus that were being treated surgically. When I went to the surgical theater, I noticed that globes were recycled: They didn't use new gloves but recycled the old ones. Operation rooms weren't as clean as today, and the patients were in poor condition. Yet they had less mortality and much less morbidity than you report today as well as much less leakage and no postoperative infections. Your rates and percentages are the same as what we have in Sweden. How do you explain these discrepancies?

Dr. Merigliano: We have rebuilt our institute and so operated for 1 year in a transitory operating room created in the area where there were patient rooms with no special protections or filters. We had the same results then that we get with new operating room with the laminar filters. So I think that the results depend on many things. First, we have many residents who are still learning, we attribute, some increment of complications to what we call the learning curve. That is the price we pay to develop better surgeons. Second, we have a computerized database in which any complication, even a day of fever, is considered a complication. It is the same for leakage. We consider a leakage even if during a barium swallowing test you see even a small discrepancy without any clinical significance; we call it radiological leakage, and we wait 7 days until restarting meals. This is leakage for us, but it is not a leakage for many. Therefore, it depends on the surgeons, not on the area.

Dr. Baba (Kagoshima University, Japan): Do esophageal tumors located from the upper mediastinum to the lower mediastinum metastasize to the cervical region, recurrent laryngeal nodes, and gastric paracardiac nodes? You indicated that preoperative chemoradiation is useful when the patient has no LN metastasis. If you are giving preoperative radiation, do you change the radiation fields depending on the LN status obtained by CT scan or EUS?

Dr. Merigliano: Yes, we do. The radiotherapy fields depend on the following: First is where we think positive LNs are, according to the CT scan or EUS; and it depends on the level of the tumor. If there is a lower esophageal cancer, we include paragastric and splenic LNs in the radiation fields. If there is an upper esophageal cancer, we irradiate the neck.

Dr. Baba: When the patient has extensive disease, can the main tumor be located in the lower esophagus but the LN metastases in the abdominal LNs and in the cervical area? Are these patients excluded from neoadjuvant chemoradiation therapy?

Dr. Merigliano: There are very few of those patients. In some extreme situations we used to do what we call the "test." We start with the first cycle of chemotherapy, and if the patient shows regression we change it to complete and personalized therapy. If there is no change after the first or the second chemotherapy cycle, we stop.

Strategy for Treatment of Superficial Esophageal Cancer

Misao Yoshida[1], Kumiko Momma[2], Tomoko Hanashi[1], Yosuke Izumi[1], Nobuhiro Sakaki[3], Yoshiya Yamada[3], Kenichi Oohashi[4], and Nobuaki Funada[4]

Introduction

The number of patients with superficial esophageal cancer has increased during the last 25 years in Japan, and the clinical result has been excellent. At the same time, the pathological characteristics of mucosal cancer are different from those of submucosal cancer and therefore there is a difference in the treatment. We studied the clinical results of patients with superficial esophageal cancer treated at our hospital, and the strategy for treating superficial esophageal cancer is discussed.

Subjects

A total of 323 patients with superficial esophageal cancer (mucosal cancer 206, submucosal cancer 117) were included in this study. Endoscopic mucosal resection (EMR) was carried out in 168 patients and esophagectomy in 116.

Clinicopathological Indications for Treatment

Clinicopathological characteristics should be considered when selecting treatment. The incidence of lymph node metastasis among 136 patients with superficial esophageal cancer who underwent radical esophagectomy with lymph node dissection was studied. In cases with mucosal cancer ($n = 37$), the incidence of lymph node metastasis was low (2.7%), and it was significantly high among patients with submucosal cancer (43%). These results strongly suggest that esophagectomy with lymph node dissection is appropriate for submucosal cancer of the esophagus, whereas any localized treatment that can eradicate the lesion, such as EMR, is a good choice for mucosal cancer (Table 1).

Departments of [1]Surgery, [2]Endoscopy, [3]Gastroenterology, and [4]Pathology, Tokyo Metropolitan Komagome General Hospital, 3-18-22 Hon-komagome, Bunkyo-ku, Tokyo 113-8677, Japan

TABLE 1. Lymph node metastasis in superficial esophageal cancer

Depth of invasion	No. of cases	Vascular invasion (%)	Lymph node metastasis (%)
m	37	24	2.7
sm	99	74	43
Total	136	60	32

TABLE 2. Superficial esophageal cancer: gross findings of mucosal cancer ($n = 350$)

Cancer type	No. of lesions	sm (%)	m (%)
0-I	49	92	8
0-II	277	15	85
0-III	24	96	4

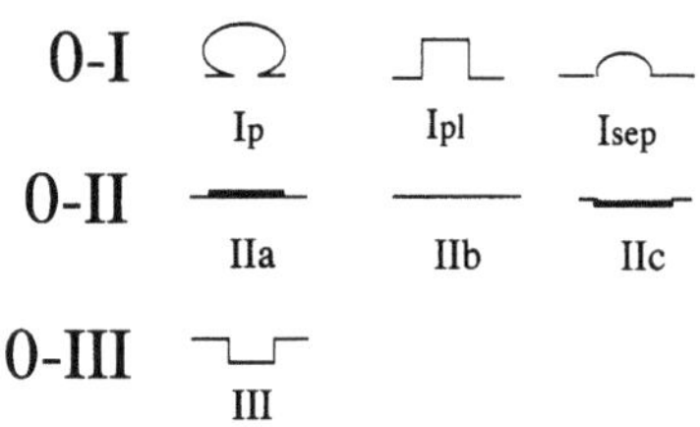

FIG. 1. Gross classification of superficial esophageal cancer. (From 1992.3 Japanese Society for Esophageal Diseases)

Clinical Estimation of Depth of Invasion

The clinical estimation of the depth of cancer invasion is indispensable for deciding on the treatment. The macroscopic classification of superficial esophageal cancer is useful for differentiating mucosal from submucosal cancer (Fig. 1). Superficial esophageal cancers can be classified into three types: type 0-I, with distinct protrusion; type 0-II, with minimal elevation or depression; type 0-III, with deep depression. With type 0-I and 0-III cancers the invasion probably reaches the submucosa, whereas 85% of all type 0-II lesions are mucosal cancer (Table 2). Type 0-II lesions can be classified into three subtypes: type IIa (slightly elevated), type IIb (flat), type IIc (slightly depressed) (Table 3). The clinical estimation of the depth of invasion is accurate for 91% of all mucosal cancers when aided by conventional endoscopy, an endoscopic staining technique, and endoscopic ultrasonography (Table 4).

Clinical Results

For patients with mucosal cancer ($n = 206$) the overall survival rate after EMR and esophagectomy was 84% at 5 years and 57% at 10 years. In those with submucosal cancer, radical esophagectomy was undertaken in somewhat more than 80% of cases.

TABLE 3. Gross findings of mucosal cancer ($n = 277$)

Cancer type	No. of lesions	sm (%)	m (%)
IIa	41	15	85
IIb	58		100
IIc	178	20	80

TABLE 4. Superficial esophageal cancer: clinical estimation of depth of invasion

Depth of invasion	No. of cases	Accuracy rate (%)
m	193	91
sm	92	71
Total	285	85

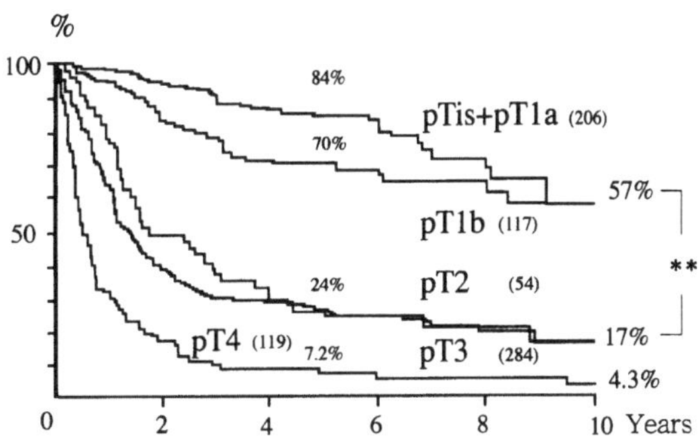

FIG. 2. Survival curves of esophageal cancer ($n = 780$). ** $P < 0.001$ (Kaplan-Meier)

The overall survival rate was 70% at 5 years and 57% at 10 years. These clinical results are significantly better than those for patients with advanced cancer, suggesting the efficacy of radical esophagectomy (Fig. 2).

Endoscopic Mucosal Resection

EMR Procedures

Progress in the detection and estimation of mucosal cancer allowed us to establish the procedure for EMR. Our first paper on the use of EMR to treat mucosal cancer of the esophagus appeared in 1989. Our procedure for EMR is as follows: (1) Delineate mucosal cancer as a yellowish white unstained area against dark brown normal mucosa by endoscopic iodine staining. (2) Puncture the submucosa close to the unstained area and inject normal saline. This makes the submucosa thicken and allows us to remove the mucosal lesion with a sufficient amount of the lining submucosa. A squamous cell carcinoma of the esophagus frequently proceeds to the duct of the esophageal gland and reaches the submucosa. (3) Grasping forceps for EMR and a wire snare should be introduced through working channels of a video-endoscope that has two working channels. The unstained area should be grasped with a narrow stripe of dark brown normal mucosa close to the unstained area by a grasping forceps. The wire snare is then applied, and the lesion is resected by high-frequency electric current.

Results

Complete resection was confirmed in 94% of the patients. Complications were recognized in 14%; and conservative treatment for bleeding at EMR ulcers, mediastinitis, and strictures were effective. All patients recovered promptly (Table 5). The 10-year survival rate for patients with mucosal cancer ($n = 168$) was 69%; and for those with mucosal cancer treated by esophagectomy ($n = 37$) it was 49%. There was no significant difference between the two groups. The quality of life after EMR was excellent. EMR is one of the standard treatments for mucosal cancer of the esophagus today (Fig. 3).

Local Recurrence and Metachronous Cancer after EMR

Local recurrence was identified in 5.6% of all patients with a clinically complete resection. Endoscopic surveillance aided by iodine staining once a year was recommended, as all the local recurrences detected by endoscopic surveillance were mucosal cancer. EMR was also effective for treating local recurrence after EMR. We must also be aware of metachronous cancers after EMR. Esophageal cancer at another site of the esophagus was found in 10% of all cases. The incidence of malignancies in other organs such as head and neck, stomach, and colon was 16%. Metachronous cancer of the esophagus was 10 times more frequent among patients who had many unstained areas

TABLE 5. Endoscopic esophageal mucosal resection: complications due to EMR ($n = 185$)

Complication	Incidence (%)
Perforation	0
Ulcer bleeding	2.2
Mediastinitis	3.8
Stricture	7.0
Others	0.5
Total	14.0

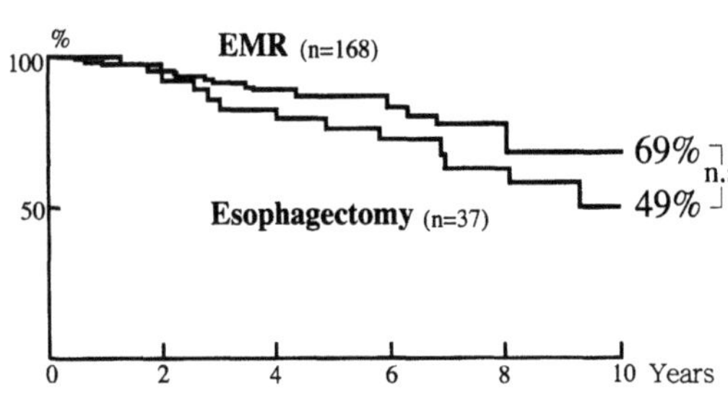

FIG. 3. Survival curves of mucosal cancer of the esophagus. *EMR*, endoscopic mucosal resection

TABLE 6. Endoscopic esophageal mucosal resection: metachronous esophageal cancers and unstained area after iodine staining

No. of unstained areas at first EMR	Incidence of metachronous cancer No.	%		
One	3/80	3.8	$P = 0.05$ (One vs. Several)	$P = 0.01$ (One vs. Many)
Several	8/47	17.0		
Many	5/13	38.5		

in the background esophageal mucosa after iodine staining compared with patients who have only one unstained area for EMR. Surveillance should be planned taking these facts into account (Table 6).

Conclusions

Treatment for superficial esophageal cancer should be chosen considering the clinical estimation of the depth of cancer invasion. EMR is indicated for mucosal cancers, and radical esophagectomy is recommended for submucosal cancers.

References

1. Japanese Society for Esophageal Diseases (1999) Guidelines for the clinical and pathologic studies on carcinoma of the esophagus, 9th edn. Kanehara, Tokyo
2. Hanashi T, Yoshida M, Takenami T, Momma K, Sakaki N, Takizawa T, Koike M (1995) Clinical evaluation on treatments for mucosal cancer of the esophagus. In: Peracchia A, Rosati R, Bonavina L, Fumagalli U, Bona S, Chella B (eds) Diseases of the esophagus, Monduzzi editore, Bologna, pp 203–207
3. Endo M, Ide H (eds) (1991) Endoscopic staining in early detection of esophageal cancer. Japan Scientific Societies Press, Tokyo
4. Iwasaki Y, et al (1993) Pathological basis of endoscopic mucosectomy of superficial esophageal carcinoma. Stomach Intestine 28:125–132
5. Ide H, et al (1993) Endoscopic mucosectomy of superficial esophageal carcinoma evaluated by surgical results. Stomach Intestine 28:133–139
6. Momma K, et al (1993) Endoscopic mucosectomy for early esophageal cancer. Stomach Intestine 28:141–151
7. Makuuchi H, et al (1993) Endoscopic mucosal resection for early esophageal cancer by the EEMR-tube method. Stomach Intestine 28:153–159
8. Inoue H, et al (1993) Endoscopic mucosal resection of early esophageal cancer: EMRT and EMRC techniques. Stomach Intestine 28:161–169
9. Goseki N, et al (1987) A definition of "early esophageal cancer": histopathological comparative study with so-called "early gastric cancer." Stomach Intestine 22:1429–1337
10. Endo M, et al (1993) Endoscopic classification of superficial esophageal cancer. Stomach Intestine 22:11343–1349
11. Yoshida M, et al (1990) Endoscopic evaluation of intraepithelial or mucosal cancer of the esophagus. Stomach Intestine 25:1059–1066
12. Unakami M, et al (1992) Macroscopic evaluation of the depth of invasion in superficial esophageal cancer. Stomach Intestine 27:139–156

Q & A after Dr. Yoshida's presentation

Dr. Hölscher (University of Cologne, Germany): You pointed out that the 5-year survival rate in mucosal cancer after mucosal resection was about 50%, with the lymph node infiltration rate about 4% and the local recurrence rate about 7%. What is the cause of death in these patients if the 5-year survival was only 50%?

Dr. Yoshida: We have no patients with superficial mucosal cancer lost to recurrence of the esophageal cancer, but about 15% were lost because of something other than the esophageal cancer. About half of them were lost to benign diseases such as cardiac disease, penumonia, and so on. Another half of the patients were lost to malignant disease in other organs, such as the stomach, colorectum, and urinary organs. So all causes of death were included.

Dr. Jankowski (University of Birmingham, UK): What were the synchronous and metachronous cancers associated with your esophageal cancer? Do the synchronous cancers of the stomach arise in the proximal or distal part of the stomach?

Dr. Yoshida: We could to find any difference between the stomach cancer that arose after esophageal cancer and the usual gastric cancer. The most frequent site of the gastric cancer was the middle part of the stomach.

Dr. Hölscher: You said that you have an endoscopic accuracy rate for submucosal cancer of about 70%. Therefore if your diagnosis was not right after mucosal resection, do you perform the esophagectomy or do you leave the patient and just observe?

Dr. Yoshida: When we perform EMR for submucosal cancer invading the middle or sometimes a deeper part of the submucosa, they have some characteristics of infiltration. They invade deeper only at the narrowest point, which probably influences the prognosis. They rarely have LN metastasis. Hence we seldom add chemotherapy or irradiation. When we find massive infiltration after EMR, we have to add some treatments, including esophagectomy.

Dr. Bumm (Technische University, München, Germany): Is there any defined safety margin when you do your operation? For instance, is it 1 mm to each side or some other parameter?

Dr. Yoshida: That's an important question. When we employ EMR, there is some limitation imposed by the size of the mucosa. We try to keep as much of the free margin as possible, but sometimes we have to resect with a narrow surgical margin. Even if there is a narrow margin (for instance, only 1 mm), it's enough to avoid local recurrence. We can delineate the lesion clearly by iodide staining, so we can easily keep a free margin. If it is too narrow, we have to perform two or three resections, but that is enough for treatment.

Dr. Kato (Cancer Institute, Tokyo, Japan): You presented a "decision tree" for treatment. Concerning the carcinoma with an m3 invasion depth, it appears there is only a one-way direction to the EMR. The other possibility is surgical resection. Do you have any criteria by which to decide on this point?

Dr. Yoshida: It is a difficult question. The decision tree was constructed in such a manner because about 8% of the patients with m3 lesions have LN metastases. When cancer invasion before treatment is estimated to be sm1 we usually recommend esophagectomy to the patient because there is a small number of patients who have sm2 cancer; the clinical findings are similar to those of sm1, and sometimes EUS cannot exclude sm2 invasion in such cases. So in these patients we say that it's probably an sm1 cancer but we cannot exclude sm2 invasion. In such cases we recommend that these patients undergo esophagectomy.

Dr. Kato: So the decision is made after endoscopic resection?

Dr. Yoshida: There are few studies on LN metastasis and macroscopic findings of m3 and sm1 cancers, but we know that m3 cancers with LN metastasis have massive invasion into the muscularis mucosae, and it resembles submucosal cancer. Therefore, for the patient with m3 cancer that has a somewhat distinct elevation and depression characteristic of submucosal cancer, we usually do not apply EMR. We recommend esophagectomy. It is difficult to estimate the depth of the lesion and decide on the treatment.

Surgical Experience of Superficial Squamous Cell Carcinoma in Thailand

APINOP CHANVITAN

Introduction

In Thailand, esophageal cancer is most prevalent in the south. Songkhla Province in southern Thailand has the highest incidence of esophageal cancer in Thailand, with a world population standardized rate of 9.7 per 100000 in males and 3.1 per 100000 in females. In this registry, it is the third most common cancer in men. More than 90% of cases with a histological diagnosis were squamous cell carcinoma [1-3]. Esophageal cancer is a significant public health problem in southern Thailand. About 80-100 patients with esophageal cancer are treated each year at Songklanagarind University Hospital. In 1984 the Department of Surgery set up a unit to undertake research into this disease. Lines of investigation that we have followed so far include descriptive epidemiology, exploration of potential risk factors, trials of a screening test for early detection, and improvement of therapy with special emphasis on using of multimodality treatment.

Superficial cancer of the esophagus, defined as a tumor limited to the mucosa or submucosa, seems to have the best prerequisites for complete cure by surgery. Up to now large series of superficial esophageal cancer have not been reported from Thailand. Consequently, the objectives of the current study were to: (1) evaluate the prognosis of superficial squamous cell carcinoma of the esophagus in a series of Thai patients; and (2) determine prognostic factors of cancer by analyzing the pathological staging and patterns of lymph node metastasis.

Patients and Methods

Patients

From January 1982 to December 1998 a total population of 934 patients with esophageal cancer were treated at the Department of Surgery, Prince of Songkla University. Altogether, 878 cases were squamous cell carcinoma and 56 were adenocarci-

Khaengkoi Medical Center, 36 Vorasawasdi Road, Khaengkoi, Saraburi, 18110, Thailand

noma. All of these cases were in advanced stages. In 1991 Chanvitan and associates [4] developed a balloon cytology method with silk mesh to improve the cytologic detection of early esophageal cancer. Between 1993 to 1998, among the total population of 462 patients with squamous cell carcinoma, 18 patients (3.9%) had a carcinoma limited to intramucosal or submucosal tissues. All of the tumors were resected with curative intention.

The routine preoperative staging included endoscopy, percutaneous ultrasonography, computed tomography, and endoscopic ultrasonography. Histopathologic examination of all resected specimens consisted of thorough evaluation of tumor stage, grade, and number of resected lymph nodes [5]. According to the TNM (supplement 1993), T1 tumors were subclassified further as T1a (limited to the mucosa and muscularis mucosae) and T1b (limited to the submucosa) [6]. Follow-up was performed regularly in the tumor clinic of the Department of Surgery. Follow-up was completed for all 14 patients, with a median duration of 2.2 years (range 0.5–5.8 years). The median age of the 18 patients with superficial squamous cell carcinoma of the esophagus was 54.1 years (range 36–73 years). The male/female ratio was 4:1.

Method

The treatment of choice was subtotal en bloc esophagectomy using a right transthoracic approach; it included two-field lymphadenectomy of the mediastinal and abdominal nodes [7, 8]. The reconstruction was usually accomplished by stomach interposition.

Statistics

The survival function was calculated according to the Kaplan-Meier method. The 5-year survival rate was computed using 95% confidence interval (CI) statistics including the Peto-Wilcoxon test with a significance limit of $P < 0.05$. Survival curves were calculated including the postoperative mortality. Statistical analysis was performed with BMDP Statistical Software, Revision 1990 (Cork, Ireland) using program modules 1L and 2L.

Results

In 3.9% of the 462 patients (n = 18) the carcinoma was limited to the mucosa or submucosa in 10 cases and to the submucosa in 8 cases. All patients underwent complete resection without microscopic or macroscopic tumor residuals. None of the 10 patients with mucosal carcinoma showed lymphatic infiltration, whereas 3 of 8 patients (37.5%) with submucosal involvement had lymph node metastasis (Table 1). Deaths among the 18 patients during the first 90 days postoperatively occurred in one patient with a submucosal tumor; two patients had a recurrence. The 5-year survival rate for the 18 patients with resected superficial squamous cell carcinoma of the esophagus was 72% (Fig. 1). Among the patients with complete resection there was no significant difference in outcome between the groups with mucosal or submucosal tumor infiltration. The 5-year survivals of patients with either stage 0 lesions or stage I–IV lesions were significantly different (Fig. 2; Table 2).

TABLE 1. Lymph node involvement in patients with superficial squamous cell carcinoma of the esophagus

Tumor type	Lymph node involvement[a]
Intramucosal	0 (0/10 cases)
Submucosal	37.5% (3/8 cases)

[a] Paraesophageal and paratracheal nodes

TABLE 2. Survival analysis of squamous cell carcinoma of the esophagus in various stages

Stage	5-Year survival (%)
0	72.0
I + II	35.4
III	2.9
IVa	1.9
IVb	0

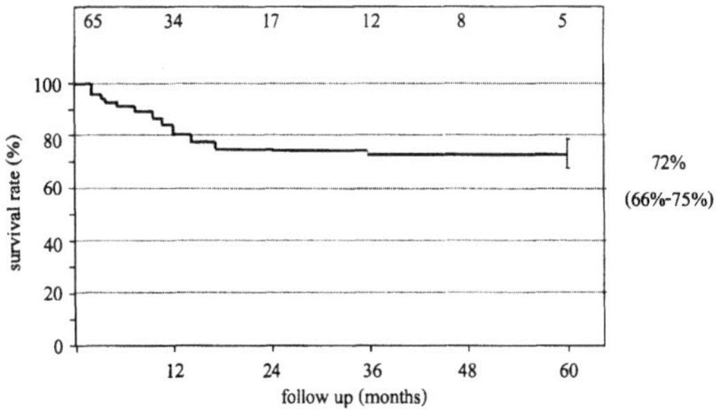

FIG. 1. Five-year survival of patients with resected early squamous cell carcinoma of the esophagus ($n = 18$)

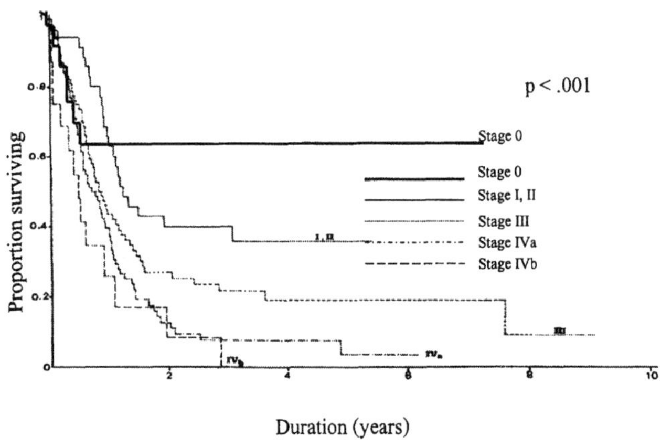

FIG. 2. Five-year survival of patients with complete resection at various stages. Stage 0 and stage I–IV show a significant difference ($P < 0.001$)

Discussion

In the present study, a survival advantage was noted in patients undergoing transthoracic esophagectomy, and the incidence of local recurrence was significantly lower in this patient subgroup. However, when the patients were stratified based on the depth of tumor infiltration, the survival advantage of transthoracic esophagectomy was evident only in those with a submucosal tumor. Although it could be argued that this is an effect of selection bias, the data suggest that mediastinal lymphadenectomy is beneficial when submucosal invasion is suspected. An enlarged three-field lymphadenectomy can improve staging, but the potential benefits of this technique on long-term survival are far from proven [9]. Transhiatal esophagectomy may be sufficient in patients with mucosal tumors, but the regional extent of the disease can be underestimated. When this operation is planned, splitting the anterior hiatus and dissection of the esophagus under direct vision allows us to achieve satisfactory mediastinal clearance up to the carina [10].

The presence and localization of lymph node metastases is another important parameter that influences the type of surgical resection to be performed. None of the patients with a carcinoma limited to the mucosa, including those with infiltration of the muscularis mucosae had lymph node metastases. This finding is in accordance with the reports of others concerning early squamous cell carcinoma [11–13]. If the submucosa was infiltrated, lymph node involvement had already occurred in 37.5% of the patients. As reliable preoperative classification of the depth of infiltration (mucosal/submucosal) of T1 cancer is not yet possible, patients with early squamous cell carcinoma should be treated with radical lymphadenectomy, as for advanced cancer. Endoscopic mucosectomy can be considered sufficient only when treating mucosal cancer; this local excision would be inadequate in approximately one-quarter of the patients with submucosal cancer because of the presence of lymph node metastasis. Perhaps further refinement of the high-frequency ultrasonographic probes can lead to better preoperative differentiation of the T1 stages of these patients [14].

References

1. National Cancer Institute (1987) Cancer statistics 1982. Ministry of Public Health, Bangkok, pp 108–112
2. Chanvitan A, Ubolcholket S, Chuprapawan C (1991) Surveillance of oesophageal carcinoma in southern Thailand in 1998. J Med Assoc Thai 74:3–8
3. Vatanasapt V, Martin N, Sriplung H, et al (1993) Cancer in Thailand 1998–1991. IARC Techical Report No. 16. IARC, Lyon, pp 61–130
4. Chanvitan A, Geater AF, Ubolcholket S, Huang GI (1990) Detection of oesophageal cancinoma in southern Thailand. J Med Assoc Thai 73:565–570
5. UICC (1992) TNM classification of malignant tumors, 5th edn. Springer, Berlin Heidelberg NewYork
6. UICC (1993) TNM supplement 1993. Springer, Berlin Heidelberg NewYork, 1993
7. Siewert JR (1989) Esophageal cancer from the German point of view. Jpn J Surg 19: 11–20
8. Siewert JR (1991) Breitner Chirurgische Operationslehre, vol IV: Chirurgie des Abdomens 2. Urban & Schwarzenberg, Munich

9. Kato H, Tachimori Y, Mizobuchi S, Igaki H, Ochiai A (1993) Cervical, mediastinal, and abdominal lymph node dissection (three-field dissection) for superficial carcinoma of the esophagus. Cancer 72:2879–2882
10. Peracchia A, Bonavina L, Segalin A, Ruol A, Fumagalli U (1994) Esophagectomy without thoracotomy or transmediastinal endodissection for esophageal carcinoma. Dis Esophagus 7:36–38
11. Nishimaki T, Tanaka O, Suzuki T, Aizawa K, Watanabe H, Muto T (1993) Tumor spread in superficial esophageal cancer: histopathologic basis for rational surgical treatment. World J Surg 17:766–772
12. Gayet B, Vons C, Molas G, Belghiti J, Fekete F (1990) Superficial squamous cell carcinoma of the esophagus: an early lesion of good prognosis? A report of 58 patients resected. In: Ferguson NK, Little AG, Skinner DB (eds) Diseases of the esophagus, vol 1: Malignant diseases. Futura, Mount Kisko, NY, pp 161–169
13. Yoshinaka H, Shimazu H, Fukumoto T, Baba M (1991) Superficial esophageal carcinoma: a clinicopathological review of 59 cases. Am J Gastroenterol 86:1413–1417
14. Murata Y, Ota M, Suzuki S, Hayashi K, Yamada H, Ide H (1995) How to discriminate between mucosal cancer and submucosal cancer according to depiction of muscularis mucosae. Presented at the 6th world congress of the ISDE, Milan

Q & A after Dr. Chanvitan's presentation

Dr. Udagawa (Toranomon Hospital, Japan): Your experience is similar to ours. We know that the truly superficial carcinoma of the esophagus does not need radical surgery. Do you know any special program for excluding such early-stage tumors from your standard operation?

Dr. Chanvitan: Mucosal cancer is first experienced because I have no way to detect superficial cancers. Submucosal cancer is still in the learning curve in my hospital.

Dr. Udagawa: So now is the time for you to begin to exclude such early cancers from your standard operations.

Dr. Hölscher (University of Cologne, Germany): We heard the presentations on superficial adenocarcinoma and SCC of the esophagus. There are some new items concerning the pathology. In regard to Dr. Meligriano's presentation, he noted that patients who have chemoradiation therapy and afterward are classified as T1 now have a completely different entity than patients who have a primary T1 cancer. It is difficult to comprehend the discussions about chemoradiotherapy and down-staging, but I think you would agree with me on this item: There must be another congress to talk about new adjuvant chemoradiotherapy and down-staging. We have also learned a lot from the various prsentations here and about the endoscopic findings important for making judgments about mucosal resection or complete resection.

Histocytologic Criteria for Squamous Cell Carcinoma In Situ of the Esophagus

CARLOS A. RUBIO

Introduction

Squamous cell carcinoma has been regarded for many years to be the most common malignant tumor of the esophagus in Western [1] and Asian [2] countries. Studies have shown, however, that the time trend incidence of esophageal carcinoma is subjected to geographical variation [3]. In fact, the incidence of esophageal carcinoma has increased in some countries, has remained stable in others, and has decreased in yet others [3].

The frequency of adenocarcinoma is rapidly increasing in Western countries [4] without a parallel increase in the incidence of squamous cell carcinoma; and it has now surpassed the frequency of squamous cell carcinoma. The causes for the increased incidence of esophageal adenocarcinoma in Western countries remains elusive. Enigmatically, Asian patients have not experienced a similar change in the histology of esophageal carcinoma, and squamous cell carcinoma continues to be the most common malignant tumor in that organ [2].

Frequency of Squamous Cell Carcinomas in Sweden

In Sweden the ratio of squamous cell carcinoma/adenocarcinoma (SCC/ADC) of the esophagus is rapidly decreasing. Twenty years ago, squamous carcinomas of the esophagus accounted for 82.1% (1242/1512) of all esophageal carcinomas reported to the Swedish National Cancer Registry Office during a 6-year period (1975–1980). Almost 20 years later, during another 6-year period (1993–1998) only 68.7% (1335/1942) of all esophageal carcinomas reported to the same Registry were squamous cell carcinomas. When only the last year with available data is considered (1998), squamous carcinomas accounted for only 61.6% (213/346) of all esophageal carcinomas in Sweden.

It should be pointed out that between the two aforementioned 6-year periods (1975–1980 and 1993–1998, respectively) the number of squamous cell carcinomas

Gastrointestinal and Liver Pathology Research Laboratory, Karolinska Institute, 171 76 Stockholm, Sweden increased by only 93 cases, whereas the number of esophageal adenocarcinomas increased with 337 cases. Thus, squamous cell carcinoma accounted for only 21.6% (93/430) of all esophageal carcinomas reported in Sweden between the two aforementioned periods, almost 20 years apart.

Similar to squamous cell carcinomas in other organs, overt esophageal squamous cell carcinomas are preceded by a series of cellular and epithelial aberrations, starting with low-grade dysplasia followed by high-grade dysplasia, before adenocarcinoma ensues. Adenocarcinomas display a sequence of histologic steps from intraepithelial carcinoma (i.e., carcinoma in situ) to intramucosal carcinoma (invading the lamina propria mucosae) to submucosal carcinoma. The latter three levels of carcinomatous growth are considered superficial carcinomas [2].

Histological Criteria Used to Diagnose Squamous Intraepithelial Neoplasias of the Esophagus by Western and Japanese Pathologists

Much discussion has centered around the histological criteria used to diagnose squamous intraepithelial neoplasias of the esophagus by Western and Japanese pathologists. Using the definition of Western pathologists, high-grade dysplasia includes carcinoma in situ [5]. In Japan, however, carcinoma in situ is considered not a dysplastic change but a carcinomatous growth, and the presence of specific cytologic aberrations are considered essential criteria for differentiating dysplasias from carcinoma among Japanese pathologists [6].

At our hospital, histocytologic criteria similar to those applied in Japan have been used to differentiate esophageal squamous dysplasia from carcinoma. The aim of the present work is to describe and illustrate the criteria used in our department to classify squamous cell carcinoma of the esophagus in the absence of invasion (i.e., carcinoma in situ).

Squamous Cell Carcinoma In Situ: Histocytological Criteria

The diagnosis of squamous cell carcinoma in situ of the esophagus is based on several microscopic alterations of the epithelium. These alterations may be grouped into three main categories: structural, internuclear, and intranuclear aberrations.

Structural Aberrations

Squamous cell carcinoma in situ of the esophagus often shows expanding epithelial buds of neoplastic cells pushing downward into the lamina propria mucosae (Fig. 1). The top of the lamina propria mucosae surrounding the neck of the buds is centered by a vascular core. The latter is part of a tridimensional network of vessels that runs horizontally, parallel to the luminal aspect of the epithelium. Between that vascular network, the squamous epithelial buds of carcinoma in situ protrude into the lamina propria mucosae.

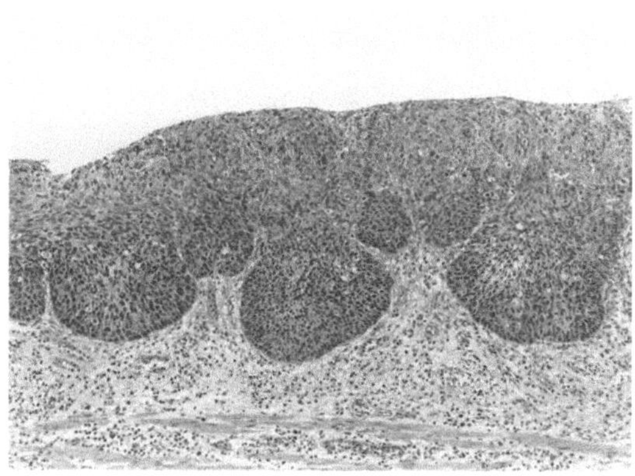

FIG. 1. Epithelial buds of squamous cell carcinoma in situ of the esophagus. Note the remnant palisade arrangement in basal cells. (H&E, ×5)

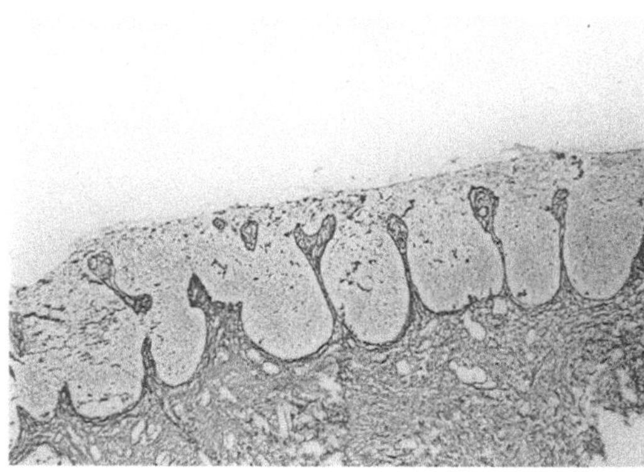

FIG. 2. Epithelial buds of squamous cell carcinoma in situ of the esophagus. Note the sharp epithelial-lamina propria mucosa border. (Gordon-Sweet, ×3.75)

These epithelial buds create an extensive interphase between the neoplastic epithelium and the underlying lamina propria mucosae. The increased contact surface between the proliferating neoplastic epithelial buds and the underlying "host" may be one of the important factors involved in the progression from a highly proliferating carcinoma in situ toward invasive carcinoma. The epithelium-lamina propria mucosae border in squamous cell carcinoma in situ is sharp (Fig. 2).

Internuclear Aberrations

Internuclear alterations are distinguished by squamous cell (nuclear) pleomorphism (Fig. 3). The pleomorphism includes anisocytosis (cells varying in size), anisokaryosis (nuclei varying in size), anisochromatosis (nuclear chromatin deposits varying in size among cells), and aberrant (multidirectional) nuclear polarity. In some cases of squamous cell carcinoma in situ the nuclear polarity is unidirectional (Fig. 4). There is a focal increased number of mitotic figures that may embrace the superficial layers of the neoplastic epithelium.

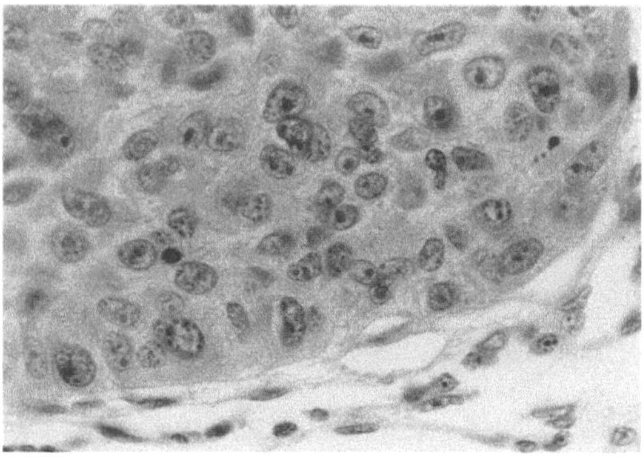

FIG. 3. Basal aspect of one bud with squamous cell carcinoma in situ of the esophagus. Note the cell-nuclear pleomorphism (anisocytosis, anisokaryosis, anisochromatosis) and multidirectional nuclear polarity. (H&E, ×50)

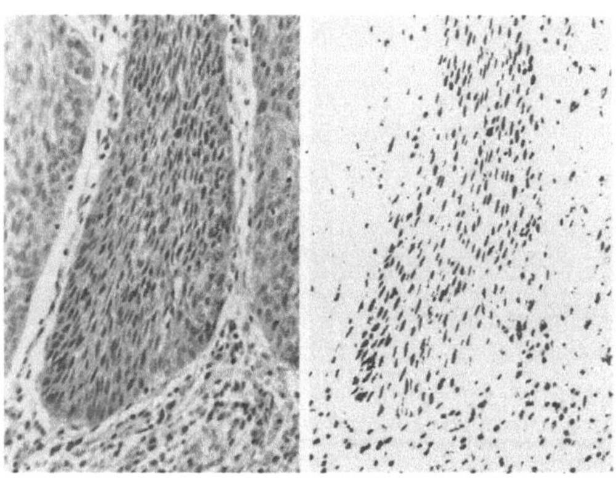

FIG. 4. **Left** Epithelial buds of squamous cell carcinoma in situ of the esophagus demonstrate the unidirectional nuclear polarity of the neoplastic cells. (H&E, ×6). **Right** The H&E-stained picture was scanned and manipulated in Photo-shop (Adobe 4.0) to enhance the polarity of the nuclei. For that purpose, eosin and background impurities were deleted. (Photo-shop, ×6)

Intranuclear Aberrations

Neoplastic cells show large, irregular, single or multiple eosinophilic nucleoli, or irregular single or multiple basophilic nucleolus-associated chromatin, with irregular chromatin deposits (chromocenters) in the nuclear area or along the nuclear membrane (Fig. 3). The nuclear membrane is often irregular, jagged, and indented. Chromatin bands connect irregular chromocenters to each other, to the nucleolus-associated chromatin, or to the chromatin deposits present along the nuclear membrane. Atypical mitosis (Fig. 5) may be recorded during each of the five mitotic phases (prophase, prometaphase, metaphase, anaphase, telophase).

Abnormal Pattern of Cell Proliferation

When sections exhibiting esophageal carcinoma in situ are challenged with MIB1 monoclonal antibody, which recognizes the proliferation-related antigen Ki-67, large irregularly labeled nuclei are seen in the parabasal, intermediate, and superficial cell layers. The MIB1 nuclei contain dark, coarse granules varying in size (anisogranulocytosis).

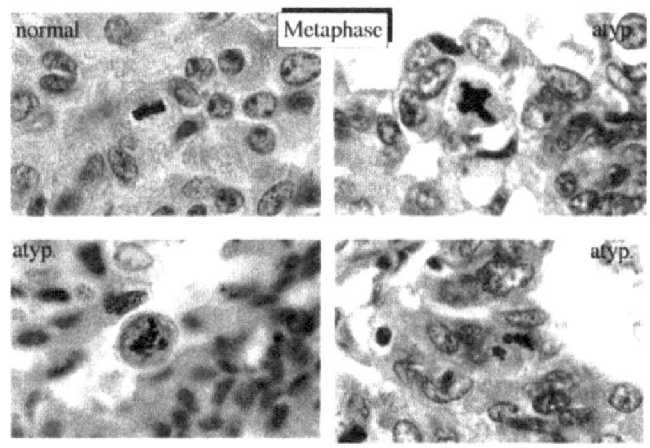

FIG. 5. Normal metaphase plate (**top left panel**) and examples of atypical metaphases in squamous cell carcinoma in situ of the esophagus. (H&E, reduced from ×125)

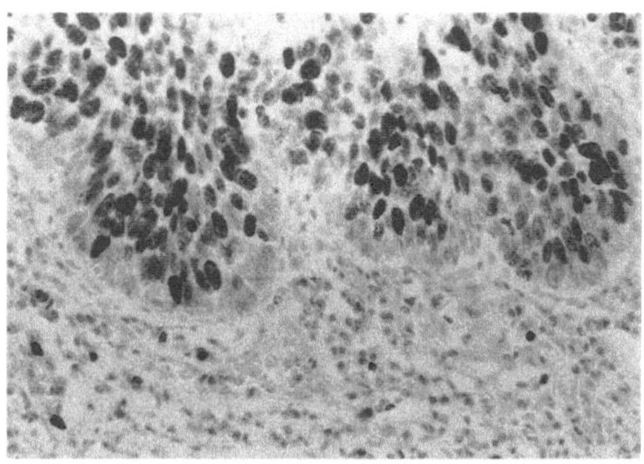

FIG. 6. Section of squamous cell carcinoma in situ of the esophagus challenged with the proliferating monoclonal antibody MIB1. Note the large, irregular, labeled nuclei in the parabasal, intermediate, and superficial cell layers. Labeled nuclei contain dark, coarse granules varying in size (anisogranulosis). Note the absence of labeling in the basal cell layers. (MIB1, ×25)

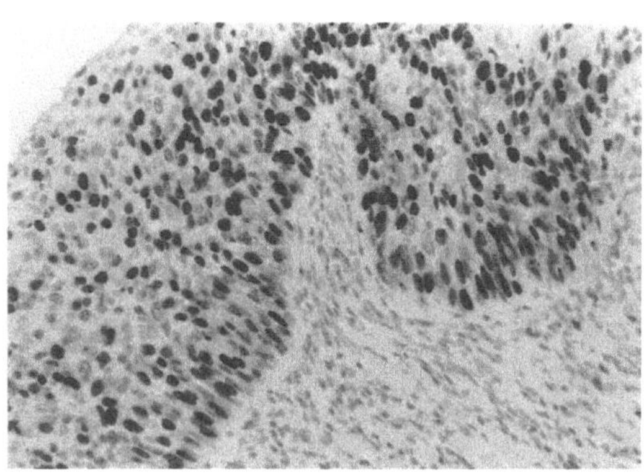

FIG. 7. Squamous cell carcinoma in situ of the esophagus challenged with the proliferating monoclonal antibody MIB1. Note the labeling of the basal cell layer. (MIB1, ×25)

Abnormal Pattern of Basal Cell Proliferation

In carcinoma in situ the basal cell layer usually remains unlabeled with the MIB1 stain (Fig. 6). Nonetheless, part of or the entire basal cell layer may appear labeled in some carcinomas in situ (Fig. 7).

Discussion

Esophageal squamous cell carcinoma in situ is histologically characterized by abnormal maturation and architectural distortion of the normal squamous epithelium with formation of proliferating epithelial buds. Increased contact surface between those proliferating neoplastic epithelial buds and the underlying tissues may be one of the important factors involved in the possibility of in situ carcinoma invading the host. Interestingly, similar epithelial bud formation has been demonstrated in carcinoma in situ in other organs also covered by squamous epithelium, such as the uterine cervix of humans [7] and rodents [8] and the squamous metaplastic epithelium of the bronchial mucosa.

Carcinoma in situ cells show aberrant, usually multidirectional nuclear polarity, anisokaryosis, anisochromatosis, irregular chromatin pattern, large nucleoli, connecting chromatin bridges, atypical mitosis, and irregular nuclear membranes. The nuclear polarity in a few cases may remain unidirectional. Whether unidirectional cell arrangement heralds synchronous behavior of carcinoma in situ cells before the host becomes invaded remains to be elucidated.

A marker of cell proliferation (MIB1) shows clear nuclear aberrations, with large labeled nuclei displaying anisogranulomatosis reaching the superficial layers. Whereas the basal layer in carcinoma in situ usually remains unlabeled, it may be entirely labeled in other cases. The latter suggests active proliferation in the basal cells. The question arises whether the labeling of otherwise unlabeled basal cells mirrors downward progression (intraepithelial) of the carcinoma in situ cells. This possibly aggressive behavior seems to be substantiated by the fact that areas of carcinoma in situ abutting microinvasive squamous cell carcinomas often show proliferating basal cells.

That neoplastic budding is an event of paramount importance in esophageal carcinogenesis is substantiated by the fact that invasive squamous cell carcinoma has

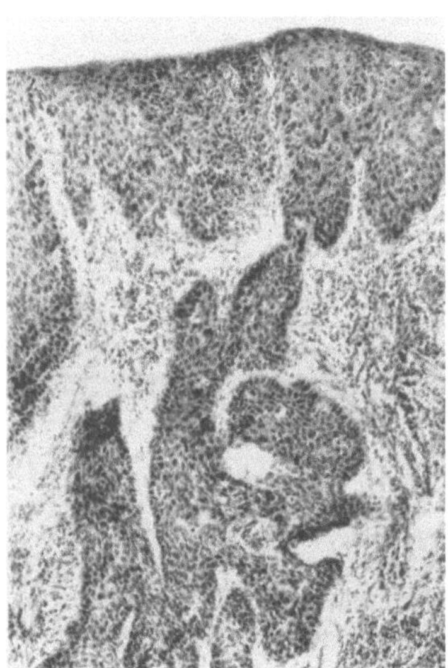

FIG. 8. Invasive squamous cell carcinoma of the esophagus originating at the tip of a squamous epithelial bud with carcinoma in situ. (H&E, ×3.75)

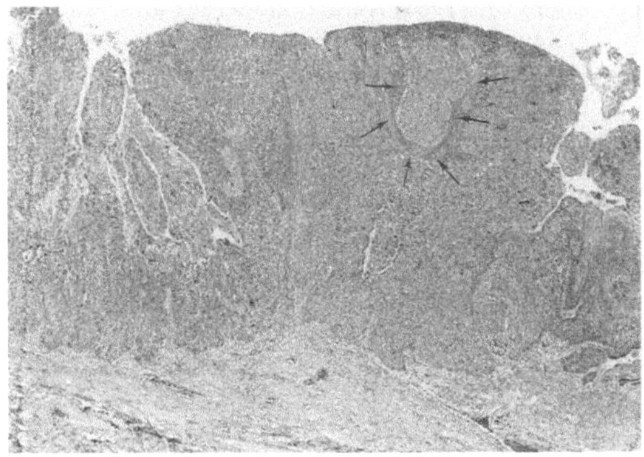

FIG. 9. Invasive squamous cell carcinoma of the esophagus. Note the uninvolved squamous epithelial bud with carcinoma in situ at the *arrows*. (H&E, ×3.75)

been seen to originate in the deeper part of one or more neoplasic buds with in situ carcinoma not only in the human esophagus [9] (Figs. 8, 9) but also in the esophagus from rodents [10] and chickens [11].

Because similar buds of nonneoplastic squamous epithelium develop in those with chronic reflux esophagitis, the possibility that nondysplastic epithelial buds (evolved through proliferation initiated by chronic inflammation) are eventually "replaced" by dysplastic cells and subsequently by carcinoma in situ cells has been entertained. In other cases of chronic gastroesophageal reflux, however, the squamous epithelium becomes columnar metaplastic and may eventually follow the adenomatous dysplasia-adenocarcinoma pathway. The factors responsible for those two alternative behavioral responses in the human esophagus remain poorly understood.

Acknowledgment. Thanks are due to Mr. Mats Talbäck from the Center of Epidemiology, Cancer Registry, National Board of Health and Welfare, Stockholm.

References

1. Allen JW, Richardson JD, Edwards MJ (1997) Squamous cell carcinoma of the esophagus: a review and update Surg. Oncology 6:193–200
2. Takubo K (2000) Pathology of the esophagus. Educa, Tokyo, pp 131–132
3. Muñoz N, Day D (1996) Esophageal cancer. In: Schottenfeld D, Fraumeni J Jr (eds) Cancer epidemiology and prevention, 2nd edn. Oxford University Press, Oxford, pp 681–690
4. Mueller J, Werner M, Siewert JR (2000) Malignant progression in Barrett's esophagus: pathology and molecular biology. Recent Results Cancer Res 155:29–42
5. Van Sandick JW, van Lanschott JJ, ten Kate FJ, Offerhaus GJ, Fockens P, Tygat GN, Obertop H (2000) Pathology of early invasive adenocarcinoma of the esophagus or esophagogastric junction: implications for therapeutic decision making. Cancer 88:2429–2437
6. Schlemper R, Dawsey S, Itabashi M, Iwata A, Kato Y, Koike M, Lewin K, Riddell R, Shimoda T, Sipponen P, Stolte M, Watanabe H (2000) Differences in diagnostic criteria for esophageal squamous cell carcinoma between Japanese and Western pathologists. Cancer 88:996–1006
7. Rubio CA (1974) Autoradiographic studies of dysplasia and carcinoma in situ in cervical cones Acta Pathol Microbiol Scand A 82:161–168

8. Rubio CA (1983) Animal model for SEM studies on cervical carcinogenesis. In: Hafez E, Kenemans P (eds) SEM atlas on human reproduction in three dimensions. Elsevier, Amsterdam, pp 305–309
9. Rubio CA, Liu FS, Zaho HZ (1983) Histological classification of intraepithelial neoplasias and micro-invasive squamous carcinoma of the esophagus. Am J Surg Pathol 1989;13:685–690
10. Rubio CA (1985) Experimental models. In: DeMeester T, Levin BT (eds) Cancer of the esophagus. Grune & Stratton, Orlando, pp 21–42
11. Rubio CA, Liu FS (1989) Spontaneous squamous carcinoma of the esophagus in chickens. Cancer 64:103–106

Part 4
Presentation of Patients and Discussion on the Pathological Diagnosis of Superficial Esophageal Neoplasms

Carcinoma In Situ of the Esophagus: Case Report

Takashi Nishigami, Masayuki Oe, Tadaaki Takanashi, Akira Okimura, Keiji Nakasho, and Kunio Uematsu

Introduction

Because the prognosis of esophageal cancer is generally poor, it is important to detect the disease at an early stage. Although iodine staining is an excellent method for finding early esophageal cancer by endoscopy, it is almost impossible to spray iodine in all patients. We fortunately have detected a tumor without iodine staining because of its white color. We report here a flat-type esophageal tumor with controversial histopathology.

Case Report

A 55-year-old woman had been suffering from epigastric pain for 8 years. She was followed up endoscopically. In May 1993 endoscopic examination revealed a flat lesion with a white surface. It measured approximately 1.5 cm in diameter and was located in the distal portion of the esophagus (Fig. 1). Endoscopic mucosal resection (Fig. 2) was carried out in July 1993.

Histologically, atypical cells were seen in the mucosal surface epithelium, but they had not spread into deeper layers of the wall (Fig. 3). The border between the lesion and normal mucosa was clear (Fig. 4). On immunohistochemical examination, p53-positive cells were seen only in the atypical cell group (Fig. 5). There were no papilloma viruses in the atypical cells.

Discussion

The most important point at issue is whether this lesion is cancer. Many European pathologists who attended the Kyoto symposium on esophageal cancer diagnosed this lesion as viral infectious disease, whereas many Japanese pathologists diagnosed it as

---

Second Department of Pathology, Hyogo College of Medicine, 1-1 Mukogawa-cho, Nishinomiya, Hyogo 663-8501, Japan

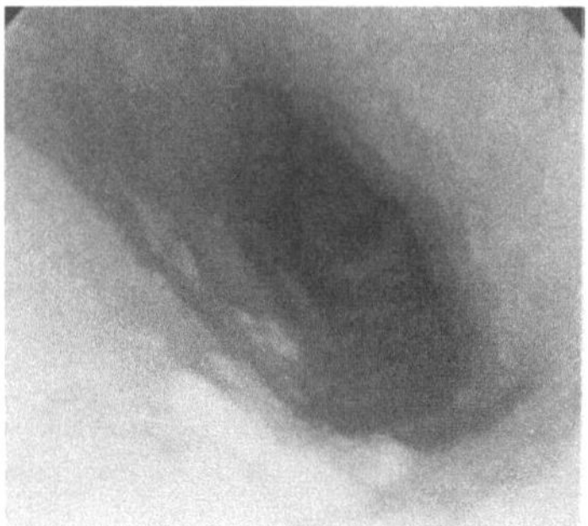

FIG. 1. Flat lesion with a whitish surface is noted on a conventional endoscopic examination

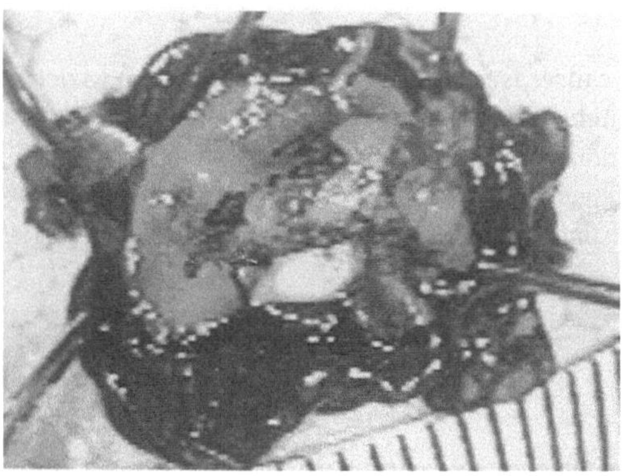

FIG. 2. Mucosectomy specimen with iodine staining. There is an unstained area at the center of the specimen surrounded by normal mucosa

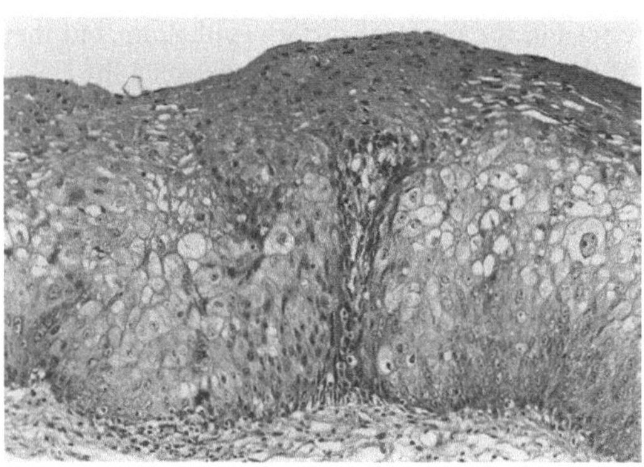

FIG. 3. Atypical cells are seen in the mucosal surface epithelium without spreading into deeper layers of the wall. (H&E, ×20)

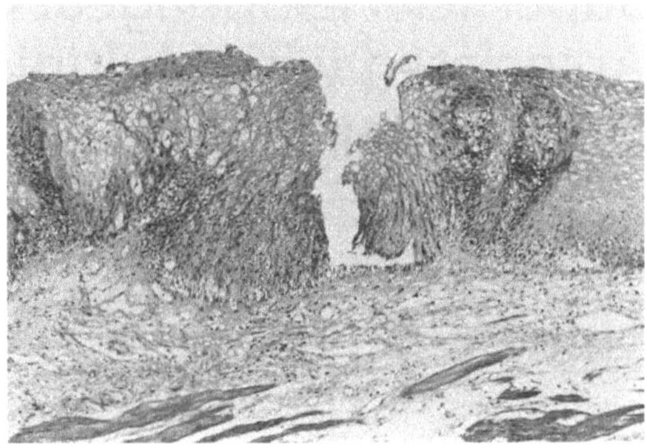

FIG. 4. Border between atypical cells and normal mucosal cell layer is clear. (H&E, ×10)

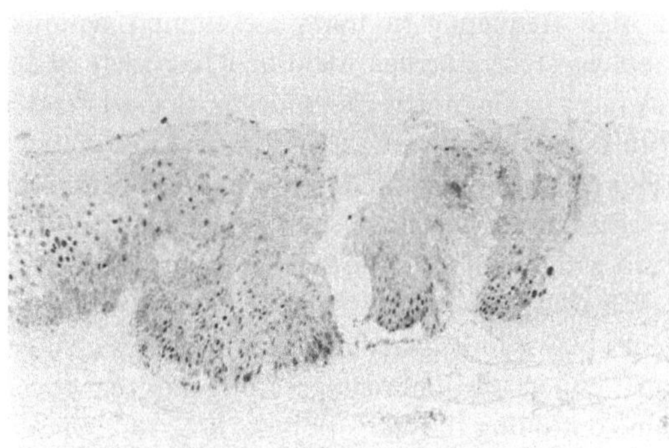

FIG. 5. The p53-positive cells are seen only in the atypical cell group. (H&E, ×10)

carcinoma in situ (except two who diagnosed it as a regenerative lesion). We believe the confusion of diagnosis of this case is the koilocytosis-like finding. The bases of support for a diagnosis of cancer are as follows.

1. The lesion was macroscopically seen in a limited portion of the esophagus.
2. The lesion had a clear border between atypical cells and the normal mucosal cell layer.
3. The p53 positivity was limited to the atypical cells.
4. Atypical cells showed negativity for papilloma virus staining.

Superficial Esophageal Carcinomas Associated with Multiple Lesions that Do Not Stain with Iodine

Minako Yoshikawa, Hiroyuki Kato, Tatsuya Miyazaki, Masanobu Nakajima, Youichi Kamiyama, Yasuyuki Fukai, Kouhei Tajima, Norihiro Masuda, Hitoshi Ojima, Katsuhiko Tsukada, and Hiroyuki Kuwano

Introduction

Esophageal cancer is a relatively common neoplasm throughout the world but is found at high frequency in many developing nations [1]. The number of superficial esophageal carcinomas identified has increased rapidly in recent years owing to advances in diagnostic methods, particularly endoscopy [2, 3]. Small areas unstained with Lugol's iodine are often observed in the mucosa surrounding esophageal squamous cell carcinoma (SCC). In patients in whom this type of esophageal SCC has been resected and where the esophageal mucosa shows multiple small areas that do not stain with Lugol's iodine, there is often multicentric cancer of the esophagus [4].

It is well known that strong expression of oncogenes and loss of tumor suppressor genes play important roles in tumorigenesis. Alterations of the *p53* gene (one of the most important tumor suppressor genes that encodes a 53-kDa nuclear phosphoprotein controlling the transition of G_0/G_1 to S phase [5]) are the most common genetic changes detected in various human cancers [6, 7]. These changes are pivotal in the complex process of carcinogenesis. The incidence of *p53* gene mutations has been reported to correlate with a high level of p53 protein overexpression in esophageal cancers [8–11]. It is thought that alteration of *p53* is an early event in esophageal carcinoma [8–13], and approximately 50% of esophageal carcinomas contain *p53* mutations [14, 15]. However, there have been few studies of the relation between multiple small areas unstained by iodine and *p53* expression in tumors [16].

We compared surgical cases of superficial esophageal carcinoma with and without additional multiple lesions that do not stain with iodine to investigate the difference in carcinogenesis between these two groups. We also assessed the correlation between pathological factors and *p53* expression.

Department of Surgery I, School of Medicine, Gunma University, 3-39-22 Showa-machi, Maebashi, Gunma 371-8511, Japan

Patients and Methods

Surgically resected specimens of superficial esophageal carcinoma from 21 male patients were collected from our hospital since 1990. These patients with an age range of 40–76 years (mean 61.90 ± 1.69 years) had undergone esophageal resection without any preoperative cancer treatment. The tumor stage and disease grades were classified according to the fifth edition of the TNM classification of the International Union Against Cancer (UICC). Group 1 consisted of four patients with superficial esophageal carcinoma associated with multiple lesions that did not stain with iodine, in addition to the main tumor mass. We defined "multiple lesions" as those where there were more than 20 areas unstained by iodine in the surrounding mucosa. In this group, the main tumor was mucosal in two cases and submucosal in the other two cases. Group 2 comprised 17 patients with a solitary tumor without major additional lesions in the mucosa. Tissue samples were collected during surgery, fixed in 10% buffered formalin, and embedded in paraffin for histochemical study.

Immunohistochemical Detection of p53 Protein

Sections 4 μm thick cut from paraffin blocks were deparaffinized and treated with a 0.3% H_2O_2-methanol solution for 30 min at room temperature to block endogenous peroxidase activity. After rehydration through a graded ethanol series, the sections were microwaved in 10 mM phosphate citrate buffer (pH 8.0) at 90°C for 15 min and then cooled to 30°C. After rinsing in 0.1 M phosphate-buffered saline (PBS), pH 7.4, nonspecific binding sites were blocked by incubating with 10% normal horse serum for 30 min. The sections were then incubated with primary antibody overnight at 4°C. The primary antibody raised against p53 (DO-7; Novocastra Laboratories, Newcastle, UK) was diluted 1 : 100. Immunohistochemistry was performed using the ABC system (Vector Laboratory, Burlingame, CA, USA). Incubation with the secondary antibody, biotinylated anti-mouse immunoglobulin G (IgG), was carried out for 30 min. The chromogen utilized was 3,3′-diaminobenzidine tetrahydrochloride, applied as a 0.02% solution containing 0.005% H_2O_2 in 50 mM ammonium acetate-citric acid buffer (pH 6.0). The sections were lightly counterstained with hematoxylin. Negative controls were established by replacing the primary antibody with buffered saline PBS or normal horse serum.

Evaluation of p53 Staining

Immunohistochemistry for p53 was graded as negative if fewer than 10% of cells were stained, or positive if more than 10% of cells were stained.

Statistical Analysis

Statistical analysis was performed using the χ^2 test and Fisher's exact test. Differences at $P < 0.05$ were considered significant.

TABLE 1. Pathological characteristics in patients

Parameters	No.	Group 1 ($n = 4$)	Group 2 ($n = 17$)	P
Tumor status: T1				
m	5	2	3	0.172
sm	16	2	14	
Nodal status				
N0	14	3	11	0.694
N1	7	1	6	
Pathological stage				
I	14	3	11	0.694
II	7	1	6	
Histological grade				
Well differentiated	6	1	5	0.453
Moderately differentiated	10	3	7	
Poorly differentiated	5	0	5	
Total	21	4	17	

m, mucosal carcinoma; sm, submucosal carcinoma

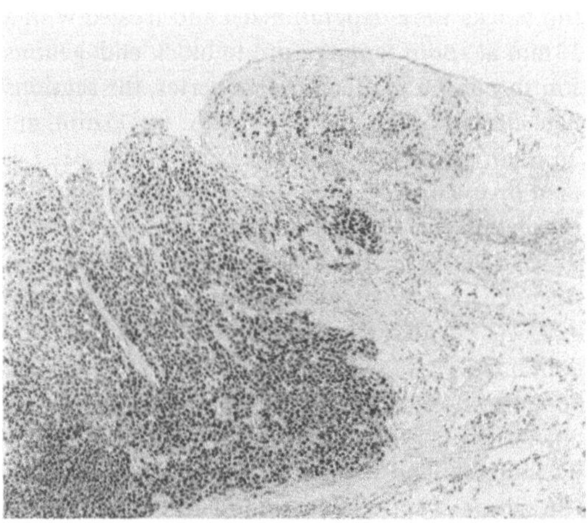

FIG. 1. Strong immunoreactivity for p53 was detected in the nuclei of cancer cells

Results

Group 1 comprised four patients with multiple superficial esophageal squamous cell cancers (SCCs) with multiple lesions unstained by iodine. We found a total of 10 satellite tumors in the mucosal cancers. The detailed pathological features of the 21 patients in groups 1 and 2 are summarized in Table 1. There were no significant differences between the two groups in terms of depth of tumor invasion, lymph node metastasis, pathological stage, or histology; and no patient had distant metastasis.

TABLE 2. Relation between p53 expression and patients

Group	Expression of p53		P
	Negative	Positive	
1 ($n = 4$)	0	4	0.081
2 ($n = 17$)	8	9	

Immunostaining of p53 was seen in the nuclei of cancer cells (Fig. 1). Table 2 shows the expression of p53 in the two groups. In group 1, the main tumor in all four cases (100%) was p53-positive. In addition, 10 satellite tumors were also defined as p53-positive. In group 2, only 9 of 17 cases (52.9%) were p53-positive. There was no statistically significant difference between the two groups.

Discussion

In this study we found four patients (group 1) with superficial esophageal SCC associated with multiple lesions unstained by iodine. There were a total of 10 satellite tumors in addition to the main tumor, and most of these multiple lesions contained dysplastic cells. In all of these group 1 cases there was p53 overexpression in all of the main and additional tumors. Patients with multiple areas unstained by iodine had multiple tumors and abnormal expression of p53 in these tumors. Based on our results, we suggest that p53 expression is related to the "field cancerization" theory [17] of esophageal SCC carcinogenesis.

Others have reported similar observations of frequent development of additional cancer in patients where esophageal SCC is associated with multiple small areas unstained by iodine. Nakanishi et al. reported that among 147 resected esophageal carcinoma specimens 78 (53%) had multiple (more than 11) small areas unstained by Lugol's iodine, and 45 (30.6%) patients had multicentric cancer in the esophagus [4].

The effects of tobacco and alcohol on carcinogenesis of esophageal SCC have been well demonstrated [18]. In our studies, patients in group 1 tended to have a higher daily consumption of tobacco and alcohol than those in group 2 (data not shown). It has previously been reported that when there is a high incidence of small areas unstained by iodine in the mucosa surrounding resected esophageal carcinoma it is significantly correlated with heavier alcohol consumption and the development of multiple primary tumors in the esophagus [4].

It is well known that strong expression of oncogenes and loss of tumor suppressor genes play important roles in tumorigenesis. Alteration of the *p53* gene, one of the important suppressor genes, is the most common genetic change detected in various human malignancies [6]. These changes play a critical role in the complex process of carcinogenesis. The sporadic distribution of p53-positive cells and the distribution and frequency of p53-positive precursor lesions support the view that accumulation of p53 protein is multifocal and occurs in precursor lesions at an early stage of esophageal carcinogenesis [19]. The pattern and frequency of p53 protein accumulation in precursor lesions and tumors of the esophagus are consistent with the field cancerization theory.

Conclusions

We have found that abnormal expression of the *p53* gene is closely related to multiple lesions unstained by iodine. We suggest that esophageal SCC involves both multifocal and field carcinogenesis. Clinically, we recommend that there should be careful preoperative examination and frequent postoperative follow-up to enable early detection of multiple tumors.

References

1. Flood WA, Furastiere AA (1995) Esophageal cancer. Curr Opin Oncol 7:381–386
2. Endo M, Kawano T (1997) Detection and classification of early squamous cell esophageal cancer. Dis Esophagus 10:155–158
3. Yokoyama A, Ohmori T, Makuuchi H, et al (1995) Successful screening for early esophageal cancer in alcoholics using endoscopy and mucosa iodeine staining. Cancer 76:928–934
4. Nakanishi Y, Ochiai A, Yoshimura K, et al (1998) The clinicopathologic significance of small areas unstained by Lugol's iodine in the mucosa surrounding resected esophageal carcinoma: an analysis of 147 cases. Cancer 82:1454–1459
5. Mercer WE, Avignolo C, Beserga R (1984) Role of the p53 protein in cell proliferation as studied by microinjection of monoclonal antibodies. Mol Cell Biol 4:276–282
6. Hollstein M, Sidransky D, Volgelstein B, et al (1991) P53 mutations in human cancer. Science 253:49–53
7. Baker SJ, Fearon ER, Nigro JM, et al (1989) Chromosome 17 deletions and p53 gene mutations in colorectal carcinomas. Science 244:217–221
8. Wang LD, Zhou Q, Hong JY, et al (1996) P53 protein accumulation and gene mutations in multifocal esophageal precancerous lesions from symptom free subjects in a high incidence area for esophageal carcinoma in Henan, China. Cancer 77: 1244–1249
9. Gao H, Wang LD, Zhou Q, et al (1994) P53 tumor suppressor gene mutation in early esophageal precancerous lesions and carcinoma among high-risk populations in Henan, China. Cancer Res 54:4342–4346
10. Kuwano H, Sadanaga N, Watanabe M, et al (1996) Oesophageal cancer composed of mixed histological types. Eur J Surg Oncol 22:225–231
11. Kuwano H, Sumiyoshi K, Sonoda K, et al (1997) Expression of p53 protein in glandular differentiation admixed with squamous cell carcinoma of the esophagus. Hepatogastroenterology 44:170–174
12. Sasano H, Goukon Y, Nishihara T, et al (1992) In situ hubridization and immunohistochemistry of p53 tumor suppressor gene in human esophageal carcinoma. Am J Pathol 141:545–550
13. Bennett WP, Liang L, He AG, et al (1996) Circulating anti-p53 antibodies in esophageal cancer patients are found predominantly in individuals with p53 core domain mutations in their tumors. Cancer Res 56:4917–4921
14. Kato H, Yoshikawa M, Fukai Y, et al (2000) An immunohistochemical study of p16, pRb, p21 and p53 proteins in human esophageal cancers. Anticancer Res 20:345–350
15. Suwiwat S, Oda H, Shimizu Y, et al (1997) Prevalance of p53 mutations and protein expression in esophageal cancers in southern Thailand. Int J Cancer 72:23–26
16. Kitamura K, Kuwano H, Yamada M, et al (1996) What is the earliest malignant lesion in the esophagaus? Cancer 77:1614–1619

17. Slaughter DP, Southwick HW, Smejkal W (1953) "Field cancerization" in oral stratified squamous epithelium. Cancer 6:963–968
18. Blot WJ (1994) Esophageal cancer trends and risk factors. Semin Oncol 121:403–410
19. Yokoyama A, Muramatsu T, Ohmori T, et al (1996) Multiple primary esophageal and concurrent upper aerodigestive tract cancer and the aldehyde dehydrogenase-2 genotype of Japanese alcoholics. Cancer 77:1986–1990

Case of Superficial Esophageal Adenocarcinoma in Short-Segment Barrett's Esophagus

Noriya Uedo[1], Hiroyasu Iishi[1], Masaharu Tatsuta[1], Ryu Ishihara[1], Hiroyuki Narahara[1], Toru Otani[1], Tsutomu Hashimoto[2], Toshiyuki Kabuto[3], Masayuki Mano[4], and Shingo Ishiguro[4]

Case Study

A 64-year-old man with a history of myocardial infarction presented with heartburn and abdominal fullness that he had had for a month. He visited a primary physician, and barium radiography and esophagogastroduodenoscopy revealed a tumor in the distal esophagus. He was referred to our institute for surgical treatment. Vital status and physical examination revealed no abnormality. Except a mild elevation of the fasting plasma glucose level, blood cell count, blood chemistries, and serum carcinoembryonie antigen (CEA) level were all normal.

Barium radiography showed an irregularly lobulated 1.5-cm polypoid tumor in the lower thoracic esophagus. There was no ulceration on the tumor or lateral deformity, suggesting the absence of wall invasion (Fig. 1).

Endoscopic examination revealed a protruded tumor with a multinodular surface 35 cm distant from the upper incisor teeth (Fig. 2a). After spraying Lugol's solution, tongue-like Lugol-unstained columnar epithelium was seen around the tumor (Fig. 2b). Biopsy specimens from the tumor revealed a papillotubular growth pattern of the atypical gland, and it was diagnosed as adenocarcinoma.

The patient underwent esophagectomy. In the resected specimen, Barrett's mucosa, which consisted mainly of atrophic gastric-fundic-type epithelium and partly scattered specialized columunar epithelium, extended at its longest projection 1.5 cm from the esophagogastric junction. Most of the intestinal metaplasia stained with MUC2 was prevalent in specialized columunar epithelium (Fig. 3). The main tumor was moderately differentiated adenocarcinoma of a superficial protruding plateau type and measuring 19×24 mm. It invaded the submucosa, with lymphatic and blood vessel invasion as well (Fig. 4). A small intramucosal adenocarcinoma, measuring 6×4 mm, existed apart from the main tumor (Fig. 5). There was a metastasis in a lymph node. No distant metastasis was detected at the time of the operation.

Departments of [1]Gastroenterology, [2]Radiology, [3]Surgery, and [4]Pathology, Osaka Medical Center for Cancer and Cardiovascular Diseases, 3-3 Nakamichi 1-chome, Higashinari-ku, Osaka 537-8511, Japan

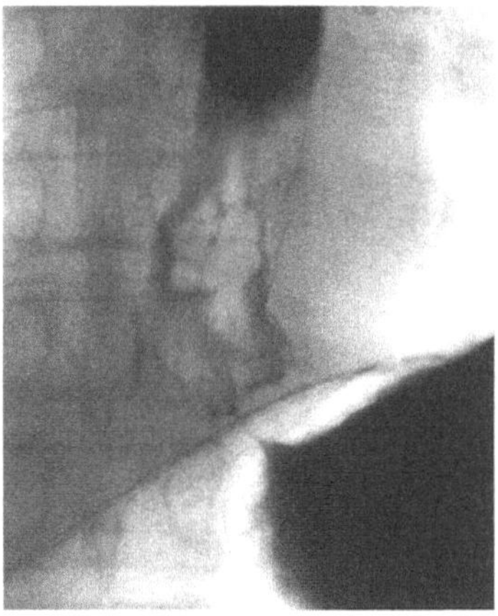

FIG. 1. Barium esophagography. An irregularly lobulated 1.5-cm polypoid tumor was found in the lower thoracic esophagus

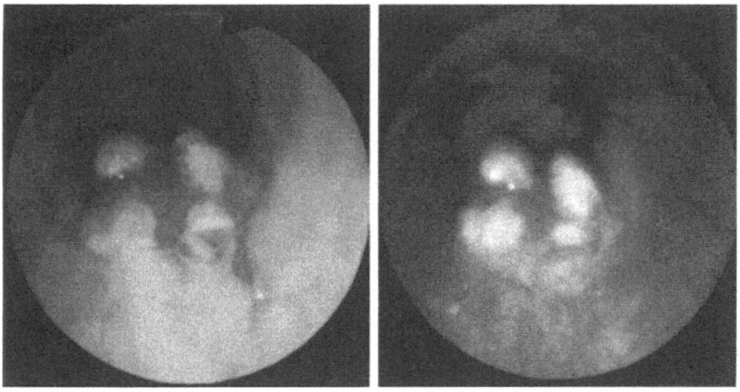

FIG. 2. **a** Esophagoscopy of a multinodular protruding tumor 35 cm from the upper incisor teeth. **b** Chromoendoscopy. After spraying Lugol's solution, squamous epithelium was stained dark brown. The tumor was within Lugol-unstained columnar epithelium

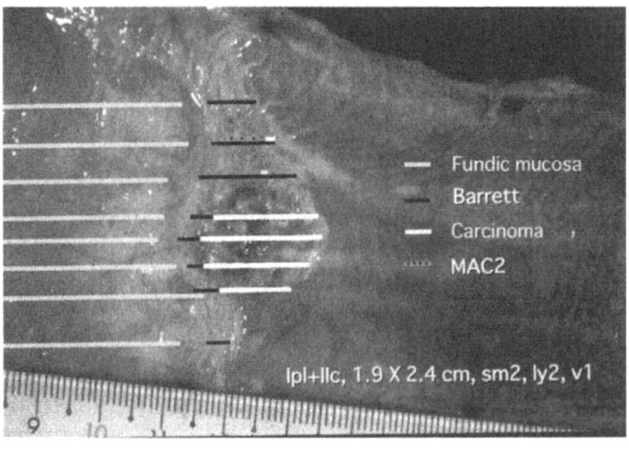

FIG. 3. Macroscopic appearance of the resected specimen. Metaplastic Barrett's esophagus extended, at its longest projection, 1.5 cm from the esophagogastric junction. Superficial protruding plateau-type and small flat intramucosal carcinomas existed within it

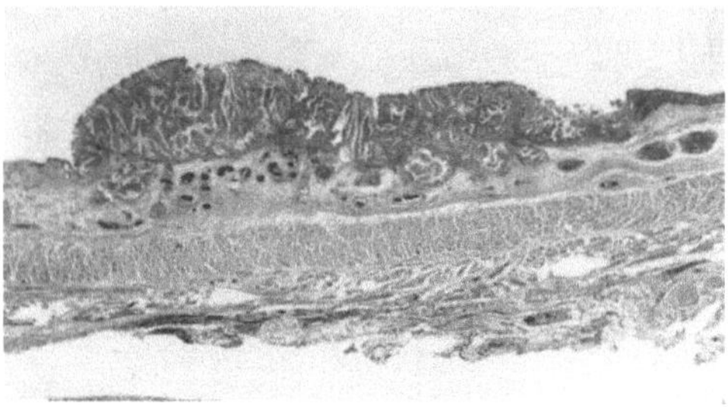

FIG. 4. Main tumor invaded the submucosa, with lymphatic and blood vessel invasion as well. (H&E, ×10)

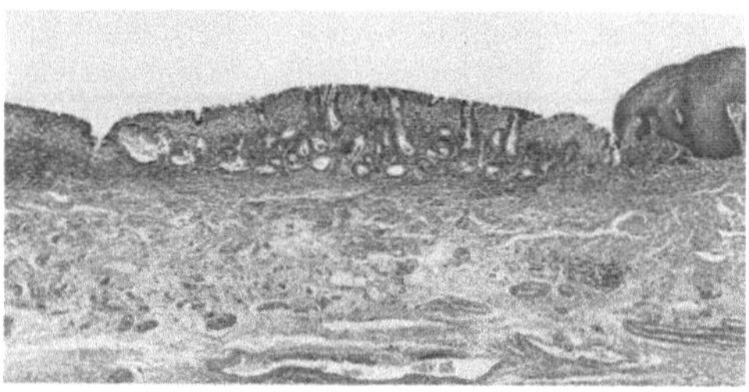

FIG. 5. A flat intramucosal well differentiated adenocarcinoma coexisted apart from the main tumor. (H&E, ×10)

Two years after esophagectomy, a lung metastasis was detected in the right upper lobe. The patient underwent right upper lobectomy, but he died of multiple lung metastases 2 years later.

Discussion

The incidence of adenocarcinoma of the esophagus and gastric cardia is rapidly increasing in the United States and western Europe [1]. In Japan, however, adenocarcinoma accounts for less than 5% of esophageal carcinomas. It is generally accepted that Barrett's esophagus, a lesion caused by gastroesophageal reflux disease, is the major risk factor for adenocarcinoma of the esophagus. The prevalence of Barrett's esophagus is also lower in Japan than in Western countries. Nishi et al. [2] reported that the incidences of traditional Barrett's esophagus, defined as circumferential columnar-lined esophagus involving tissues more than 3 cm from the esophagogastric junction [2], and short-segment Barrett's esophagus are 0.3% and 5.8%, respectively, among Japanese people who undergo health check screening endoscopy [3]. Differences of prevalence rates and strains [4] of *Helicobacter pylori* as well as ethnicity explain the lower incidence of Barrett's esophagus related to gastroesophageal reflux disease and associated esophageal adenocarcinoma in Japan [5].

We have reported a case of multiple adenocarcinomas arising in short-segment Barrett's esophagus. A small, flat intramucosal carcinoma coexisted with the protruded submucosal carcinoma. Neither lesion had a dysplasia component. The dysplasia–carcinoma sequence has been thought to be a main source of carcinogenesis of esophageal adenocarcinoma in Barrett's esophagus. However, we believe that not all Barrett's adenocarcinomas are involved in that pathway. New methods for detecting high-grade dysplasia and adenocarcinoma in Barrett's esophagus have been introduced [6-8]; and these new techniques and histological assessment of en bloc specimens obtained during endoscopic mucosal resection may change the diagnosis in patients with Barrett's esophagus and lesions with endoscopic features that suggest neoplasia [9].

References

1. Orlando RC (1999) Reflux esophagitis. In: Yamada T, Alpers DH, Laine L (eds) Textbook of Gastroenterology, 3rd ed. Lippincott Williams & Wilkins, Philadelphia, pp 1235-1262
2. Nishi T, Makuuchi H, Machimura, et al (1997) Incidence of Barrett's esophagus and Barrett's mucosa in Japan (*in Japanese*). Syokaki Naishikyo 9:891-896
3. Skinner DB, Walter BC, Riddle RH, et al (1983) Barrett's esophagus: comparison of benign and malignant cases. Ann Surg 198:554-566
4. Campbell S, Fraser A, Holliss B, et al (1997) Evidence for ethnic tropism of *Helicobacter pylori*. Infect Immun 65:3708-3712
5. El-Serag HB, Sonnenberg A (1998) Opposing time trends of peptic ulcer and reflux disease. Gut 43:327-333
6. Messmann H, Knuchel R, Baumler W, et al (1999) Endoscopic fluorescence detection of dysplasia in patients with Barrett's esophagus, ulcerative colitis, or adenomatous polyps after 5-aminolevulinic acid-induced protoporphyrin IX sensitization. Gastrointest Endosc 49:97-101
7. Reid BJ, Blount PL, Feng Z, et al (2000) Optimizing endoscopic biopsy detection of early cancers in Barrett's high-grade dysplasia. Am J Gastroenterol 95:3089-3096
8. Bourg-Heckly G, Blais J, Padilla JJ, et al (2000) Endoscopic ultraviolet-induced autofluorescence spectroscopy of the esophagus: tissue characterization and potential for early cancer diagnosis. Endoscopy 32:756-765
9. Nijhawan PK, Wang KK (2000) Endoscopic mucosal resection for lesions with endoscopic features suggestive of malignancy and high-grade dysplasia within Barrett's esophagus. Gastrointest Endosc 52:328-332

Superficial Esophageal Cancer Treated by Radical Surgery: Case Study

Hideo Shimada, Yoshifumi Kise, Osamu Chino, Hikaru Tanaka, Takahiro Kenmochi, and Hiroyasu Makuuchi

Introduction

The diagnostic criteria for intraepithelial cancer of the esophagus are different between Western countries and Japan. In Western countries only the malignant tumor invading the lamina propria mucosae seems to be regarded as cancer [1]. We report a case of esophageal cancer invading the submucosal layer diagnosed by typical upper gastrointestinal and endoscopic findings. It was treated by radical surgery.

Case Report

A 70-year-old woman complaining of postprandial sternal pain and dysphagia was transferred from a local hospital for further evaluation after an endoscopic biopsy diagnosis of esophageal cancer. She had a history of smoking 20 cigarettes a day for 45 years and used to be an alcohol abuser. There was no remarkable past history other than hypertension. Physical examination and laboratory studies showed no abnormalities. Esophagography showed a small barium fleck on the posterior wall of the middle thoracic esophagus. In the enlarged image, this esophagogram showed an approximately 15-mm depressed lesion surrounded by a crest. There were no abnormal findings in the area surrounding the lesion (Fig. 1).

Endoscopic examination showed a protruding lesion with a depression at the center 31 cm from the incisors; it progressed to being slightly depressed with granular change 30 cm from the incisor, indicating intraepithelial invasion. Nearer the lesion the rough surface of the summit of the protruding lesion was more clearly seen. The right side of the tumor was covered by normal whitish epithelium.

When toluidine blue staining was employed, this irregular surface in the center and the extended slightly depressed area stained purple. When both toluidine blue and

Department of Surgery, Tokai University School of Medicine, Boseidai, Isehara, Kanagawa 259-1193, Japan

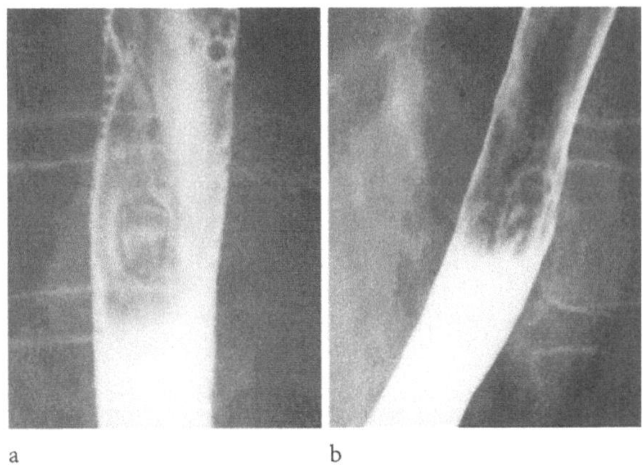

FIG. 1. Upper gastrointestinal series revealed a small barium fleck extending for 2 cm on the posterior wall of the middle thoracic esophagus. **a** Front position. **b** Second oblique position

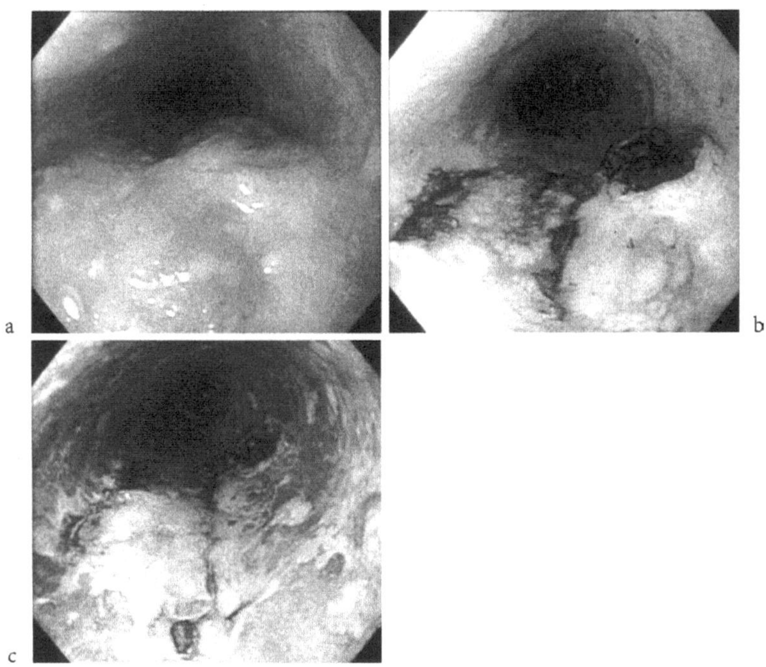

FIG. 2. Endoscopy showed a protruding lesion with a depression in the center 31 cm from the incisors and intraepithelial spread on the left side detected by double staining. **a** Conventional observation. **b** Toluidine blue staining. **c** Toluidine blue-iodine double staining. With toluidine blue staining the depressed portion of the lesion was stained blue, and the cancer area became clearer by color contrast

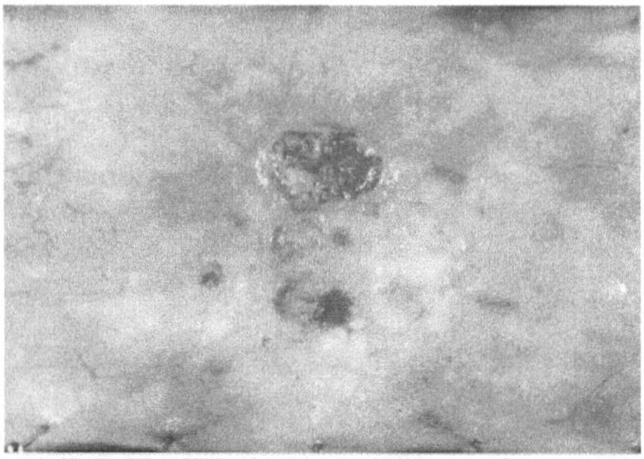
a

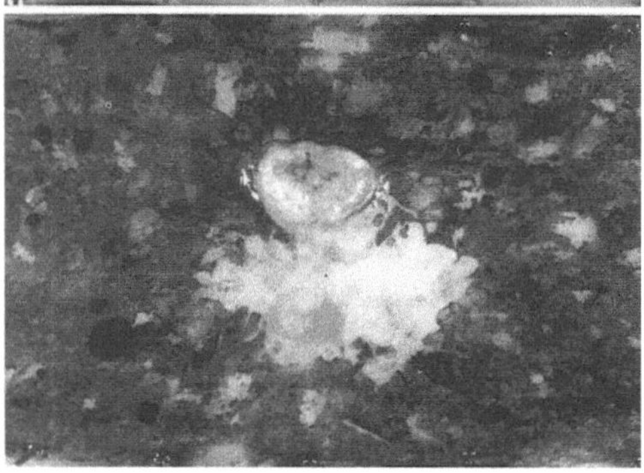
b

FIG. 3. Resected specimen of this case. **a** Fresh specimen without staining. **b** Staining with iodine

iodine double staining were performed, the surrounding normal epithelium appeared brown, and the border of the lesion was delineated (Fig. 2).

A diagnosis of esophageal cancer invading the shallow submucosal layer was based on these findings. Chest computed tomography and endoscopic ultrasonography demonstrated no apparent lymph node metastasis, and there were no serious risks for operation.

The resected specimen, before fixation, showed an approximately 30 × 30 mm combined-type superficial protrusion with a slight depression in the center; it was located in the middle of the esophagus. After iodine staining the lesion became clear as an unstained area. There were also multiple tiny unstained lesions in the surrounding area (Fig. 3).

Histological examination revealed moderately differentiated squamous cell carcinoma (Fig. 4) characterized by proliferation of carcinoma cells with disordered nuclear polarity and irregular keratinization. Concerning the depth of invasion, the deepest point was at the center of the protruding area, and it was limited to the upper one-third of the submucosal layer. The irregular depressed area on the oral side of the protrusion was found to be a cancer invading the lamina propria. There was no lymphatic or blood vessel permeation, and all 52 of the removed lymph nodes were found to be free of metastasis. The patient was discharged following an uneventful recovery.

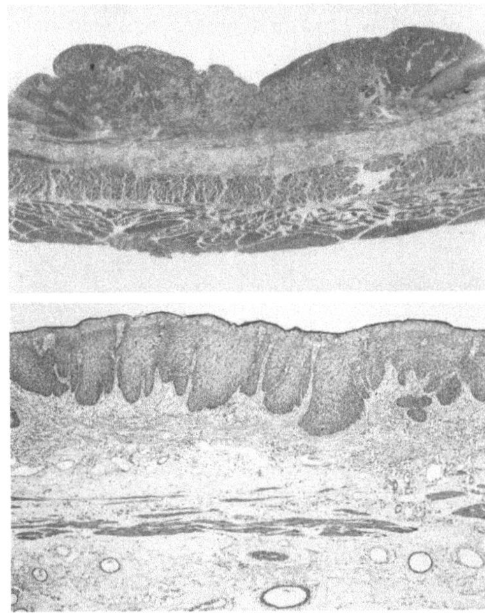

FIG. 4. **a** Histological findings showed moderately differentiated squamous cell carcinoma invading the submucosal layer. **b** Surrounding slight irregular surface revealed mucosal cancer invading the lamina propria mucosa

Discussion

The depth of invasion relative to vascular invasion and lymph node metastases was investigated in patients who underwent surgery for superficial esophageal cancer in Japan. The results showed that esophageal cancers limited to the proper mucosal mucosae have extremely low rates of lymph node metastasis and vascular invasion [2]. The recent development of endoscopic techniques with iodine staining has improved the diagnosis of early esophageal cancer, and endoscopic esophageal mucosal resection is widely used as the treatment of choice in such cases [3].

In this present case, we diagnosed a superficial esophageal cancer invading the submucosal layer based on endoscopic findings of a protruding lesion with a markedly depressed area that stained deeply with toluidine blue. Superficial esophageal cancers invading the submucosal layer, are regarded as having a more than 30% rate of lymph node metastasis. Therefore, subtotal esophagectomy with three-field lymph node dissection using the gastric roll for reconstruction is the standard procedure for cancer of the thoracic esophagus. We consider it necessary to use three-field lymph node dissection in such a cases, when the preoperative diagnosis of lymph node metastasis is not clear [4].

References

1. Schlemper RJ, Dawsey SM, Itabashi M, et al (2000) Difference in diagnostic criteria for esophageal squamous cell carcinoma between Japanese and Western pathologists. Cancer 88:997–1006

2. Kodama M, Teruo K (1998) Treatment of superficial cancer of the esophagus: a summary of responses to a questionnaire on superficial cancer of the esophagus in Japan. Surgery 123:432–439
3. Hiroyasu M (1996) Endoscopic mucosal resction for early esophageal cancer: indication and techniques. Dig Endosc 8:175–179
4. Hideo S, Osamu C, Hikaru T, et al (1999) Significance of lymph node dissection of neck and upper mediastinum according to metastatic analysis of 3-field dissection for cancer of the thoracic esophagus (in Japanese). Nishogekashi

Patient Presentation and Pathologic Diagnosis of Superficial Carcinoma of the Esophagus: High-Grade Dysplasia and Mucosal Carcinoma from the Japanese Standpoint

KAIYO TAKUBO[1], TOMIO ARAI[2], and SHINGO ISHIGURO[3]

In Japan, people should consider whether *Stomach and Intestine*, which is probably the best journal for learning about early neoplasms of the gastrointestinal tract, should not be published in English as well as Japanese. Additionally, we Western pathologists should avail ourselves more of the great hospitality of our Japanese colleagues than we have done so far, to gain training in their departments with their large collections of early gastric carcinomas.—Stolte [1]

Nomenclature Problems in the West and Japan

It is well known that there are large differences between Western and Japanese pathologists regarding the criteria used for the histologic diagnosis of dysplasia and carcinoma with no or minimal invasion in the gastrointestinal tract [2–5]. Many of these discrepancies arise from differences in the nomenclature used to describe gastrointestinal tract cancers.

Adenoma of the Stomach and Colorectum

The entity "adenoma" of the stomach is well established among Japanese pathologists, and the lesion is regarded as distinct from mucosal well-differentiated tubular adenocarcinoma [6]. Adenomas usually consist of atypical tubular structures lined by relatively uniform cells in the upper half of an intramucosal lesion and dilated pyloric-type glands in the lower half. These tumors are usually a few centimeters in diameter.

The histologic criteria for both adenoma and intramucosal adenocarcinoma of the colorectum, however, have recently become matters of considerable debate among Japanese pathologists, as no clear histologic criteria for either have been proposed in

[1]Department of Clinical Pathology, Tokyo Metropolitan Institute of Gerontology, [2]Department of Clinical Pathology, Tokyo Metropolitan Geriatric Hospital, 35-2 Sakaecho, Itabashi-ku, Tokyo 173-0015, Japan
[3]Department of Pathology, Osaka Medical Center of Cancer and Adult Diseases, 1-1-3 Nakamichi, Higashinari-ku, Osaka 537-0025, Japan

Japan. In fact the criteria used for the diagnoses of adenoma and mucosal carcinoma of the colorectum vary even among Japanese pathologists.

Nomenclature Problems with the Esophagus

Dysplasia or adenomatous change has been reported to occur in both nonmetaplastic esophageal mucosa and Barrett's mucosa. High-grade dysplasia is also frequently associated with invasive adenocarcinoma arising in Barrett's esophagus and in the stomach. High-grade dysplasia of Barrett's mucosa and the stomach are considered in Western countries to be precursors of adenocarcinoma, whereas in Japan these lesions are considered to be very well-differentiated or well-differentiated intramucosal adenocarcinomas; in other words, the lesions are thought to be the intramucosal well-differentiated components of invasive adenocarcinomas of Barrett's esophagus and the stomach. This is analogous to invasive ductal carcinoma of the breast, which often has a component of ductal carcinoma in situ.

Textbooks of Gastrointestinal Pathology

Differences in terminology can also be found in some textbooks of surgical pathology. Textbooks of gastrointestinal pathology recently published in America and Europe show photographs of squamous and glandular dysplasia in the esophagus. Many of the examples described as severe or high-grade dysplasia of the esophagus, and even some of those described as mild dysplasia, would be regarded as squamous cell carcinoma in situ or intramucosal well-differentiated adenocarcinoma by many Japanese histopathologists. In particular, whereas the high-grade dysplasia of Barrett's esophagus (even if there is no clear stromal invasion) is considered a type of intramucosal well-differentiated adenocarcinoma in Japan, in Western countries the term "high-grade dysplasia" is generally used when there is no clear stromal invasion, as is the case for all sites in the gastrointestinal tract.

Kyoto Symposium on Esophageal Cancer

It is important for both Western and Japanese pathologists to be able to recognize high-grade dysplasia and intramucosal well-differentiated adenocarcinoma of the esophagus and to be aware of the differences in diagnostic criteria used for mucosal epithelial neoplasms in the West and Japan. The Kyoto Symposium on Esophageal Cancer was held in July 2000, and its president was Masayuki Imamura (Department of Surgery and Surgical Basic Science, Graduate School of Medicine, Kyoto University). Eleven interesting esophageal carcinomas were presented at the symposium. The data presented included the patients' clinical courses, endoscopic findings (including chromoendoscopy), esophagography, histopathology, and immunohistochemistry. As part of this examination, the histopathology of 17 neoplastic foci (including primary tumors and other associated lesions detected histologically in the resection or biopsy specimens) was reviewed by 4 Western and 12 Japanese pathologists (listed in the Acknowledgments section). A 2-h histologic review session was held one evening and a discussion with microscopy was held for 2 h the following morning. These sessions provided an excellent opportunity to discuss differences in tumor classification. We

TABLE 1. Vienna Classification of Gastrointestinal Epithelial Neoplasia

Category 1:	negative for neoplasm/dysplasia	
Category 2:	indefinite for neoplasia/dysplasia	
Category 3:	noninvasive low-grade neoplasia (low-grade adenoma/dysplasia)	
Category 4:	noninvasive high-grade neoplasia	
	4.1:	high-grade adenoma/dysplasia
	4.2:	noninvasive carcinoma (carcinoma in situ)[a]
	4.3:	suspicious for invasive carcinoma.
Category 5:	invasive neoplasia	
	5.1:	intramucosal carcinoma[b]
	5.2:	submucosal carcinoma or beyond

[a] Noninvasive indicates absence of evident invasion
[b] Intramucosal indicates invasion into the lamina propria or muscularis mucosa

describe here the results of the pathologists' review of the histologic sections. The Vienna Classification of Gastrointestinal Epithelial Neoplasia was used by both groups (Table 1) [7, 8].

Data and Comments on the Case Presentations

We reviewed the histologic sections and discussed the results from the standpoint of Japanese pathologists. Data on the histopathologic diagnoses of the cases are shown in Table 2. The lesions were divided into three groups (groups 1–3) according to the histologic diagnosis and are discussed below.

Group 1

Patient 1, lesions 1 and 2; patient 2, lesions 1 and 2; patient 3, lesions 1 and 2; patient 4, lesion 1; patient 5; patient 6, lesions 1 and 2; patient 7, lesions 1 and 2; and patients 8 to 11 were mainly diagnosed as category 4 (noninvasive high-grade neoplasia) or category 5 (invasive neoplasia) by both Western and Japanese pathologists, with few exceptions. These results suggest that histologic evidence of invasion is difficult to identify in the esophageal mucosa, and that high-grade dysplasia, as described by Western pathologists, and well-differentiated carcinoma, as described by Japanese pathologists, can be placed in the same categories in the Vienna classification. Patients with category 4 or 5 disease are deemed, in both Western countries and Japan, to require some form of therapy.

In this group the agreement between Western and Japanese pathologists was good when the Vienna classification system was used, as noted above. This was to be expected because the Vienna Classification was devised only to gain superficial consistency of the categories of histologic diagnosis used by Western and Japanese pathologists, not to resolve problems with classification [3]. High-grade dysplasia (mainly diagnosed by Western pathologists) and squamous cell carcinoma in situ and intramucosal well-differentiated adenocarcinoma (mainly diagnosed by Japanese pathologists) should all be placed in the same category. However, these lesions were classified as category 4 or 5 by both Western and Japanese pathologists, suggesting that invasion is difficult to recognize histologically by both the Western and Japanese systems.

TABLE 2. Histologic diagnoses of the 17 foci presented at the Kyoto Symposium by Western and Japanese pathologists classified using the Vienna Classification of Gastrointestinal Epithelial Neoplasia

	Western pathologists (n = 4)					Japanese pathologists (n = 12)				
Case	C-1	C-2	C-3	C-4	C-5	C-1	C-2	C-3	C-4	C-5
1				3	1				11	1
2 (1)[a]				2	2				9	3
2 (2)				1	3	1			6	5
3 (1)				4					11	1
3 (2)					4					12
4 (1)				3	1		1		10	1
4 (2)			3	1			2	8	2	
5			1	1	2				4	8
6 (1)				1	3				2	10
6 (2)				1	3				2	10
6 (3)		2	2				2	2	6	1
7 (1)			1	3				1	11	
7 (2)				1	3				5	6
8				3					11	1
9			2	2		2		1	8	1
10				4					9	3
11				3	1		2			10

C-1: category 1; C-2: category 2; C-3: category 3; C-4: category 4; C-5: category 5
[a] Numbers in parentheses are the number of lesions

Group 2

Lesion 2 in patient 4 was mainly diagnosed as category 3 by both Western and Japanese pathologists. The participants agreed that category 3 lesions can be managed clinically by endoscopic treatment or follow-up.

Group 3

Patient 6, lesion 3 and patient 9 were diagnosed as category 4 or 5 by most Japanese pathologists but as category 2 or 3 by most Western pathologists. This is in keeping with the fact that some patients described in Western textbooks of gastrointestinal pathology as having mild dysplasia would be regarded to have squamous cell carcinoma in situ or intramucosal well-differentiated adenocarcinoma by many Japanese histopathologists; such lesions would be diagnosed as category 3 by Western pathologists but as category 4 or 5 by Japanese pathologists. This difference poses a problem for subsequent management. Although follow-up and endoscopic treatment are the most appropriate options for category 3 patients, those with category 4 and category 5 disease need more intensive treatment, which may range from endoscopic mucosal resection to major surgery. Thus, these patients would not be treated in Western countries but would be treated in Japan. Some agreement on diagnostic criteria is obviously needed for this group of lesions.

Histopathologic Basis of the Japanese Criteria for Mucosal Well-Differentiated Carcinoma

Western pathologists rely heavily on demonstrating invasion into underlying or adjacent stroma to determine if a tumor is cancer, whereas Japanese pathologists examine cytologic features and base their opinion on such features as nuclear enlargement, hyperchromatism, and pleomorphism [2–4]. Most Japanese pathologists agree that the terms intramucosal or mucosal well-differentiated tubular adenocarcinoma can and should be used for lesions in the stomach and esophagus that have cytologic features of cancer but that lack clear stromal invasion. Intraepithelial spreading carcinoma often coexists with invasive squamous cell carcinoma, and Japanese pathologists consider such intraepithelial spread to be histologic evidence of an esophageal primary [5]. Intraepithelial spread can be subdivided histologically into a total-layer type (in which the whole epithelium is replaced by tumor cells) and a basal-layer type (in which the basal half is predominantly replaced by tumor cells). Tumor cells infiltrate between the basement membrane and the normal squamous epithelium at the interface between an intraepithelial spreading carcinoma and the normal epithelium. Degenerated cancer and epithelial and mesenchymal cells can be seen on light and electron microscopic examination of the interface; there are also small spaces at the interface, and tumor cells are sometimes directly attached to normal epithelial cells by desmosomes [5, 9, 10]. The basal layer type of intraepithelial spread also shows these changes at the interface. Japanese pathologists do not diagnose this type of spread as squamous dysplasia. An intraepithelial neoplasm that is histologically similar to an intraepithelial spreading carcinoma but that has retained its basement membrane would usually be diagnosed as a squamous cell carcinoma in situ by Japanese pathologists, rather than as squamous dysplasia. Both Western and Japanese pathologists have difficulty with the histologic recognition of invasion, but the distinction between intraepithelial squamous cell carcinoma and squamous cell carcinoma invading only the lamina propria is not clinically important because neither of these lesions metastasizes to lymph nodes and both are curable by endoscopic mucosal resection [5].

Although we encounter few cases of Barrett's adenocarcinoma in Japan and the incidence of adenocarcinoma is usually less than about 2% of all esophageal malignancies [11], we have much more experience with adenocarcinoma of the stomach than most Western pathologists [1]. Judging from experience gained by the pathologic observation and clinical follow-up of many gastric cancers in Japan, virtually all lesions classified as high-grade dysplasia by Western pathologists, but as intramucosal well-differentiated tubular (or papillary) adenocarcinoma by Japanese pathologists, later develop into submucosal invasive carcinomas. One case of a mucosal carcinoma that remained confined to the mucosa for more than 11 years 8 months has been reported, but it has been found that most of these tumors invade the submucosa within 3 years [12]. Invasive adenocarcinoma of the stomach occasionally gives rise to an extensive intramucosal spreading component of well-differentiated carcinoma. In Japan we are able to diagnose intramucosal carcinomas because they have histologic features similar to those of widely spreading intramucosal carcinomas adjacent to deeply invasive carcinomas. Japanese pathologists scrutinize cytologic features and assess the presence or absence of such indicators as nuclear enlargement, hyperchromatism, and pleomorphism when making this diagnosis.

Rosen cited Broders (1932) in a chapter on in situ (intraepithelial) carcinoma in his textbook *Rosen's Breast Pathology* [13].

> A condition in which malignant epithelial cells and their progeny are found in or near the positions occupied by their ancestors before the ancestors underwent malignant transformation. At least they have not migrated beyond the juncture of the epithelium and connective tissue or the so-called basement membrane. The diagnosis of carcinoma in situ, as of carcinoma in general, is based chiefly on altered cellular characteristics in contradistinction to the cellular situation. If, in a specimen obtained for biopsy, carcinoma in situ is associated with infiltrating carcinoma, there is little chance of missing the diagnosis of carcinoma.—Broders [14]

Rosen noted that although Borders' study dealt with neoplastic changes in the oral mucosa it was applicable to other organs.

Conclusions

Our conclusions are neatly summarized in the quotation from Stolte [1] cited at the beginning of this chapter. We add only that if high-grade glandular dysplasia by Western criteria (the same category as mucosal well-differentiated adenocarcinoma by Japanese criteria) is diagnosed from an esophageal biopsy specimen, treatment must involve endoscopic or surgical removal rather than follow-up alone. This is because studies have shown that these lesions usually become deeply invasive within 3 years or occasionally have invasive components into the submucosa or deeper. Also, some lesions classified as low-grade dysplasia by Western pathologists are regarded as intramucosal carcinoma by Japanese pathologists, and these lesions can give rise to invasive foci.

Acknowledgments. Many thanks are due to Dr. R. J. Schlemper, Department of Internal Medicine, Fukuoka University School of Medicine, Fukuoka, Japan, for his kind advice and Dr. N. K. Lambie, Department of Anatomic Pathology, Canterbury Health Laboratories, Christchurch Hospital, Christchurch, New Zealand, for proofreading the manuscript. The histopathologists who attended the Kyoto Symposium on esophageal cancer are as follows: Parakrama Chandrasoma, M.D.; Rebecca H. Harrison, M.D.; Jeremy R. Jass, M.D.; Carlos A. Rubio, M.D.; Tomio Arai, M.D.; Shingo Ishiguro, M.D.; Masayuki Itabashi, M.D.; Yo Kato, M.D.; Masayuki Mano, M.D.; Yasuaki Nakanishi, M.D.; Takashi Nishigami, M.D.; Kenichi Ohashi, M.D.; Tadakazu Shimoda, M.D.; Kaiyo Takubo, M.D.; Shinya Toyokuni, M.D.; and Hirohiko Yamabe, M.D.

References

1. Stolte M (1999) Diagnosis of gastric carcinoma: Japanese fairy tales or Western deficiency? Virchows Arch 434:279–280
2. Schlemper RJ, Itabashi M, Kato Y, et al (1997) Differences in diagnostic criteria for gastric carcinoma between Japanese and Western pathologists. Lancet 349:1725–1729
3. Jass JR (1999) Discrepancies between East and West. Cancer 88:969–970

4. Schlemper RJ, Dawsey SM, Itabashi M, et al (2000) Differences in diagnostic criteria for esophageal squamous cell carcinoma between Japanese and Western pathologists. Cancer 88:996–1006
5. Takubo K (2000) Pathology of the esophagus. Educa, Tokyo, pp 131–168
6. Sekine H, Shibuki S, Ohara H, et al (1994) Issues of gastric biopsy for diagnosis of benign/malignant borderline lesion: from the viewpoint of long-term clinical follow-up. I to Cho 29:143–151 (in Japanese with English abstract)
7. Schlemper RJ, Kato Y, Riddell RH, et al (1999) New consensus Vienna Classification of Gastrointestinal Epithelial Neoplasia. I to Cho 34:1043–1049 (in Japanese)
8. Schlemper RJ, Riddell RH, Kato Y, et al (2000) The Vienna Classification of Gastrointestinal Epithelial Neoplasia. Gut 47:251–255
9. Takubo K, Takai A, Takayama S, et al (1987) Intraductal spread of esophageal squamous cell carcinoma. Cancer 59:1751–1757
10. Takubo K, Nishimura H, Taniguchi Y, et al (1984) Junctions between intraepithelial carcinoma and non-neoplastic tissue of the esophagus: light and electron microscopic studies. Act Pathol Jpn 34:785–796
11. Registration Committee for Esophageal Cancer of The Japanese Society for Esophageal Diseases (2000) Comprehensive registry of esophageal cancer in Japan (1988–1994), 1st edn. Japanese Society for Esophageal Diseases, Chiba-city, pp 19–39
12. Nisizawa M, Nomoto K, Ueno M, et al (1992) Natural history of gastric cancer in a fixed population with emphasis on depressed sm cancer. I to Cho 27:16–24 (in Japanese with English abstract)
13. Rosen PP (1997) In situ (intra-epithelial) carcinoma: an overview. In: Rosen's Breast Pathology. Lippincott-Raven, Philadelphia, pp 219–221
14. Broders AC (1932) Carcinoma in situ contrasted with benign penetrating epithelium. JAMA 99:1670–1674

Part 5
Molecular Biology of Esophageal Neoplasms

Oncogene Amplification and Oncoprotein Overexpression in Superficial Esophageal Cancer

Mario Sarbia

Introduction

The depth of tumor penetration is a crucial factor determining the prognosis of esophageal carcinoma patients [1, 2]. Any carcinoma that extends no deeper than the submucosa is referred to as superficial esophageal carcinoma regardless of lymph node metastasis [3]. Patients with superficial esophageal carcinomas, especially those limited to the mucosa, have significantly more favorable outcome than those with advanced cancer. On the other hand, the risk of nodal metastasis of submucosal carcinomas is about 35%, and the prognosis of these patients does not differ significantly from that of patients with advanced carcinoma. Whereas the frequency of superficial esophageal carcinomas in Western countries is still low [4], in Japan, because of intensified screening, the rate of superficial cancer has been increasing in recent years [3]. Nevertheless, the features of superficial esophageal carcinoma, especially its molecular biologic aberrations, are poorly studied so far. In the current study we therefore investigated the frequency of oncogene amplification and oncoprotein overexpression in the two histological main types of esophageal cancer: squamous cell carcinoma (SCC) and adenocarcinoma (ADC). To determine if the molecular biology of superficial carcinoma differs significantly from that of advanced carcinoma, we compared our findings with a series of advanced esophageal SCCs and ADCs.

Materials and Methods

Patients

The current study included esophagectomy specimens from 40 patients who underwent resection without preoperative chemotherapy or irradiation between January 1, 1987 and December 31, 1999 for superficial ADC (group I, $n = 20$) or superficial SCC (group II, $n = 20$). A group of 40 patients with advanced esophageal ADC (group III, $n = 20$) or SCC (group IV, $n = 20$) were included as controls.

Department of Pathology, University of Düsseldorf, Postach 101007, 40001 Düsseldorf, Germany

The esophagectomy specimens were fixed in 4% buffered formaldehyde, embedded in paraffin, sectioned, and stained with hematoxylin and eosin. The grading of invasive carcinomas was performed according to the World Health Organization (WHO) criteria [5], and the pTNM classification was performed according to the International Union against Cancer (UICC) criteria [6].

Group I consisted of 4 female and 16 male patients with an age range of 30 to 81 years. Altogether, 7 carcinomas were limited to the mucosa, and 13 tumors invaded the submucosa. One tumor showed lymph node metastasis, but the others were lymph node-negative. Of these tumors, 11 were graded as G2, 8 as G3, and 1 as G4. Group II included 7 female and 13 male patients with an age range of 45 to 65 years. Of these 20 tumors, 2 were confined to the mucosa and 18 to the submucosa; 6 tumors showed lymph node metastasis, and 14 were lymph node-negative. Among them, 2 tumors were graded as G1, 6 as G2 and 12 as G3. Group III consisted of 20 male patients with an age range of 36 to 73 years. There were 5 tumors in category pT2 and 15 in category pT3; 14 tumors were lymph node-positive and 6 were lymph node-negative. There were 8 tumors graded as G2 and 12 as G3. Group IV included 7 female and 13 male patients with an age range of 24 to 71 years. Altogether, 6 tumors were in category pT2, 13 in category pT3 and 1 in category pT4; 14 tumors were in category pN1 and 6 in category pN0. Of these tumors, 1 was graded as G1, 9 as G2, and 10 as G3.

One representative paraffin block per case, comprising central and peripheral portions of the tumor, was selected for subsequent molecular genetic and immunohistochemical investigations.

DNA Preparation

Two 10-µm slices from the selected paraffin blocks were deparaffinized for DNA preparation. One corresponding block with tumor-free gastric tissue from the distal resection margin was added, representing normal tissue. The sections were lightly stained with hematoxylin to identify the areas of interest, which were subsequently scraped off the slides under light microscopic control. For DNA extraction, the microdissected tissue specimens were placed in reaction cups containing TE buffer (10 mM Tris-Cl pH 7.5, 0.1 mM EDTA) and treated overnight at 55°C with proteinase K (Merck, Darmstadt, Germany) at a concentration of 2.5 mg/ml. The samples were subsequently heated at 94°C for 8 min to inactivate proteinase K, and 2–5 µl of this template solution was used for the polymerase chain reaction (PCR) without further DNA purification.

Differential Polymerase Chain Reactions

Differential PCR was carried out to detect amplification at the c-*myc*, c-*erb*-b2, and *EGFR* gene loci. Fragments from each of these genes were amplified with fragments of a reference gene, which was either an 82-bp fragment of the interferon-γ (*IFNG*) gene located on chromosome 12 or a 134-bp fragment of the adenosine phosphoribosyl transferase (*APRT*) gene located on chromosome 16. The optimal primer concentrations and the PCR parameters were first established for each primer pair, so selective amplification of one PCR fragment at the expense of the other was eliminated. Also, the number of cycles was maintained as low as possible to ensure that the

PCR did not proceed beyond the exponential phase of amplification, thereby not obscuring any potential amplification. In addition, a set of positive controls were amplified along with the tested probes. They consisted of DNA extracted from cell lines COLO 320DM for *c-myc* [7], A431 for *EGFR* [8], and SKBR-3 for *c-erb*-b2 [9] as well as DNA extracted from paraffin-embedded tumor tissues with known amplification for the tested gene loci. Placental tissue served as the reference tissue with normal copy number.

The PCR at the three oncogene loci proceeded in a 50-μl volume containing 3 units Taq-DNA-polymerase, 200 μM of each dNTP, 5 μl of PCR buffer (10×) containing 15 mM $MgCl_2$, 40 pmol of each forward and reverse primers (*c-erb*-b2 *c-myc* or *EGFR*) along with 20 pmol of each reference gene primer (*IFNG* or *APRT*). The primer concentration for *c-myc* gene amplification were 60 pmol along with 30 pmol *IFNG* or 30 pmol with 60 pmol *APRT*. The primer sequences and details of the PCR parameters are presented in Table 1.

Assessment of gene amplification was carried out on the digitized agarose gels by densitometric quantification of the signal intensity using ScanPack 2 software (Biometra, Göttingen, Germany). A minimum threefold increase in the target gene/

TABLE 1. Primer sequences and polymerase chain reaction parameters

Gene loci	Primer sequence	PCR conditions
c-myc		
Upstream	CCT CAA CGT TAG CTT CAC CAA C	Initial denaturation 94°C, 5 min
Downstream	CTG CTG GTA GAA GTT CTC CTC	(denaturation 94°C, 1 min; annealing: 56°C, 1 min; polymerization: 72°C, 1 min) × 31 cycles
		Final elongation: 72°C, 4 min
c-erb-B2		
Upstream	CCT CTG ACG TCC ATC ATC TC	Initial denaturation 94°C, 5 min
Downstream	ATC TTC TGC TGC CGT CGC TT	(denaturation 94°C, 1 min; annealing 56°C, 1 min; polymerization 72°C, 1 min) × 30 cycles
		Final elongation 72°C, 4 min
EGFR		
Upstream	AGC CAT GCC CGC ATT AGC TC	Initial denaturation 94°C, 5 min
Downstream	AAA GGA ATG CAA CTT CCC AA	(denaturation 94°C, 1 min; annealing 56°C, 1 min; polymerization 72°C, 1 min) × 31 cycles
		Final elongation 72°C, 4 min
APRT		
Upstream	TGG GAA AGC TGT TTA CTG CG	As for *c-erbB2*, *c-myc*, and *EGFR*
Downstream	CAG GGA ACA CAT TCC TTT GC	
IFNG		
Upstream	GCA GAG CCA AAT TGT CTC CT	As for *c-erbB2*, *c-myc*, and *EGFR*
Downstream	GGT CTC CAC ACT CTT TTG GA	

reference gene ratio in tumor tissue relative to corresponding normal tissue was taken to be evidence of gene amplification [10]. Suspected gene amplification was verified by repeating the PCR experiment, and it was confirmed with a third PCR using another reference gene.

Immunohistochemistry

Overexpression of c-erb-b2 and EGFR proteins was investigated using 4 μm thick sections of formalin-fixed paraffin-embedded blocks mounted on silaned slides. Following deparaffinization with xylene and ethanol, the sections were rehydrated through decreasing concentrations of ethanol, and endogenous peroxidase activity was eliminated by incubation in 3% H_2O_2. After microwave pretreatment in 10 mM citrate buffer for 5 min in a pressure cooker (c-erb-B2) or incubation in 0.1% Pronase E solution for 20 min (EGFR), endogenous biotin was blocked with avidin and biotin (0.02% in TBS buffer) (Sigma, St. Louis, MO, USA) for 15 min at room temperature. Slides were then incubated with either a rabbit anti-c-erb-b2 polyclonal antibody (Dako, Golstrup, Denmark) (1:1000, 40 min, 37°C) or a murine monoclonal anti-EGFR antibody (clone E30; Merck, Darmstadt, Germany) (1:150, overnight, 4°C). After a second incubation with an appropriate biotin-conjugated secondary antibody, slides were incubated with an avidin-biotin-peroxidase reagent (both from Sci Tek, Logan, USA). Reaction products were visualized by immersing slides in diaminobenzidine tetrachloride and then counterstained with hematoxylin. As a positive control, paraffin-embedded breast cancer with known c-erb-b2 overexpression and an esophageal SCC with known EGFR overexpression was used. The immunohistochemical staining was evaluated by investigators blinded for the results of the molecular genetic analyses and vice versa.

The expression of c-erb-b2 was determined semiquantitatively following the manufacturer's protocol.

0: no staining or membrane staining in fewer than 10% of the cells
1+: faint or barely perceptible membrane staining in more than 10% of the cells; they are stained on only part of their membrane
2+: weak to moderate complete membrane staining in more than 10% of the cells
3+: strong complete membrane staining in more than 10% of the cells

Overexpression of c-erb-b2 protein is considered negative when no or faint staining (0 and 1+) was seen. Moderate or strong staining (2+ and 3+) is considered positive. Overexpression of EGFR was considered present if at least 10% of the tumor cells showed distinct membrane expression.

Results

c-erb-b2 Protein Overexpression and Gene Amplification

Immunohistochemical investigations showed c-erb-b2 protein overexpression in none of the superficial SCCs, but it was present in 3 of 20 advanced SCCs (15%). Among the ADCs, overexpression was found in 3 of 20 superficial carcinomas (15%) and 6 of 20 advanced carcinomas (30%).

Amplification of c-*erb*-b2 gene was present in none of the superficial SCCs but was found in 2 of 18 advanced SCCs (11%; two cases were not analyzable by means of differential PCR). Among the ADCs, c-*erb*-b2 amplification was found in 2 of 19 superficial carcinomas (11%; one case not analyzable) and in 4 of 20 advanced carcinomas (20%).

Correlation of the findings for gene amplification and protein overexpression shows a congruent result between differential PCR and immunohistochemistry in 94% of the samples. Thus, 85% of the cases presented neither gene amplification nor protein overexpression, and 9% showed gene amplification and protein overexpression. In contrast, 5% of the cases displayed protein overexpression without simultaneous gene amplification. Additionally, in one case gene amplification was detectable without protein overexpression.

EGFR Protein Overexpression and Gene Amplification

EGFR protein overexpression was detected in 9 of 20 superficial SCCs (45%) and in 3 of 20 advanced SCCs (15%) but in none of the analyzed ADCs. In contrast to the positive controls, no EGFR gene amplification was detected in any of the 80 analyzed tumor specimens.

c-myc Gene Amplification

Amplification of the c-*myc* gene was found in 5 of 20 superficial SCCs (25%) and in 5 of 18 advanced SCCs (28%; two cases not analyzable). Among the superficial ADCs, c-*myc* amplification was present in 6 of 19 tumors (32%; one case was not analyzable), whereas 11 of 20 advanced ADCs (55%) showed such amplification (Fig. 1).

Discussion

The current study compares the frequency of molecular aberrations between superficial and advanced esophageal carcinomas in three oncogenes frequently involved in the molecular carcinogenesis of esophageal ADC and SCC [11]. The aim of this study

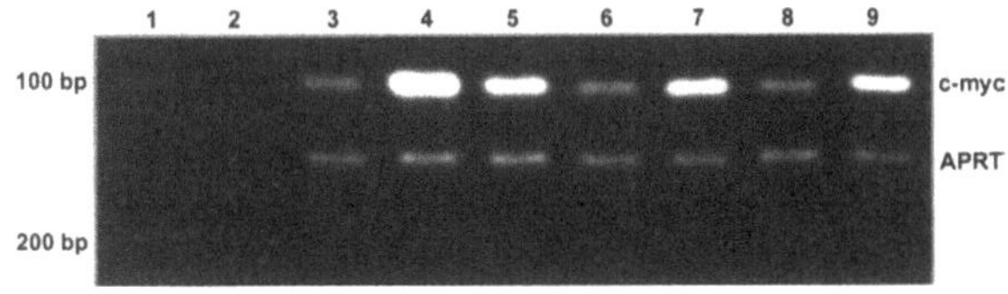

FIG. 1. Ethidium bromide-stained agarose gel of a differential polymerase chain reaction (PCR) for the c-*myc* gene and the *APRT* gene, including tissue samples from two paired samples of carcinoma tissue and corresponding normal tissue. Note amplification of the c-*myc* gene in lanes *7* (carcinoma 1) and *9* (carcinoma 2) and no c-*myc* amplification in lanes *6* (normal 1) and *8* (normal 2). Lane *5* (formalin-fixed samples of an esophageal squamous cell carcinoma with known c-myc amplification) and lane *4* (cell line COLO320DM) are positive controls; lane *3* is a constitutive control (placental tissue); lane *2* is a no template; lane *1* is a size marker

was to determine whether superficial esophageal cancer significantly differs from advanced cancer on the molecular level. Several interesting observations were made concerning this question. For two of the three oncogenes investigated (i.e., c-*erb*-b2 and c-*myc*) there was a tendency for aberrations (gene amplification, protein overexpression, or both) to appear more frequently in advanced cancer than in superficial cancer. This was true for both SCCs and ADCs.

Molecular biologic aberrations in superficial esophageal cancer have rarely been investigated. In an immunohistochemical investigation of superficial SCCs Natsugoe et al. [12] found an accumulation of p53 protein in 54% of cases, a figure that does not differ significantly from previously reported data on advanced SCCs. This probably indicates that there are no significant differences in p53 status between superficial and advanced SCCs, although this point must be clarified in future investigations that should also include studies at the DNA level. However, those data would fit well in the current concept that aberrations of p53 are an early event in esophageal carcinogenesis, occurring before the development of invasive cancer [11]. The timing of aberrations in c-*erb*-b2, c-*myc*, and *EGFR* investigated by us is less well defined. Concerning c-*erb*-b2, however, previous studies indicate that gene amplification is a late event in the molecular carcinogenesis of esophageal ADCs [13, 14], which means that amplification of the c-*erb*-b2 gene may occur at the transition from superficial to advanced ADC in a subset of cases. Detailed investigations on the frequency of c-*myc* or *EGFR* amplification in precursor lesions of esophageal carcinoma have not been reported. Therefore, definitive conclusions on the timing of their appearance during carcinogenesis cannot yet be drawn.

Conclusions

Our results indicate that amplification of the oncogenes c-*myc* and c-*erb*-b2 and overexpression of the c-erb-b2 protein are more frequent in superficial than in advanced esophageal cancer. This finding may indicate that these aberrations are late events in the molecular carcinogenesis of esophageal ADC and SCC.

References

1. Jizuka T, Isono K, Kakegawa T, et al (1989) Parameters linked to ten-year survival in Japan of resected esophageal carcinoma. Chest 96:1005–1011
2. Hermanek P (1995) pTNM and residual tumor classifications: problems of assessment and prognostic significance. World J Surg 19:184–190
3. Lewin KJ, Appelman HD (1995) Tumors of the esophagus and stomach, third series, fascicle 18. Armed Forces Institute of Pathology, Washington, DC
4. Hölscher AH, Bollschweiler E, Schröder W (1997) Prognostic differences between early squamous-cell and adenocarcinoma of the esophagus. Dis Esophagus 10:179–184
5. World Health Organisation (1990) Histological typing of oesophageal and gastric tumors, 2nd edn. Berlin, Springer
6. Sobin LH, Wittekind CH (1997) TNM classification of malignant tumors, 5th edn. Wiley-Liss, New York
7. Schwab M, Alitalo K, Klempnauer KH (1983) Amplified DNA with limited homology to myc cellular oncogene is shared by human neuroblastoma cell lines and a neuroblastoma tumor. Nature 305:245–248

8. Yamamoto T, Kamata N, Kawano H (1986) High incidence of amplification of the epidermal growth factor receptor gene in human squamous carcinoma cell lines. Cancer Res 46:414–416
9. An H, Niederacher D, Beckmann MW, et al (1995) ErbB2 gene amplification detected by fluorescent differential polymerase chain reaction in paraffin-embedded breast carcinoma tissues. Int J Cancer 64:291–297
10. Sarbia M, Loberg C, Wolter M (1999) Expression of Bcl-2 and amplification of c-myc are frequent in basaloid squamous cell carcinomas of the esophagus. Am J Pathol 155:1027–1032
11. Montesano R, Hainaut P (1998) Molecular precursor lesions in oesophageal cancer. Cancer Surv 32:53–68
12. Natsugoe S, Nakashima S, Kijima F, et al (1999) Analysis of macroscopic appearance and p53 expression in superficial esophageal carcinoma. Hepatogastroenterology 46:1398–2404
13. Al-Kasspooles M, Moore JH, Orringer MB, et al (1993) Amplification and overexpression of the EGFR and erbB-2 genes in human esophageal adenocarcinomas. Int J Cancer 54:213–219
14. Chiang P-W, Beer DG, Wei W-L, et al (1999) Detection of c-erbB-2 amplifications in tumors and sera from esophageal carcinoma patients. Clin Cancer Res 5:1381–1386

Q & A after Dr. Sarbia's presentation

Dr. Ozawa (Keio University, Japan): I have been involved in a study of *EGFR* and several oncogenes in esophageal cancer. In our data, which we have published, *EGFR* amplification in both superficial and advanced cancer has shown overexpression of *EGFR* protein in both superficial and advanced cancers. In contrast to our data, you showed that *EGFR* amplification was not detected in all samples. How do you explain that amplification and expression?

Dr. Sarbia: Are your data based on squamous cell carcinoma mainly?

Dr. Ozawa: Yes.

Dr. Sarbia: I am aware that our data on *EGFR* gene amplifications are in contrast to some in literature, and I have no explanation for it. I think there are sufficient data that this amplification occurs in SCCs, and we have some other cases not included in this study where there is *EGFR* amplification. As far as I know, *EGFR* amplification in adenocarcinoma is not well established.

Dr. Jankowski (Birmingham University, UK): We have shown that *EGFR* is strongly expressed in adenocarcinoma, and I am quite sure that our data are correct because we've used many methods, including in situ tests, various antibodies, flow cytometry, Western blotting, and functional assays to show autophosphorylation of the EGFR receptor. What is your explanation for your own results?

Dr. Sarbia: I can only comment on our own findings. As I said, I just interpreted the membrane staining pattern, and I am not sure if everyone believes in the membrane staining pattern. If you investigate EGFR immunohistochemically, you often see cytoplasmic staining, which in my opinion is not a good representation of overexpression. I think that some of the differences might be explained by differences in the interpretation of immunostaining.

Dr. Mori (Kyushu University, Japan): Have you ever studied the messenger RNA level of the gene?

Dr. Sarbia: No, we couldn't do it because it is formalin-fixed material.

Dr. Mori: I think that messenger RNA status is important because the protein expression level is controlled by DNA methylation and histone deacetylation rather than DNA amplification.

Dr. Sarbia: I am aware that there are various ways to control protein expression. We didn't stop at the DNA level; as mentioned, we focused on formalin-fixed material, and I think if immunohistochemistry is validated, as I demonstrated for *erb-B2*, it is the best way to go for functional studies.

Dr. Aikou (Kagoshima University, Japan): What kind of superficial tumors show *erb-B2* amplification? Is there any relation between the macroscopic appearance and expression of this gene?

Dr. Sarbia: I did not investigate this particular point. The point I was most interested in was if there was any correlation with LN metastasis because I think it is the most important clinical issue; as you have seen, we had only a few cases with LN metastasis, and there was no correlation with any of the investigated parameters. I don't know if there was a correlation with macroscopic findings, as I did not examine this question.

Dr. Nakamura (Tokyo Women's Medical College, Japan): I studied c-*erb-B2* expression in Barrett's esophageal cancer when I was in Munich, with Professor Holscher. I concluded that c-*erb-B2* expression is a prognostic factor in Barrett's esophageal cancer. What is the prognostic value of c-*erb-B2* expression in your study?

Dr. Sarbia: We did not investigate prognostic issues. It was too small a study group. The aim of my study was just to determine if there are any differences in superficial and advanced carcinoma.

Patterns of *TP53* Mutations in Cancers of the Esophagus and Esophagogastric Junction: Correlation with Risk Factors and Functional Implications

PHILIPPE TANIÈRE, KATARIINA CASTREN, and PIERRE HAINAUT

Introduction

Mutation of *TP53* is the most frequent genetic event in squamous cell carcinoma (SCC) and adenocarcinoma (ADC) of the esophagus. These mutations differ for SCC and ADC. In SCCs mutation patterns also differ from one geographic area to another. These mutations provide clues on the mutagenic mechanisms involved and confirm that SCC has multiple, region-specific causes.

Inactivation of *TP53* results in loss of coordination between cell cycle, apoptosis, DNA repair, and differentiation. Fas (CD95/APO1), a cell-death receptor regulated by *p53*, and its ligand FasL are expressed in a differentiation-related manner in normal esophagus. This pattern of expression is perturbed in precancerous and cancerous lesions. Furthermore, apoptosis induced by a Fas-agonist antibody is enhanced in esophageal cancer cell lines exposed to cholesterol sulfate, an inducer of keratinocyte differentiation. This result suggests that differentiation-inducing drugs may help improve the response to cytotoxic therapy.

Cancers of the esophagogastric junction have an ill-defined status. Tumors occurring at the junction with no evidence of Barrett's mucosa show differences from Barrett's adenocarcinoma in the prevalence of *TP53* mutations and *MDM2* amplifications and in the pattern of cytokeratin expression. These results suggest that ADC of the cardia is a distinct pathological entity.

Etiopathogenesis of Esophageal Cancers

The two main forms of esophageal cancer, SCC and ADC, show opposite epidemiological trends. SCC is the most prevalent form worldwide, particularly in developing countries. SCC develops along a classical hyperplasia–dysplasia–carcinoma sequence. Its geographic distribution shows spectacular variations, with regions of extremely high incidence in northern Iran (Caspian littoral) and central China (Henan and

Group of Molecular Carcinogenesis, International Agency for Research on Cancer, World Health Organization, 150 Cours Albert Thomas, 69372 Lyon cedex 08, France

Shanxi provinces). In these regions the incidence exceeds 100 per 10^5 per year in both males and females. Other, less-defined areas of high incidence include southeastern Africa and parts of South America. In Europe and the United States the overall incidence does not exceed 10 per 10^5 per year in males and 1–2 per 10^5 in females but with considerable variation from one area to another. In western Europe, two areas of high incidence (more than 30 males and 5 females per 10^5 per year) have been identified in western France (Normandy and Brittany) and in northeastern Italy. This heterogeneous distribution is thought to reflect the heterogeneity of the exogenous factors involved in the pathogenesis of SCC. Tobacco and alcohol are considered the main risk factors in developed countries; and a number of cultural habits (betel chewing, opium consumption, hot tea drinking) and dietary factors (high levels of nitrosamine in diet, contamination by mycotoxins, vitamin and mineral deficiencies) have been implicated in developing countries. However, the factors responsible for the differences between high- and low-incidence areas are still unknown [1].

In contrast to SCC, ADC develops in the lower esophagus from a pre-neoplastic lesion in which squamous epithelium is replaced by columnar, glandular epithelium (Barrett's mucosa) [2, 3]. The highest incidence of ADC is observed in the United States, Australia, New Zealand, and several European countries (most notably the United Kingdom) [4]. In these countries ADC now appears to be the most common form of esophageal cancer. In addition, the frequency of ADC is rapidly increasing throughout Europe and North America [5]. Japan appears to be an exception, with the lowest incidence of ADC of all industrialized countries [4]. The main risk factors for ADC are chronic gastroesophageal reflux (which causes the initial injury leading to the formation of Barrett's mucosa), tobacco smoking, and alcohol consumption.

Genetic alterations in genes involved in the control of cell cycle transition from G_1 to S phase are frequent in both forms of esophageal cancer. These alterations include mutations in *TP53*, amplification or overexpression of *cyclin* D and *cyclin* E, amplification of *myc*, down-regulation of *p16/CDKN2A* by several molecular mechanisms, and loss of *RB1*. In addition, the progression of both SCC and ADC is accompanied by multiple loss of heterozygosity (LOH) at loci known to contain tumor suppressor genes (including *FHIT*, *APC*, *MSH2*, *MLH1*, *DCC*) [6, 7]. However, none of the genetic alterations identified so far appears to be restricted to either ADC or SCC. In 1996 we proposed that the frequent involvement of G_1–S cell cycle regulators may reflect the fact that these genes play an important role as integrators of signals involved in the regulation of the growth, differentiation, and survival of cells of the esophageal mucosa [6]. The molecular mechanisms of G_1–S cell cycle control may be compared to a "decisional switchboard" determining whether cells divide, engage in terminal differentiation, or undergo apoptosis. Cancer may arise from a defect in this decision-making process in the context of the selection pressure exerted by physical and chemical stresses that attack the esophageal mucosa.

In this review, we focus on the *TP53* gene, which is the most frequently altered of all G_1–S cell cycle regulators in esophageal cancers. First, we describe how a comparison of mutation patterns in SCC and ADC provides clues to the mutagenic mechanisms involved. Second, we summarize evidence from our laboratory indicating that induction of squamous cell differentiation may modulate apoptotic responses in SCC. Third, we discuss molecular differences between the ADC on Barrett's mucosa and the

ADC that appears at the esophagogastric junction without any evidence of preexisting metaplasia.

Patterns of *TP53* Mutation in Esophageal Cancers

TP53 encodes a transcription factor that regulates genes involved in the control of the cell cycle, DNA repair, apoptosis, and differentiation. It plays a central role in inhibiting the growth of cells exposed to chemical or physical stress, including cancer cells. Thus, inactivation of *TP53* promotes the growth of cells under stress conditions that suppress the proliferation of normal cells. Most *TP53* mutations are missense mutations and differ by their chemical nature and their position. In several cancers, mutation patterns carry molecular "fingerprints" of exogenous mutagens or endogenous mutagenic processes [8].

In esophageal cancers, *TP53* is mutated in at least 50% of in situ or invasive carcinomas. However, in ADC the mutations are detectable in Barrett's metaplasia prior to cancer [9]. In SCCs we have found mutations in the mucosa of individuals with chronic esophagitis in a region of high cancer incidence (Normandy) [10]. These observations indicate that *TP53* mutation is an early, if not the earliest, genetic event in esophageal cancers.

The data available on the diversity of *TP53* mutations in esophageal cancers are summarized in Fig. 1. In ADC the mutation prevalence is 60%–80%, and most of the mutations are transitions at CpG dinucleotides, a type of mutation thought to be primarily caused by endogenous mutational mechanisms (deamination of methylated cytosines within CpG dipyrimidine repeats) [11, 12]. In SCCs the mutation prevalence varies between 35% and 80%, and mutation patterns are highly heterogeneous, with important geographic variations suggesting the involvement of different mutagens. In China and in a region of moderate incidence in southern Thailand, most of the muta-

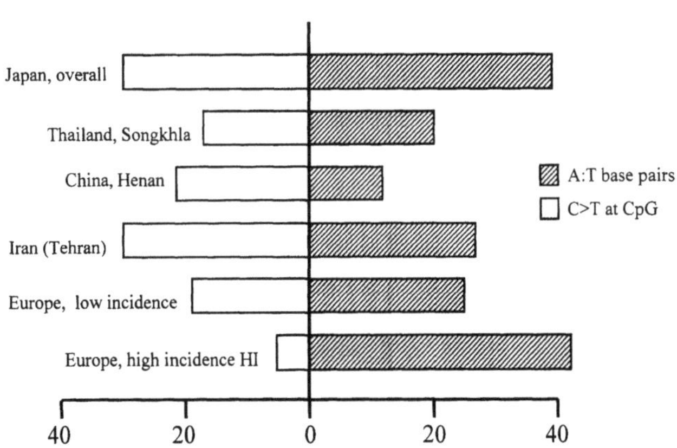

FIG. 1. Prevalence of two common mutations in squamous cell carcinoma (SCC): mutations at A:T basepairs and transitions (C to T) at CpG dinucleotides. The prevalence of mutations in various parts of the world is shown. Data are from the International Agency for Research on Cancer (IARC) *TP53* mutation database (www.iarc.fr/p53) and unpublished data

tions are either transitions (at non-CpG sites) or transversions at C:C basepairs [13]. In Iran, the most prevalent mutation type is transition at CpG sites (similar to ADC). In Europe, different patterns are found in tumors from high- and low-incidence areas. In high-incidence areas (western France, northern Italy) many mutations occur at A:T base pairs and are consistent with the mutagenic effect of acetaldehyde, a metabolite of ethanol. However, this phenomenon is not observed in regions of low incidence (Lyon area in France). In Japan, the data available suggest that the mutation pattern is close to that of the low-incidence areas in Europe. At the genetic level, an increased risk of SCC in the Japanese population (and of cancer of the oral cavity) is associated with a polymorphism in *ALDH2*, the gene responsible for the metabolism of acetaldehyde [14]. Recently, it has been shown that the bacterial microflora of the oral cavity was an important source of acetaldehyde production [15]. Thus, the composition of this microflora might also be an important determinant of individual risk.

Overall, these observations are useful in two respects. First, they help narrow the list of candidate causative factors in SCC and ADC. Second, they allow us to propose a biological Darwinian model for the occurrence of esophageal cancer based on the selection of cellular populations with altered *TP53* function.

As far as causative factors are concerned, the evidence available suggests that most *TP53* mutations in ADC (C to T transitions at CpG) may be due to a purely endogenous mutagenic process that does not require an external mutagen. However, it is interesting to note that the same type of mutation is often detected in cancer cells derived from glandular mucosa of the digestive tract (particularly colon cancer). In experimental systems, the rate of spontaneous deamination of 5′-methylcytosine into thymine is enhanced by exposure to nitric oxide (NO) [16, 17]. This important mediator of inflammation may be produced endogenously by overexpression of inducible nitric oxide synthase (NOS2) [18]. We propose that in Barrett's mucosa glandular cells exposed to physical and chemical stress due to chronic reflux may contain high levels of NO, increasing the risk for formation of a CpG transition in *TP53*.

In SCCs the variations in mutation patterns are related to the geographic heterogeneity of risk factors. However, it should be noted that in all cases the mutation patterns are complex and cannot be assigned to a single causative agent or mechanism. Overall, the trends revealed by these spectra are consistent with an important role of dietary nitrosamines as mutagens in eastern Asia (except Japan) and of metabolites of alcohol in most industrialized countries. The spectrum observed in Iran is peculiar. The similarities with the spectrum of ADC suggests that the chemical basis of mutagenesis may be the same, with a crucial role for NO donors. However, we suspect that in Iran this excess NO may result directly from exposure to some unidentified, exogenous risk factors.

In mechanistic terms, inactivation of *TP53* may alter the G_1–S "decisional switchboard" in esophageal cells exposed to physical or chemical stress. In the stressful conditions that prevail in the esophagus of most precancer patients, loss of *TP53* function may allow cells to escape the *p53*-dependent growth suppression that occurs in normal cells. Expansion of these mutant cells may then form clones with deficient repair capacity, with a high risk of acquiring further genetic lesions during the progression to neoplasia. Thus, exogenous risk factors are involved at two critical steps in esophageal carcinogenesis: first as candidate mutagens and then as effectors of a selection pressure that favors the expansion of cells with mutations.

Enhanced Apoptotic Response in Esophageal Cells Exposed to Differentiating Agents

In 1998 Ohgaki and her collaborators found that APO1/Fas/CD95, a cell-surface receptor of the "death receptor" family, was expressed exclusively in esophageal mucosal cells undergoing terminal differentiation. In contrast, the Fas ligand (FasL) was expressed in the basal and suprabasal layers. In dysplastic lesions there was an increase in cells expressing FasL and a decrease in cells expressing Fas. In SCCs there was a quasidisappearance of cells expressing Fas, whereas most cancer cells expressed FasL [19].

These results have several implications. First, they show that expression of Fas and FasL is dependent on cell differentiation in the esophageal mucosa. Second, they support the hypothesis that disruption of normal differentiation is an early event in the pathogenesis of SCC. Third, they suggest that loss of apoptotic response by down-regulation of Fas may play a role in enhancing the survival of esophageal cancer cells.

To better understand the role of Fas and FasL, we analyzed the expression of these factors in a series of nine cell lines derived from SCCs [20]. Surprisingly, we found that most cell lines co-expressed Fas and FasL, the latter in the soluble form. Co-culture experiments with FasL-sensitive and FasL-resistant Jurkatt cells indicated that FasL was functional [19]. In vitro experiments with Fas agonist antibodies revealed that cells had poor sensitivity to killing through the Fas pathway. These results led us to postulate that this pathway was somehow down-regulated in SCC cell lines, and that its reactivation may render cells more sensitive to cytotoxic treatments.

As Fas and FasL expression appears to be differentiation-dependent in vivo, we exposed cultured esophageal cancer cells to cholesterol sulfate, an agent that specifically stimulates the terminal differentiation of squamous epithelial cells [21]. Although it did not induce consistent changes in the level of Fas expression, choles-

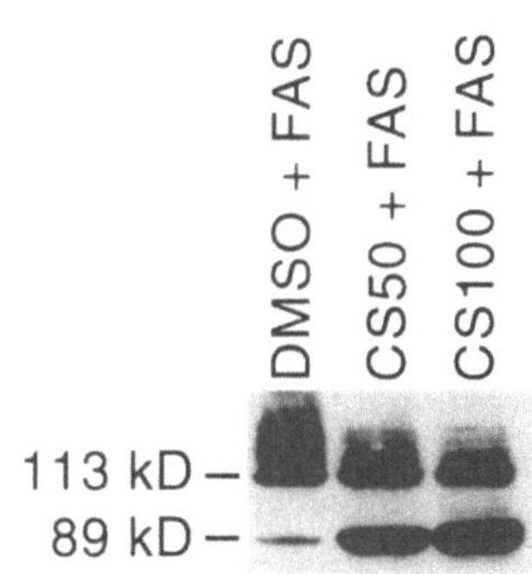

FIG. 2. Effect of cholesterol sulfate (*CS*) on apoptosis induced by Fas-agonist antibody in the TE-6 SCC cell line. Cultured cells were exposed to either dimethylsulfoxide (DMSO) (vehicle) or CS at 50 or 100 μM, followed by treatment with a Fas-agonist antibody. Apoptosis was detected by finding cleavage of poly-ADP ribose-polymerase (PARP), a substrate of caspase 3 that generates two fragments of 89 kDa and 24 kDa upon cleavage. No significant cleavage of PARP was detected without CS. CS alone did not induce PARP cleavage (data not shown)

terol sulfate increased the apoptotic effect of Fas agonists by one to two orders of magnitude (Fig. 2). We also observed an increased cytotoxic effect with various DNA-damaging agents. These results suggest that differentiation may restore the Fas pathway in esophageal cancer cells, improving responses to cytotoxic treatments. A similar mechanism has been postulated to explain the resistance of renal cell carcinomas to apoptosis [22, 23].

To conclude, we interpret these in vivo and in vitro results as an indication of the role of Fas and its ligand in the maturation of normal esophageal mucosa. FasL expressed by basal and suprabasal cells may diffuse to upper layers of the epithelium and bind to Fas expressed by cells located there to induce their terminal differentiation, death, and desquamation. Interestingly, expression of Fas is under transcriptional control by *p53*. Therefore, it is conceivable that inactivation of *TP53* may contribute to the deregulation of this important differentiation pathway.

Cancers of the Esophagogastric Junction: Distinct Entity?

The exact status of the adenocarcinomas that arise at the esophagogastric junction is a matter of debate [12, 24]. The cardia corresponds to a small area lined by special glandular mucosa at the junction between the squamous esophageal epithelium and the gastric mucosa [25–27]. A short segment of this type of mucosa (average 1.8 mm) is consistently detectable in pediatric autopsy material, indicating that it is present from birth as a normal structure [24, 25]. However, there is also evidence that the length of cardiac mucosa increases with aging, perhaps as a consequence of reflux [27, 28].

In a recent study we selected a series of adenocarcinomas that appeared at the esophagogastric lesion without any gross or microscopic evidence of preexisting Barrett's mucosa. The tumors were defined as adenocarcinomas of the cardia (ADCC) and were analyzed for *TP53* mutations, amplification of *MDM2* (a gene that encodes a p53 regulator amplified in some tumors without *TP53* mutations [29]), and patterns of cytokeratin expression. Results were compared with a parallel series of ADCs occurring in well characterized, short- or long-segment Barrett's mucosa. We found that ADCC differed from ADC on Barrett's mucosa (ADC/B) by the prevalence of *TP53* mutations (35% in ADCC and 56% in ADC/B) and *MDM2* amplifications (19% and 4%, respectively). The two types of cancer also showed a different pattern of cytokeratin expression, with the presence of cytokeratins 7 and 13 in most ADC/B (100% and 81%, respectively) but not in ADCC (CK 7, 41%; CK13, 37%).

The two tumor groups also differed by the characteristics of the patients and the outcome of the disease. Patients with ADC/B were typically men (90%), heavy smokers, and regular drinkers, with a poor overall survival after treatment. Patients with ADCC included 40% women, with less exposure to tobacco and alcohol. Furthermore, they responded better to therapy, and their overall survival was superior to that of the ADC/B patients. Interestingly, 5 of 26 ADCC patients had a history of other neoplasms, particularly three breast adenocarcinomas. In contrast, only 1 of 28 ADC/B patients had a previous cancer history (squamous cell carcinoma of the head and neck).

Overall, these results may be interpreted in two distinct forms. The first is to consider ADCC and ADC/B as two distinct pathologies, with different risk factors, causes, and clinical courses. The second is to consider that ADCC and ADC/B represent two different sources for the development of an ADC at the esophagogastric junction (Fig. 3). In the absence of significant reflux, some individuals develop a tumor that arises within the normal mucosa of the cardia. These patients are of both genders, with no particular exposure to tobacco and alcohol; and they may carry a genetic predisposition to cancer, as suggested by the frequency of other neoplasms. However, in most cases, ADC appears in the context of a reactive, metaplastic mucosa that develops in response to extensive stress by chronic reflux disease combined with high tobacco and alcohol consumption. These patients are mostly men, with other rare neoplasms also being linked to their high exposure to tobacco and alcohol. The molecular differences we observed between the two groups are compatible with this hypothesis: *TP53* mutations are less frequent in the "low-stress" situation that results in ADCC than in the "high-stress" situation that results in ADC/B.

Perspectives

Esophageal cancers are a highly lethal collection of tumors in which inactivation of *TP53* is a critical event. How this inactivation cooperates with other genetic changes in the temporal sequence of events that lead to cancer is a matter for future investigation. In this respect, it should be kept in mind that there is growing evidence that *P63*, a member of the *TP53* family, encodes a protein expressed in the normal squamous epithelium that is involved in keratinocyte differentiation [30, 31]. This gene has been found to be amplified in several squamous carcinomas and has been termed *AIS* (amplified in squamous cell carcinoma) [24, 32, 33]. We have found it to be amplified

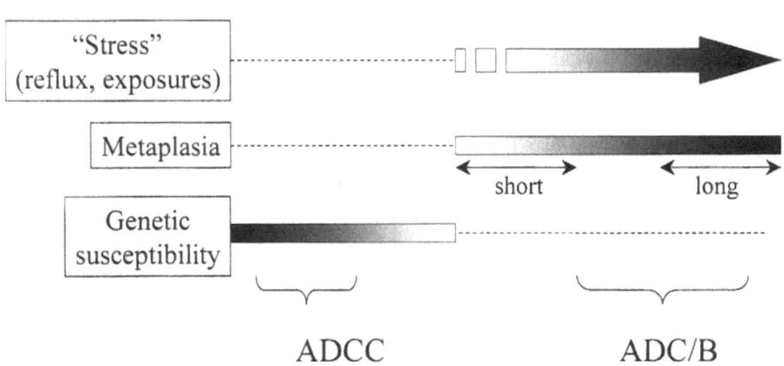

FIG. 3. Occurrence of adenocarcinomas at the esophagogastric junction: adenocarcinomas of the cardia (*ADCC*) and adenocarcinomas of Barrett's mucosa (*ADC/B*). This model takes into account three factors: stress (e.g., chronic reflux, exposure to harmful exogenous factors such as tobacco and alcohol), formation of metaplasia, and the possible existence of a genetic predisposition. In low-stress conditions, tumors may arise with no evidence of metaplasia in genetically susceptible patients. In intermediate or high stress conditions, metaplasia occurs as an adaptive response to stress and favors the occurrence of a tumor. See text for further explanations

in about 20% of SCCs collected in Europe. It is therefore essential to determine how *P63* and *TP53* cooperate in the formation and development of esophageal cancers.

Acknowledgment. K. C. was supported by an IARC Research Training Fellowship from the International Agency for Research on Cancer (1997–1998).

References

1. Muñoz N, Day NE (1996) Esophageal cancer. In: Schottenfeld D, Fraumeni JF (eds) Cancer epidemiology and prevention. Oxford University Press, Oxford, pp 681–706
2. Bytzer P, Christensen PB, Damkier P, et al (1999) Adenocarcinoma of the esophagus and Barrett's esophagus: a population-based study. Am J Gastroenterol 94:86–91
3. DeMeester SR (1997) Management of Barrett's esophagus free of dysplasia. Semin Thorac Cardiovasc Surg 9:279–284
4. Parkin DM, Whelan SC, Ferlay J, Raymond L, Young J (1997) Cancer incidence in five continents, vol VII. IARC Scientific Publication 143. IARC, Lyon
5. Devesa SS, Blot WJ, Fraumeni JFJ (1998) Changing patterns in the incidence of esophageal and gastric carcinoma in the United States. Cancer 83:2049–2053
6. Montesano R, Hollstein M, Hainaut P (1996) Genetic alterations in esophageal cancer and their relevance to etiology and pathogenesis: a review. Int J Cancer 69:225–235
7. Tanière P, Montesano R, Hainaut P (in press) The natural history of esophageal cancer. In: Shields PE (ed) Methods in cancer risk assessment: from laboratory to the clinic. Dekker, New York
8. Hainaut P, Hollstein M (2000) P53 and human cancer: the first ten thousand mutations. Adv Cancer Res 77:81–137
9. Barrett MT, Sanchez CA, Prevo LJ, et al (1999) Evolution of neoplastic cell lineages in Barrett oesophagus. Nat Genet 22:106–109
10. Mandard AM, Hainaut P, Hollstein M (2000) Genetic steps in the development of squamous cell carcinoma of the esophagus. Mutat Res 462:335–342
11. Gleeson CM, Sloan JM, McManus DT, et al (1998) Comparison of p53 and DNA content abnormalities in adenocarcinoma of the oesophagus and gastric cardia. Br J Cancer 77:277–286
12. Ireland AP, Shibata DK, Chandrasoma P, et al (2000) Clinical significance of p53 mutations in adenocarcinoma of the esophagus and cardia. Ann Surg 231:179–187
13. Tanière P, Martel-Planche G, Puttawibul P, et al (2000) TP53 mutations and MDM2 gene amplification in squamous-cell carcinomas of the esophagus in South Thailand. Int J Cancer 88:223–227
14. Muto M, Hitomi Y, Ohtsu A, et al (2000) Association of aldehyde dehydrogenase 2 gene polymorphism with multiple oesophageal dysplasia in head and neck cancer patients. Gut 47:256–261
15. Muto M, Hitomi Y, Ohtsu A, et al (2000) Acetaldehyde production by non-pathogenic *Neisseria* in human oral microflora: implications for carcinogenesis in upper aerodigestive tract. Int J Cancer 88:342–350
16. Murata J, Tada M, Iggo RD, et al (1997) Nitric oxide as a carcinogen: analysis by yeast functional assay of inactivating p53 mutations induced by nitric oxide. Mutat Res 379:211–218
17. Souici AC, Mirkovitch J, Hausel P, et al (2000) Transition mutation in codon 248 of the p53 tumor suppressor gene induced by reactive oxygen species and a nitric oxide-releasing compound. Carcinogenesis 21:281–287
18. Ambs S, Bennett WP, Merriam WG, et al (1999) Relationship between p53 mutations and inducible nitric oxide synthase expression in human colorectal cancer. J Natl Cancer Inst 91:86–88

19. Gratas C, Tohma Y, Barnas C, et al (1998) Up-regulation of Fas (APO-1/CD95) ligand and down-regulation of Fas expression in human esophageal cancer. Cancer Res 58:2057–2062
20. Barnas C, Martel-Planche G, Furukawa Y, et al (1997) Inactivation of the p53 protein in cell lines derived from human esophageal cancers. Int J Cancer 71:79–87
21. Kuroki T, Ikuta T, Kashiwagi M, et al (2000) Cholesterol sulfate, an activator of protein kinase C mediating squamous cell differentiation: a review. Mutat Res 462:189–195
22. Gerharz CD, Ramp U, Dejosez M, et al (1999) Resistance to CD95 (APO-1/Fas)-mediated apoptosis in human renal cell carcinomas: an important factor for evasion from negative growth control. Lab Invest 79:1521–1534
23. Ramp U, Dejosez M, Mahotka C, et al (2000) Deficient activation of CD95 (APO-1/Fas)-mediated apoptosis: a potential factor of multidrug resistance in human renal cell carcinoma. Br J Cancer 82:1851–1859
24. Spechler SJ, Dixon A, Genta R, Hainaut P, Lambert R, Siewert JR (2000) Adenocarcinoma of the oesophago-gastric junction. In: Hamilton S, Aaltonen L (eds) Pathology and genetics: tumours of the digestive system. IARC Press, Lyon, pp 32–36
25. Kilgore SP, Ormsby AH, Gramlich TL, et al (2000) The gastric cardia: fact or fiction? Am J Gastroenterol 95:921–924
26. Ormsby AH, Kilgore SP, Goldblum JR, et al (2000) The location and frequency of intestinal metaplasia at the esophagogastric junction in 223 consecutive autopsies: implications for patient treatment and preventive strategies in Barrett's esophagus. Mod Pathol 13:614–620
27. Chandrasoma PT, Der R, Ma Y, et al (2000) Histology of the gastroesophageal junction: an autopsy study. Am J Surg Pathol 24:402–409
28. Oberg S, Peters JH, DeMeester TR, et al (1997) Inflammation and specialized intestinal metaplasia of cardiac mucosa is a manifestation of gastroesophageal reflux disease. Ann Surg 226:522–530
29. Momand J, Jung D, Wilczynski S, et al (1998) The MDM2 gene amplification database. Nucleic Acids Res 26:3453–3459
30. DeLaurenzi V, Rossi A, Terrinoni A, et al (2000) P63 and p73 transactivate differentiation gene promoters in human keratinocytes. Biochem Biophys Res Commun 273:342–346
31. Parsa R, Yang A, McKeon F, et al (1999) Association of p63 with proliferative potential in normal and neoplastic human keratinocytes. J Invest Dermatol 113:1099–1105
32. Yamaguchi K, Wu L, Caballero OL, et al (2000) Frequent gain of the p40/p51/p63 gene locus in primary head and neck squamous cell carcinoma. Int J Cancer 86:684–689
33. Hibi K, Trink B, Patturajan M, et al (2000) AIS is an oncogene amplified in squamous cell carcinoma. Proc Natl Acad Sci USA 97:5462–5467

Q & A after Dr. Hainaut's presentation

Dr. Jankowski (Birmingham University, UK): Can you tell me why if there are two pathways for apoptosis (for example, the *p53* and Fas and Fas ligand pathways are disabled) there is still a lot of apoptosis?

Dr. Hainaut: I think there are many other possible pathways for apoptosis, in particular hypoxia.

Dr. Toyokuni (Kyoto University, Japan): Regarding *p53* activation, modification of *p53* may be another way, as Dr. Ohshima in your institute recently reported. Did you see the modification of p53 protein in regard to nitration of tyrosine?

Dr. Hainaut: We have not looked in detail at esophageal cancer. We did study nitrogenation of p53 in tyrosine residues with Dr. Ohshima, and we found that p53 could be nitrogenated on tyrosine residues after exposing the cells to nitric oxide donors in culture. We have not seen any data regarding p53 being nitrogenated in esophageal cancer.

Dr. Hagen (University of Southern California, Los Angeles, USA): I was interested by your hypothesis on the differences you saw between the true esophageal Barrett's cancers and cardia tumors. Aside from sensitivity, you might consider the possibility that it's just a time-related phenomenon because the cardiac mucosa exhibits the earliest change and metaplasia follows. Therefore unless you are looking at the gene that is actually the earliest in the process of carcinogenesis the rest of the changes may just be a manifestation of the accumulation of mutations over time.

Dr. Hainaut: In this respect, *TP53* is interesting because it's one of the richest to differentiate, if not the earliest, as it can be found in the mucosa preceding the appearance of cancer. Another point to consider is the localization of the lesion. When Barrett's mucosa creeps into the esophagus, it meets an increased amount of the mutagen coming from the top of the esophagus, particularly tobacco smoke and alcohol. You may reach a point where exposure to mutagen becomes much greater than it is at the bottom of the esophagus.

Dr. Ohashi (Tokyo, Japan): I have examined apoptosis of the superficial esophageal carcinoma and reported my findings & found that the apoptotic rate was related to the invasion and the differentiation grade of the SCC. Did you demonstrated expression of Fas and Fas ligand of the carcinoma? Are there any correlations between the expression level of Fas/Fas ligand and the existence of invasion or the differentiation of the carcinomas?

Dr. Hainaut: I do not know.

Dr. Rubio (Karolinska Institute, Sweden): You mentioned an effect of nonsteroidal antiinflammatory drugs on the change of evolution of the carcinoma of the esophagus. I worked for many years on inducing carcinoma of esophagus in mice with the help of adenonitrosamine. By giving these animals indomethacin in drinking water, I was able not only to prevent the development of the tumors but also to abrogate the development of new tumors by using indomethacin in water. This work was reported in *Cancer* about 20 years ago.

Dr. Hainaut: That is excellent to know. There are many potential problems when using drugs in the chemotherapeutic approach to disease of the gastrointestinal tract, particularly the upper digestive tract. Given the availability of highly specific inhibitors, it is worthwhile to think about such trials, particularly in areas where there are no other options for managing these cancers and where such cancers are occurring in high frequency, such as northern Iran.

Superficial Esophageal Cancer: Adenocarcinoma Related to Barrett's Metaplasia and Adenoid Cystic Carcinoma

SAUID ISHAQ, REBECCA F. HARRISON, and JANUSZ A. JANKOWSKI

Introduction

The rate of esophageal adenocarcinoma is rising, and the lesion has a poor prognosis mainly because of late presentation. Barrett's metaplasia is a major risk factor in the epidemiology of esophageal adenocarcinoma, as individuals with Barrett's metaplasia have an increased risk of adenocarcinoma of the lower esophagus [1]. Although highly curable at its early stages, esophageal cancer is usually fatal when it is more advanced [2–4]. Treatment and subsequent outcome are linked to its histology, accurate staging, and the site of the tumor [5, 6].

Given the low 1- and 5-year survival rates of patients with advanced cancer, strategies for early cancer detection have been explored. Conventional risk factors are neither sensitive nor specific enough to identify high-risk individuals. Attempts to identify tumors at an early stage with surveillance programs have not been cost-effective [7, 8], although lesions identified during surveillance programs have a better prognosis [9, 10]. There is therefore intense interest not only in primary prevention strategies aimed at inhibiting the initiation of Barrett's metaplasia but also for detecting additional risk factors so we can identify individuals at high risk of this malignant transformation. Furthermore, accurate staging has an impact on therapy options, as it might be appropriate to consider endoscopic mucosal resection for carcinoma in situ (TisN0M0) whereas surgery is still preferred for submucosal tumors (T1N0M0).

Epidemiology

The true prevalence of Barrett's metaplasia (BM) in the general population is unknown. The reported lifetime risk in the adult general population in Western countries is 1% [11] based on postmortem studies. In addition, the incidence of new cases in the at-risk population is about 0.5%–2.0% per year [12] and increasing [13–15]. It mainly occurs in caucasians, with male predominance (2.3 : 1.0) [16, 17], and is rarely

Epithelial Laboratory, Division of Medical Sciences, University of Birmingham, Edgbaston, B15 2TH, UK
email (Professor J. Jankowski): j.jankowski@bham.ac.uk

found in African-Americans [18]. BM is said to be rare in Japan and most of the Asian subcontinent [11], although there is little evidence to support this statement in the recent literature. Conversely, one study from Taiwan showed an incidence of BM similar to that in Western countries [19]. Another study also reported that there has been a tendency toward increasing prevalence of BM all over the world, including the Far East [20]. Thus there is a great need for comparative studies among geographical regions that not only can establish the incidence of BM in different countries but also might help identify risk factors prevalent in that particular region.

Adenocarcinoma of the esophagus is found to be associated with its precursor BM in at least 60% of cases [21, 22]. In parallel with BM, there has been a large increase in the incidence of esophageal adenocarcinoma during the last two decades in the Western population, increasing at a rate of up to 10% per year [23–25]. It is also more prevalent in white men than in black men and white women, although a comparable rise in the incidence has been observed particularly in white women [23, 26].

Natural History of Dysplasia and Early Barrett's Adenocarcinoma

Several histological issues are important in the progression of Barrett's adenocarcinoma.

First, when and how long does it take to develop early Barrett's adenocarcinoma from dysplasia? Second, does low-grade dysplasia (LGD) regress, stay static, or progress? Third, does high-grade dysplasia (HGD) regress, stay static, or progress? About 10% of patients with esophagitis progress to BM [27] in which the normal squamous epithelium is replaced by specialized columnar epithelium with goblet cells. BM can further evolve in three ways: regression (decreased metaplastic surface area) (7.5%), stabilization (no increase or decrease in metaplastic area) nor any dysplasia (68%), and progression (24%) to dysplasia, which may also be associated with an increase in the metaplastic area [28–30].

This dysplasia is a neoplastic, noninvasive cellular change limited to epithelium that may progress from LGD to HGD and then to Barrett's adenocarcinoma [13, 31]. Dysplasia can be graded as negative, indefinite, or positive, with the latter divided into LGD and HGD. The prevalence and natural history of dysplasia is not well known in patients with BM. In one series of BM patients the prevalence of HGD was found to be 5%, LGD 34%, indefinite dysplasia 17%, and negative dysplasia 44% [32]. Moreover LGD regresses in 50%, remains static in 30%, and progresses to HGD in 20%. We believe that the regression of LGD in studies may be artefactual, related to sampling bias and histological misclassification of regenerative changes. The interval of progression of LGD to HGD in the literature is 1.5–5.0 years [33, 34]. Some LGD remains static for 57 months before progression to cancer [34].

HGD may regress in 40%, remain static in 20%, and progress to cancer in 40%. HGD must be differentiated from intramucosal cancer and requires at least two experienced pathologists to confirm the diagnosis. The rate of progression from HGD to cancer can be as fast as 5–21 months [33, 34]. It is a progressive disorder, as suggested by findings of "prevalence" cancers in 40%–78% of the resected specimens in a group of patients who underwent esophagectomy for HGD [35]. Such patients have an early intramucosal cancer, which has a more favorable prognosis [9, 10]. Once again the reported regression of HGD may be attributed to sampling bias or misclassification. If patients with HGD are followed up by intense biopsy surveillance regimens then the occurrence of subsequent "interval" cancers is very low <20% of cases.

Adenoid Cystic Carcinoma of the Esophagus (Nonmetaplasia-Derived Esophageal Adenocarcinoma)

Adenoid cystic carcinoma of the esophagus is an unusual histologic variant of esophageal cancer that affects mainly salivary glands but other sites in the head and neck as well as the esophagus. The major interest in these lesions is because they are thought to arise directly from the esophageal glands rather than BM. Their clinical behavior and response to therapy is unclear. The neoplasm is composed of cords or islands of small epithelial cells that characteristically appear in a cribriform, trabecular, or solid histology (or a combination). Despite slow growth, this tumor is aggressively invasive locally and is associated with distant metastasis. Surgical resection is the treatment of choice in suitable patients, although the aggressiveness of the tumor may also require a chemoradiotherapeutic approach. More than 35 cases have been reported in the Japanese literature [36]. These tumors clearly arise from stem cells different from those arising from Barrett's esophagus and as such are described as nonmetaplasia-derived adenocarcinoma.

Risk Factors

Barrett's metaplasia represents an important predisposing factor for the development of esophageal adenocarcinoma [22, 37, 38]. The reported incidence of esophageal adenocarcinoma in BM ranges from 1 in 52 to 1 in 441 patients, with a mean follow-up interval of 2.9–15.0 years [39–41]. Using pooled data, the cancer risk in patients with BM is 1% per year (range 0.5%–2.0%) [12, 42]. There has been some concern that the risk might have been overestimated because of publication bias and the lack of accuracy in the prevalence data; if so, the incidence of Barrett's adenocarcinoma may be lower [43]. To balance the argument, however, it is clear that many cases of supposed BM are in reality hiatus hernia or Barrett's gastric-type metaplasia without the higher-risk intestinal metaplasia. The risk factors, incidence, histopathology, and molecular biology of Barrett's adenocarcinoma differ from those of squamous carcinoma. In particular, squamous cell carcinoma is associated with a poor diet [44], low socioeconomic status [45], and association with lung and liver as a consequence of heavy cigarette smoking and alcohol consumption, whereas adenocarcinoma is associated with obesity [46], upper socioeconomic status [23], and association with cardiovascular problems presumably related to fatty diets.

Other conventional risk factors (Table 1) include older age [11], white ethnicity [17], gender [16], obesity [46, 47], smoking [48], mucosal damage [49], absence of *Helicobacter pylori* although this has recently been questioned [50], duodeno-gastro-esophageal reflux [51, 52], chronicity of symptoms [52], presence of a hiatus hernia [53], and the length of Barrett's segment [54]. These risk factors are neither sensitive nor specific for the classification of individuals at high risk, which has led to the detection of additional risk factors that could more accurately identify the subgroup at risk of malignant transformation [55].

TABLE 1. Clinical risk factors for Barrett's adenocarcinoma

Strong clinical evidence	
	Dysplasia (low grade, high grade)
	Chronicity of symptoms (>10 years)
	Mucosal damage (ulceration/stricture in Barrett's metaplasia)
	Duodenogastric reflux[a] (acid/bile)
	Body mass index (obesity)
	Length of Barrett's segment (>8 cm)
	Gender/race (white male)
	Helicobacter pylori (absent) (Debatable)
Weak clinical evidence	
	Smoking (heavy smoker)
	Hiatus hernia (present)
	Diet (fatty food: *N*-nitrosamines)
	Drug therapy (nitrates, theophyllines, anticholinergics)

[a] More than three times per week

High-grade dysplasia in mucosal biopsies is currently accepted as the gold standard for cancer risk, as 40%–78% of the patients who have had only HGD on biopsies have invasive prevalent adenocarcinoma in the esophagectomy sample [35]. However, HGD may not be an optimal marker, as it might be subject to inter- and intraobserver error and may be missed in routine endoscopic biopsy specimens in addition in these who don't have prevalence cancers the risk of neoplasia in the subsequent years is dramatically deminished <20%. Further research is required to determine the optimal marker of cancer risk.

Molecular Biology of the Metaplasia–Dysplasia–Adenocarcinoma Sequence

Barrett's metaplasia is a predisposing condition for the development of adenocarcinoma, which occurs through a well defined series of steps from intestinal metaplasia to low-grade dysplasia to high-grade dysplasia to in situ cancer and then to carcinoma. Therefore the best predictor of Barrett's adenocarcinoma is the detection of dysplasia in BM [56–58]. Progression of BM to adenocarcinoma is associated with a wide variety of cellular and molecular abnormalities, including chromosomal deletion, aneuploidy, microsatellite instability, single gene alteration, and alteration of cellular adhesion molecules, all resulting in genetic instability that predisposes to the acquisition of abnormal clones of cells [12, 55, 59]. These changes are mirrored in the histological progression through the metaplasia-dysplasia-carcinoma sequence (Fig. 1). The prevalence of dysplasia in specialized intestinal epithelium is estimated to be 10%–20% [60]. Low-grade dysplasia is accompanied by the loss of control of stem cell proliferation with abnormal gene expression accompanied by cytokine and local growth factor stimulation [56]. Increasing dysplasia is accompanied by increasing proliferation aneuploidy, microsatellite instability, and loss of cell adhesion as high-grade dysplasia develops.

The proposed molecular changes are as follows. There is normally strict control of cell replication influenced by extracellular stimuli via cyclin-dependent receptors for

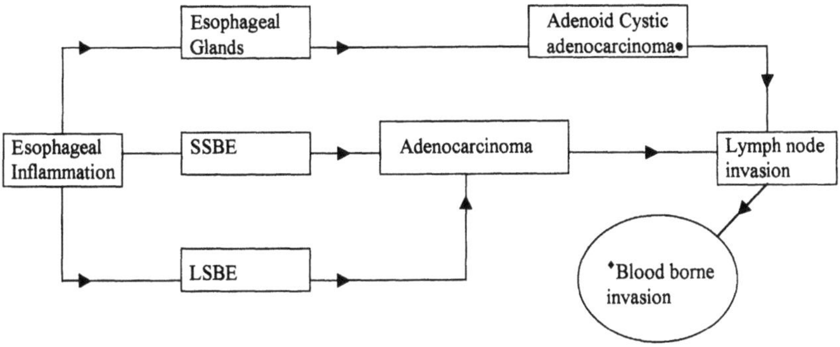

FIG. 1. Progression of esophageal cell follows the metaplasia–dysplasia–carcinoma sequence. ● Adenoid cystic carcinoma of esophagus arises from different stem cells. SSBE, short-segment Barrett's esophagus; LSBE, long-segment Barrett's esophagus. ◆ Blood-borne invasion from lymph nodes is well recognized

p15 and p16, the products of transforming growth factor-β (TGFβ), p21, and p53. Both TGFβ and p53 inhibit cell proliferation. Inactivation and loss of receptors for TGFβ and a *p53* mutation have been demonstrated in esophageal adenocarcinoma [61]. Chronic chemical damage and cell loss increases the cell proliferation and inhibition of apoptosis, which can result in a change in the genotype of this specialized lineage of columnar mucosa by clonal selection. These novel lineages have specific functions including protection against acid, bile salts repair of ulceration. Subsequent cell cycling abnormalities, including impaired DNA mismatch repair, aneuploidy, and loss of E-cadherin expression, may allow invasive Barrett's cancers to develop.

Many molecular changes in p53, p16 gene promoter methylation, cyclin D1 overexpression, decreased E-cadherin expression, and loss of heterozygosity of the adenomatosis polyposis coli (*APC*) gene have been detected in dysplastic Barrett's mucosa. These changes could be important; for example, *p53* mutation that can inhibit bile acid-induced apoptosis could initiate dysplastic growth. Tumor stage and invasiveness has been linked to reduced expression of E-cadherin [12]. These molecular changes have been evaluated in the clinical research setting and are not used routinely in clinical practice, although such genetic changes may become useful screening markers to monitor the progression of BM and to identify individuals at risk of developing malignant transformation in the future.

Diagnosis

The average age at which adenocarcinoma in the setting of Barrett's metaplasia is diagnosed is 57–63 years (range 23–96 years) [16, 17, 26, 62–64]. Early cancers of the esophagus are generally asymptomatic. The predominant presentation is with obstructive dysphagia, which occurs in 60%–90% of patients with an adenocarcinoma in Barrett's metaplasia [17, 62, 64–66]. Others present with weight loss (42%), hamorrhage (12%–36%), odynophagia [67, 68], or iron deficiency anaemia. It is interesting to note that only 5%–29% of patients with Barrett's adenocarcinoma were known to have Barrett's metaplasia before the development of cancer [63], suggesting that a significant proportion of the adult population probably have Barrett's metaplastic change that remains undetected unless carcinoma develops [39, 40, 69]. Endoscopy with biopsy is the preferred method of diagnosis for esophageal carcinoma [70–72].

For a malignant stricture, endoscopic biopsies and brush cytology have an accuracy of virtual 100% for obtaining a tissue diagnosis [73]. Tumors may grow in an infiltrative or expansive pattern, are usually moderately to poorly differentiated, and often present multifocally [74, 75]. Rarely, diffuse esophageal adenocarcinoma can occur at the gastro-esophageal junction. In all cases the family history should be obtained to exclude hereditary diffuse gastro-esophageal adenocarcinoma, which is associated with germ-line E-cadherin mutations [76].

Chemoendoscopy using topical vital dyes (Lugol's iodine, methylene blue) combined with endoscopy may improve the yield of dysplasia detection. Methylene blue stains intestinal metaplasia; an unstained area may be dysplastic. Iodine spray stains the squamous mucosa, which helps target unstained areas for biopsy [77–79]. Air-contrast barium radiology can detect small lesions, but they always require further evaluation with endoscopy and biopsy [80].

Staging Issues and Management of Superficial Barrett's Adenocarcinoma

Intramucosal or submucosal cancer: can we differentiate them? Of concern with respect to the management of patients with early cancer is the undetected extension of intramucosal tumor to the submucosa and the prevalence of lymph node (LN) metastasis. It has been reported by many surgeons that early Barrett's adenocarcinomas (T1) are less likely to have LN involvement than corresponding T1 lesions of squamous cell carcinoma, although this awaits verification. Jump metastases have been reported in 10% of patients with early Barrett's cancer (i.e., one or two distal nodes are involved, but nodes adjacent to the tumor are free of disease) [3, 67, 81, 82]. Advanced Barrett's cancers, particularly with subcarinal LN involvement, have a worse prognosis than those with involvement of gastric nodes or paraesophageal nodes.

Newer technologies are being used for accurate staging to help with selecting the treatment. The staging procedure concentrates mostly on the T category and the detection of distant metastasis. However, analysis of the N category (LN involvement in the mediastinum) is less clearly associated until surgical resection. LN involvement and vessel invasion is uncommon in intramucosal tumors compared to submucosal tumors; as a consequence, the 5-year survival for those with intramucosal lesions differs significantly from that in patients with a submucosal tumor [9, 10]. Thus another critical issue is to discriminate intramucosal cancer correctly from submucosal tumor. Endoscopic ultrasonography (EUS) has been used to improve detection of intramucosal adenocarcinoma in Barrett's metaplasia [83] and to discriminate intramucosal from submucosal tumors. The value of staging early esophageal adenocarcinoma by EUS is controversial [9; Sievert, unpublished data]. It is recognized that after EUS some 20% of tumors are staged incorrectly [9, 10], and at present there is no optimal way to determine tumor extension beyond the muscularis mucosae before its removal.

Position-emission tomography (PET) has been used to detect distant and regional LN metastasis. It has high specificity (98%) but low sensitivity (43%), and therefore its use is limited. Laproscopy is still used routinely to identify peritoneal seedings in Barrett's adenocarcinoma, but peritoneal involvement in squamous cell carcinomas is rare.

Therapy

The introduction of surveillance programs for Barrett's esophagus has led to a dramatic increase in the number of patients with HGD or tumor limited to the mucosa [9, 10]. The treatment of choice most often reported for early adenocarcinoma is surgical resection (Fig. 2), although there are many unresolved issues regarding diagnosis, staging, and selection of a particular treatment. As stated earlier, there have been difficulties differentiating HGD from intramucosal cancer [84], and to date our ability to determine submucosal extension of cancer remains uncertain. Another concern with management of these patients with early cancers is the small but consistent prevalence of LN metastasis of intramucosal cancers (up to 18% in one series) and jump metastasis in up to 10% of patients [3, 81, 82].

Recently there has been great interest in the development of new techniques for adequate local therapy of early cancer, including ablation of the mucosa by thermal or chemical methods and endoscopic mucosal resection. The basis of this treatment

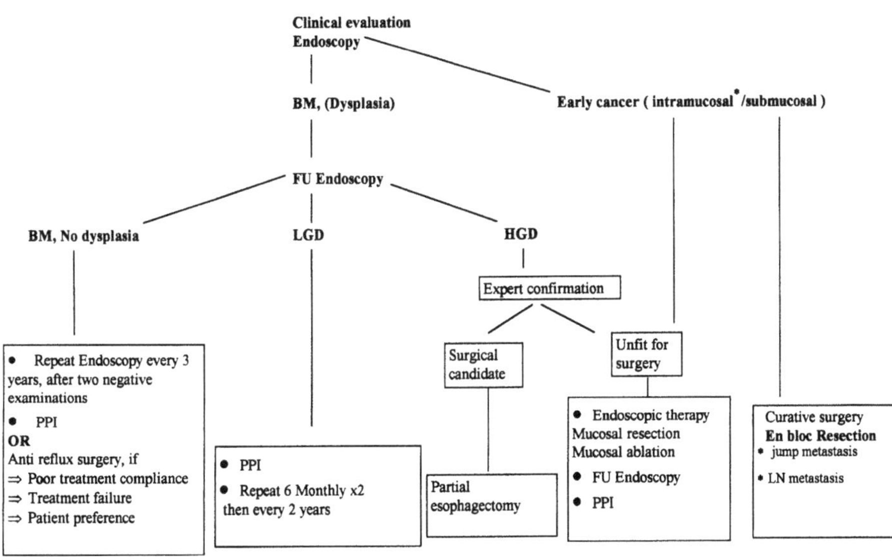

FIG. 2. Treatment options and their indications and surveillance strategies. LGD, low-grade dysplasia; HGD, high-grade dysplasia; BM, Barrett's metaplasia; PPI, proton pump inhibitor; en bloc resection, esophagectomy with dissection of mediastinal LN; F/U, follow-up. ★ Prevalence of lymph node metastasis in up to 18% and jump metastasis in up to 10% have been reported for early Barrett's adenocarcinoma (intramucosal lesions)

is to destroy the columnar epithelium, which with the help of acid suppression allows healing of the squamous epithelium [85]. The major problems with these techniques include persistence of Barrett's epithelium underneath squamous islands and recurrent tumor after an apparent initial response. Most importantly, this treatment has no impact on undetected metastasis or LN involvement. Although an attractive and novel approach aimed at eliminating dysplasia, at present these techniques have little impact on reducing mortality and should be reserved for elderly patients with co-morbid illnesses who are unfit for surgery.

For patients with BM and HGD many surgeons recommend esophagectomy [9], as more than half of these patients have been shown to have undetected intramucosal cancer in the resected specimen [37, 86]. Several authors have favoured an aggressive, frequent biopsy protocol and undertake esophagectomy only when cancer is diagnosed [58, 87].

It is important to note that our current ability to differentiate intramucosal from submucosal lesions is also questionable. Until we can resolve these issues accurately, en bloc resection with mediastinal LN dissection remains a favored option for the treatment of intramucosal (superficial) Barrett's adenocarcinomas, as these are the most curable tumors [82, 88].

Conclusions

Most patients with Barrett's adenocarcinoma present late with advanced disease and have a poor prognosis. Barrett's adenocarcinoma has been strongly linked with Barrett's metaplasia. There is great need to detect cancer at an early stage so there is better survival. How can we achieve this remains unclear, as (1) screening of all surgical fit patients with Barrett's metaplasia is neither feasible nor cost-effective, and recently its ability to detect cancer early has been questioned; and (2) conventional risk factors are neither sensitive nor specific for identifying high-risk individuals with Barrett's metaplasia. Thus, there is a great need to identify risk factors so we can target high-risk individuals for screening to detect cancer at an early stage and to develop better tools for accurately staging the disease. It certainly would improve the selection of treatment for this devastating disease. In additions strategies for chemoprevantion with proton purr inhibitors and cox-2 agents been badly needed.

Acknowledgment. Funding was provided by the Cancer Research Campaign, Imperial Cancer Research Fund, and Medical Research Council.

References

1. Stein HJ, Hoeft S, DeMeester TR (1993) Functional foregut abnormalities in Barrett's esophagus. J Thorac Cardiovasc Surg 105:163–168
2. Steup WH, DeLeyn P, Deneffe I, et al (1996) Tumors of the esophagogastric junction: long-term survival in relation to the pattern of lymph node metastasis and a critical analysis of the accuracy or inaccuracy of pTNM classification. J Thorac Cardiovasc Surg 5:S17–S26
3. Clark GW, Peters JH, Ireland AP, et al (1994) Nodal metastasis and sites of recurrence after en bloc esophagectomy of adenocarcinoma. Ann Thorac Surg 58:646–654

4. Hölscher AH, Bollschweiler E, Bumm R, et al (1995) Nodal metastasis and sites of recurrence after en bloc esophagectomy for adenocarcinoma of the esophagus. Surgery 118:845–855
5. Lightdale CJ (1994) Staging of esophageal cancer. I. Endoscopic ultrasonography. Semin Oncol 21:438–446
6. Thompson WM, Halvorsen RA Jr (1994) Staging esophageal carcinoma II: CT and MRI. Semin Oncol 21:447–452
7. Macdonald CE, Wicks AC, Playford RJ (2000) Final results from 10 year cohort of patients undergoing surveillance for Barrett's esophagitis: observational study. BMJ 321:1252–1255
8. Morales TG, Sampliner RE (1999) Barrett's esophagus: an update on screening, surveillance and treatment. Arch Intern Med 159:1411–1416
9. Peters JH, Clark GW, Ireland AP, et al (1994) Outcome of adenocarcinoma arising in Barrett's esophagus in endoscopically surveyed and non surveyed patients. J Thorac Cardiovasc Surg 108:813–821
10. Peters JH, Hoeft SF, Heimbucher J, et al (1994) Selection of patients for curative oe palliative resection of esophageal cancer based on preoperative endoscopic ultrasonography. Arch Surg 129:534–539
11. Cameron AJ, Lomboy CT, Pera M, et al (1992) Adenocarcinoma of esophagogastric junction and Barrett's esophagus. Gastroenterology 103:1241–1245
12. Jankowski J, Harrison R, Perry I, et al (2000) Barrett's metaplasia. Lancet 356:2079–2085
13. Hirota WK, Loughney TM, Lanzas DJ, Maydonovitch CL, Rholl V, Wong RKH (1999) Specialized intestinal metaplasia, dysplasia, and cancer of the esophagus and esophagogastric junction: prevalence and clinical data. Gastroenterology 116:277–285
14. Prach AT, Mohiuddin MA, Geisinger KR, et al (1997) Increasing incidence of Barrett's esophagus: education, enthusiasm, or epidemiology [letter]? Lancet 350:933
15. Sanchez RC, Santalla PF, Retamero OMD (1995) Barrett esophagus: an epidemiological study in an area of Spain. Rev Esp Enferm Dig 87:353–355
16. Sarr MG, Hamilton SR, Marrone GC, et al (1985) Barrett's esophagus: its prevalence and association with adenocarcinoma in patients with symptoms of gastroesophageal reflux. Am J Surg 149:187–193
17. Skinner DB, Walther BC, Riddell RH (1983) Barrett's esophagus: comparison of benign and malignant cases. Ann Surg 198:554–566
18. Bonelli L (1993) Barrett's esophagus: results of multicentric survey. G.O.S.P.E. (Gruppo Operativo per lo studio delle Precancerosi Esofagee. Endoscopy 25:652–654
19. Yeh C, Hsu C, Ho A, et al (1997) Erosive esophagitis and Barrett's esophagus in Taiwan: a higher frequency than expected. Dig Dis Sci 42:702–706
20. Chen PH (1997) Review: Barrett's esophagus in Taiwan. J. Gastroenterol Hepatol 12:S19–S22
21. Cameron AJ, Lomboy CT (1995) Adenocarcinoma of the esophagogastric junction and Barrett's esophagus. Gastroenterology 103:1241–1245
22. Hamilton SR, Smith RR, Camerone JL (1988) Prevalence and characteristic of Barrett's esophagus in patients with adenocarcinoma of esophagus or esophagogastric junction. Hum Pathol 19:942–948
23. Blot WJ, Devesa SS, Kneller RW, et al (1993) Rising incidence of adenocarcinoma of the esophagus and gastric cardia. JAMA 265:1287–1289
24. Haggit RC (1992) Adenocarcinoma in Barrett's esophagus: a new epidemic [editorial]? Hum Pathol 23:475–476
25. Pera M, Cameron AJ, Trastek VF, et al (1993) Increasing incidence of adenocarcinoma of the esophagus and esophagogastric junction. Gastroenterology 104:510–513
26. Jankowski J (2001) CRC cancer stats: Esophageal cancer. CRC Press, London
27. Poynton AR, Walsh TN, O'Sullivan G, et al (1996) Carcinoma arising in familial barrett's esophagus. Am J Gastroenterol 91:1855–1856

28. Fontolliet C, Ollyo JB, Brossard E (1994) Barrett's esophagus may still progress. Gut 35(suppl):A27–A27
29. Monnier P, Fontolliet C, Savary M, et al (1987) Barrett's esophagus or columnar epithelium of lower esophagus. Ballieres Clin Gastroenterol 14:769–789
30. Ollyo JB, Gonvers JJ, Froehlich F, et al (1990) Does Barrett's esophagus regress after effective treatment of gastro-esophageal reflux? Schweiz Med Wochenschr 120:716–720
31. Sampliner RE, Practice Parameters Committee of the American College of Gastroenterology (1998) Practice guidelines on the diagnosis, surveillance, and therapy of Barrett's esophagus. Am J Gastroenterol 93:1028–1032
32. Cameron AJ (1998) Management of Barrett's esophagus. Mayo Clin Proc 73:457–461
33. Barrett MT, Sanchez CA, Prevo LJ, et al (1999) Evolution in neoplastic cell lineage in Barrett's esophagus. Nat Genet 22:106–109
34. Reid BJ, Blount PL, Rubin CE, et al (1992) Flow-cytometric and histological progression to malignancy in Barrett's esophagus: prospective endoscopic surveillance of a cohort. Gastroenterology 102:1212–1219
35. Edwards MJ, Gable DR, Lentsch AB, et al (1996) The rationale for esophagectomy as the optimal therapy for Barrett's esophagus with high-grade dysplasia. Ann Surg 223:585–589
36. Morisaki Y, Yoshizumi Y, Hiroyasu S, et al (1996) Adenoid cystis carcinoma of the esophagus: report of a case and review of the Japanese literature. Surg Today 26:1006–1009
37. Pera M, Trastek VF, Carpenter HA, et al (1992) Barrett's esophagus with high grade dysplasia: an indication for esophagectomy: Ann Thorac Surg 54:199–204
38. Spechler SJ, Goyal RK (1986) Barrett's esophagus. N Engl J Med 315:362–371
39. Spechler SJ, Robbins AH, Bloomfield Rubins H, et al (1984) Adenocarcinoma and Barrett's esophagus: an overrated risk? Gastroenterology 87:927–933
40. Cameron AJ, Ott BJ, Payne WS (1985) The incidence in columnar-lined (Barrett's) esophagus. N Engl J Med 313:857–859
41. Williamson WA, Ellis FH Jr, Gibbs SP, et al (1991) Barrett's esophagus: prevalence and incidence of adenocarcinoma. Arch Intern Med 151:2212–2216
42. Drewitz DJ, Sampliner RE, Garewal HS (1997) The incidence of adenocarcinoma in Barrett's esophagus: a prospective study of 170 patients followed 4.8 years. Am J Gastroenterol 92:212–215
43. Shaheen NJ, Crosby MA, Bozymski EM, et al (2000) Is there publication bias in the reporting of cancer risk in Barrett's esophagus? Gastroenterology 119:333–338
44. Tuyns AJ (1992) Esophageal cancer in France and Switzerland: recent time trend. Eur J Cancer Prev 1:275–278
45. Day NE, Munoz N, Ghadirian P (1982) Epidemiology of esophageal cancer: a review. In: Correa P, Haenszel W (eds) Epidemiology of cancer of the digestive tract. Martinus Nijhoff, The Hague, pp 21–57
46. Brown LM, Swanson CA, Gridley G, et al (1995) Adenocarcinoma of the esophagus: role of obesity and diet. J Natl Cancer Inst 87:1104–1109
47. Chow W-H, Blot WJ, Vaughan TL, et al (1998) Body mass index and risk of adenocarcinoma of the esophagus and gastric cardia. J Natl Cancer Inst 90:150–155
48. Gray MR, Donnelly RJ, Kingsnorth JN, et al (1993) The role of smoking and alcohol in metaplasia and cancer risk in Barrett's columnar lined esophagus. Gut 34:727–731
49. Spechler SJ, Sperber H, Doos WG, et al (1983) The prevalence of Barrett's esophagus in patients with chronic peptic esophageal strictures. Dig Dis Sci 28:769–774
50. Weston AP, Badr AS, Topalovski M, et al (2000) Prospective evaluation of the prevalence of gastric *Helicobacter pylori* in patients with GERD, Barrett's esophagus, Barrett's dysplasia, and Barrett's adenocarcinoma. Am J Gastroenterol 95:387–394
51. Chow W-H, Finkle WD, McLaughlin JK, et al (1995) The relation of gastresophageal reflux disease and its treatment to adenocarcinomas of the esophagus and gastric cardia. JAMA 274:474–477

52. Lagergren J, Bergstorm R, Lindgren A, et al (1999) Symptomatic gastresophageal reflux as a risk factor for esophageal adenocarcinoma. N Engl J Med 340:825–831
53. Patti MG, Goldberg HI, Arcerito M, et al (1996) Hiatal hernia size affects lower esophageal sphincter function, esophageal acid exposure, and degree of mucosal injury. Am J Surg 94:2054–2059
54. Menke-Pluymers MBE, Hop WCJ, Dees J, et al (1993) Risk factors for the development of an adenocarcinoma in Barrett's esophagus. Cancer 72:1155–1158
55. Jankowski J, Wright NA, Meltzer S, et al (1999) Molecular evolution of the metaplasia dysplasia sequence in the esophagus. Am J Pathol 154:969–974
56. Jankowski J (1993) Gene expression in Barrett's mucosa: modulation of acute and chronic responses. Gut 34:1012–1014
57. Hamilton SR, Smith RR (1987) The relationship between columnar epithelial dysplasia and invasive adenocarcinoma arising in Barrett's esophagus. Am J Clin Pathol 87:301–312
58. Reid BJ, Weinstein WM, Lewin KJ, et al (1988) Endoscopic biopsy can detect high-grade dysplasia or early adenocarcinoma in Barrett's esophagus with or without grossly recognizable neoplastic lesions. Gastroenterology 94:81–90
59. Garewal HS, Sampliner RE, Fennerty MB, et al (1991) Flow cytometry in Barrett's esophagus: what have we learned so for? Dig Dis Sci 36:548–551
60. Boynton RF, Huang Y, blount PL, et al (1991) Frequent loss of heterozygosity at the retinoblastoma locus in human esophageal cancer. Cancer Res 51:5766–5769
61. Schneider PM, Casson AG, Levin B (1996) Mutation in p53 in Barrett's esophagus and Barrett's cancer: a prospective study of 98 cases. J Thorac Cardiovasc Surg 111:323–333
62. Sjogren RW, Johnson LF (1983) Barretts' esophagus: a review. Am J Med 74:313–321
63. Bremner RM, DeMeester TR (1991) Surgical treatment of esophageal carcinoma. Gastroenterol Clin North Am 20:743–763
64. Starnes VA, Adkins RB, Ballinger JF, et al (1984) Barrett's esophagus: a surgical entity. Arch Surg 119:563–567
65. Bytzer P, Christensen PB, Damkier P, Vinding K, Seersholm N (1999) Adenocarcinoma of the esophagus and Barrett's esophagus: a population-based study. Am J Gastroenterol 94:86–91
66. Sanfey H, Hamilton SR, Smith RRL (1985) Carcinoma arising in Barrett's esophagus. Surg Gynecol Obstet 161:57–574
67. Akiyama H (1990) Surgery for cancer of the esophagus. Williams & Wilkins, Baltimore, p 10
68. Ojala K, Sorri M, Jokinin K (1982) Symptoms of carcinoma of the esophagus. Med J Aust 1:384–385
69. Cameron AJ, Zinmeiester AR, Ballard DJ, et al (1990) Prevalence of Columnar-lined (Barrett's) esophagus. Gastroenterology 99:918–922
70. Bogomoletz WV, Molas G, Gayet B, et al (1989) Superficial squamous cell carcinoma of the esophagus: a report of 76 cases and review of the literature. Am J Surg Pathol 13:535–546
71. Goseki N, Koike M, Yoshida M (1992) Histopathologic characteristics of early stage esophageal carcinoma: a comparative study with gastric carcinoma. Cancer 69:1088–1093
72. Haruma K, Tokutomi T, Tsuda T, et al (1991) Superficial esophageal carcinoma: a report of 27 cases in Japan. Am J Gastroenterol 86:1723–1728
73. Zargar SA, Khuroo MS, Jan GM, et al (1991) Prospective comparison of the value of brushings before and after biopsy in the endoscopic diagnosis of gastroesophageal malignancy. Acta Cytol 35:549–552
74. Ohno S, Mori M, Tsutsui S, et al (1991) Growth patterns and prognosis of submucosal carcinoma of the esophagus: a pathologic study. Cancer 68:335–340
75. Thompson JJ, Zinsser KR, Enterline HT, et al (1983) Barrett's metaplasia and adenocarcinoma of the esophagus and gastroesophageal junction. Hum Pathol 14:43–61

76. Richards FM, McKee SA, Rajpar MH, et al (1999) Germ-line E-cadherin gene (CDH1) mutations predispose to familial gastric and colorectal cancer. Hum Mol Genet 4:135–144
77. Canto MI, Setrakian S, Petras RE, et al (1996) Methylene blue selectively stains intestinal metaplasia in Barrett's esophagus. Gastrointest Endosc 44:1–7
78. Weston AP, Badr AS, Hassanein RS (1999) Prospective multivariate analysis of factors predictive of complete regression of Barrett's esophagus. Am J Gastroenterol 94: 3420–3426
79. Stevens PD, Lightdale CJ, Green HR, et al (1994) Combined endoscopy with chemoendoscopy for the evaluation of Barrett's esophagus. Gastrointest Endosc 40:747
80. Roth JA, Putnam JB, Rich TA, et al (1997) Cancer of the esophagus. In: DeVita VT, Hellman S, Rosenberg SA (eds) Cancer: principles and practice of oncology, 5th edn. Lippincott-Raven, Philadelphia, pp 980–1021
81. Akiyama H, Tsurumaru M, Kawamura T, et al (1981) Principles of surgical treatment for carcinoma of esophagus; analysis of lymph node involvement. Ann Surg 194: 438–446
82. Akiyama H, Tsurumaru M, Udagawa H, et al (1994) Radical dissection for cancer of the thoracic esophagus. Ann Surg 220:364–373
83. Falk GW, Catalano MF, Sivak MV Jr, et al (1994) Endosonography in the evolution of patients with Barrett's esophagus and high grade dysplasia. Gastrointest Endosc 40:207–212
84. Ferguson MK, Naunheim KS (1997) Resection for Barrett's mucosa with high-grade dysplasia and early adenocarcinoma: comparison of endoscopic biopsy and surgical pathology findings. J Thorac Cardiovasc Surg 114:824–829
85. Overholt BF, Panjehpou M, Haydek JM (1999) Photodynamic therapy for Barrett's esophagus: followup in 100 cases. Gastrointest Endosc 49:1–7
86. Streitz JM, Andrews CW, Ellis FH Jr (1993) Endoscopic surveillance of Barrett's esophagus: does it help? J Thorac Cardiovasc Surg 105:383–387
87. Levine DS, Haggit RC, Blount PL, et al (1993) An endoscopy biopsy protocol can differentiate high grade dysplasia from early adenocarcinoma in Barrett's esophagus. Gastroenterology 105:40–50
88. Hagen JA, Peters JH, Demeester TR, et al (1993) Superiority of extended en bloc esophagogastrectomy for carcinoma of the lower esophagus and cardia. J Thorac Cardiovasc Surg 106:850–859

Molecular Biology of Adenocarcinoma Arising in Barrett's Esophagus

James D. Mueller

Introduction

The last several years have seen a rapid rise in the incidence of both Barrett's esophagus and adenocarcinoma of the distal esophagus [1]. Because most patients with these tumors present late owing to the lack of specific symptoms, the prognostic outlook for most is poor despite improvements in surgical treatment [2, 3]. For this reason it has become apparent that successful therapeutic strategies must be based on early detection and treatment. This in turn has brought heightened interest to studying the carcinogenesis of these tumors, as a better understanding of their molecular biology could provide new diagnostic and therapeutic possibilities.

Among the individuals who develop intestinal metaplasia of the distal esophagus ("Barrett's esophagus") as a result of chronic reflux, only a small proportion go on to develop carcinoma [4]. At present, the best marker to identify patients who are high risk for the development of carcinoma is the histopathologic identification of dysplasia in endoscopic biopsies [5]. However, several problems are associated with the identification of dysplasia, including improper or insufficient sampling of the area of Barrett's mucosa [6], interobserver variation among pathologists [7], and the uncertainty about the risk of subsequent carcinoma development, even when dysplasia has been definitively identified, particularly when low-grade dysplasia is diagnosed [8]. For this reason there has been a growing hope that molecular biology might soon provide us with objective parameters that could simplify and improve identification of the patients with Barrett's esophagus who are at greatest risk for the development of esophageal adenocarcinoma. It is also theoretically possible that, in the future, targets for early, specific genetic intervention might be available that would enable us to halt the development and progression of dysplasia of Barrett's esophagus in the early stages, before the carcinoma has had a chance to develop. The following is a brief overview of some of the molecular biologic changes that have been described with respect to the carcinogenesis and progression of adenocarcinoma arising in Barrett's esophagus.

Chirurgische Klinik und Poliklinik, Klinikum rechts der Isar, Technische Universität München, Ismaninger Strasse 22, D-81675 Munich, Germany

Histopathology

From the histopathologic perspective, it is well established that adenocarcinoma of the distal esophagus arises via a metaplasia–dysplasia–carcinoma sequence in which the normal stratified squamous epithelium of the esophagus is first replaced by a metaplastic, specialized intestinal epithelium that can be identified by the presence of goblet cells [9]. Dysplasia in this epithelium is recognized histologically on the basis of increasing disorder of the metaplastic glands and by increasing cytologic atypia [6]. Dysplasia is graded as high or low grade, depending on the severity of the histologic changes seen. Carcinoma is diagnosed when invasion of the lamina propria can be identified; but in many centers high-grade dysplasia is considered clinically equivalent to carcinoma owing to the high percentage of cases in which carcinoma can be identified in the resection specimen after an endoscopic diagnosis of high-grade dysplasia [10, 11]. From the molecular pathology point of view, a complicating factor for the development of carcinoma in Barrett's esophagus is that two separate but interrelated biologic processes, metaplasia and dysplasia, must be considered.

Proliferation, Ki-67 Antigen

The normal proliferative compartment of the stratified squamous epithelium of the esophagus is found at the basal layer. This zone can be visualized immunohistochemically with antibodies directed against the Ki-67 antigen (Mib1 in formalin-fixed, paraffin-embedded tissues). With establishment of the metaplastic glandular epithelium of Barrett's esophagus, a similar narrow proliferative zone can also be identified near the base of the glands. Increased proliferation appears to be an early but relatively nonspecific change in the carcinogenesis of adenocarcinoma of the distal esophagus. It has been noted that an increase in the proliferative fraction, but even more important, broadening and spreading of the proliferative zone to the surface of the epithelium, can be correlated with the onset and degree of dysplasia [12]. Morphometric measurement of proliferation in Barrett's epithelium has been proposed as a helpful adjunct for the diagnosis of dysplasia [13].

p53 Protein Overexpression

The protein p53 is probably the most intensively studied molecule in terms of its carcinogenetic role in a vast number of malignant tumors, and Barrett's esophagus is no exception. Overexpression of p53 protein usually results from a mutation that creates an abnormally stable protein molecule that accumulates so that it is visible immunohistochemically as a nuclear stain. About 60% of adenocarcinomas arising in Barrett's esophagus exhibit p53 protein overexpression [14]. Most studies have described p53 overexpression to be a relatively late event along the metaplasia–dysplasia–carcinoma sequence, so it first appears when high-grade dysplasia is already identifiable [15, 16]. However, p53 overexpression has also been found in low-grade dysplasia or even in metaplasia [17], leading to the concept that mutations of the p53 gene may be an important, early event in the loss of cell cycle control and effective DNA repair.

Cell Adhesion Molecules, E-cadherin

Cell adhesion molecules function in normal epithelia to provide attachments between cells and their matrix and to provide correct cellular orientation and polarity. Reduced or abnormal expression of various cell adhesion molecules is a relatively common event in the carcinogenesis of a variety of tumors, including Barrett's carcinoma. E-cadherin is a calcium-dependent cell adhesion molecule that plays an important role in cell–cell adhesion. Reduced E-cadherin expression is usually first visible immunohistochemically with the development of high-grade dysplasia, although subtle changes in its expression can be seen earlier using other methods, such as Western blotting [18, 19]. Reduced E-cadherin expression has been associated with a poorer prognosis for patients with esophageal adenocarcinoma [20].

Chromosomal Level, Comparative Genomic Hybridization

Comparative genomic hybridization (CGH) is a method by which the entire genome can be evaluated for chromosomal abnormalities including deletions (corresponding to the inactivation of tumor suppressor genes) and amplifications (corresponding to the activation of oncogenes). Based on a new technique in which CGH was combined with microdissection, Walch et al. were able to analyze precisely the discrete areas of metaplasia, dysplasia, and carcinoma in a group of adenocarcinomas from the distal esophagus [21]. As expected, multiple gains and losses were found in the carcinomas (gains on 8p, 20q, 2p, 7p, 10q, 6p, 15q, and 17q; losses on Y 4q, 5q, 9p, 18q, 7q, 14q); but interestingly, several changes were already evident in dysplastic and even metaplastic areas of the resected specimens adjacent to the carcinoma. It is possible that such chromosomal areas could include genes that are involved in the earliest steps of Barrett's carcinogenesis.

Microsatellite Analysis, LOH

Microsatellite analysis is a technique in which short, repetitive, highly polymorphic segments ("microsatellites") normally found scattered throughout the genome are studied. The method is extremely useful, as both microsatellite instability arising through abnormalities of DNA repair genes (e.g., hereditary monpolyposis colorectal cancer) and loss of heterozygosity (LOH) can be identified at specific chromosomal sites. Common LOH sites in adenocarcinoma of the esophagus, as in other tumors of the gastrointestinal tract, include 17p (the site of the *p53* gene), 5q (*APC* gene), and 18q (*DCC* gene).

A question that has interested our institution for some time is the nature of tumors of the gastroesophageal junction region. Because the incidence of carcinoma of the proximal stomach is increasing and these lesions have a histologic appearance similar to that of Barrett's carcinoma, some have held them to be of the same type [22]. On the other hand, because of differences in epidemiology and clinical features, others consider these tumors to be separate entities [23]. In 1999 using CGH, van Dekken et al. noted that the 14q chromosomal area might be particularly important for the carcinogenesis of esophageal adenocarcinomas because it was more often deleted in these tumors [24]. Our own study, however, using four microsatellite loci for this area failed to find a significant difference between distal esophageal and proximal gastric carcinomas [25].

Recently, however, preliminary data based on microsatellite analysis of the 17p chromosomal arm, followed by sequence analysis of the *p53* gene suggests that the pattern of *p53* mutation in adenocarcinomas of the distal esophagus may differ from that of the proximal stomach. The *p53* missense mutations are apparently much more common in distal esophageal tumors, whereas other mutation types (e.g., stop or nonsense mutations) are more common in the proximal stomach (G. Keller et al., 2000, in preparation). The meaning of these results is unclear but may indicate that the carcinogenetic mechanisms in the two sites differ.

Proteases

During the course of the development of invasive potential, tumors must become capable of digesting their surrounding extracellular matrix through the action of protease molecules. An important group of such proteases is the serine protease group. In a study of 54 completely resected tumors, Nekarda et al. showed that expression of one of the serine proteases, urokinase-like plasminogen activator (UPA), served as an independent prognostic indicator, as tumors that expressed more than 2.85 ng/mg, as determined by enzyme-linked immunosorbent assay (ELISA), had a significantly poorer prognosis [26]. Not could the tumor UPA level serve to identify a subgroups of patients with poorer prognoses who could then receive additional therapy, but it is also theoretically possible that in the future UPA might serve as a target for agents that inhibit invasive potential, thus halting tumor progression [27].

Lymph Node Micrometastases

As for other gastrointestinal tumors, lymph node metastases are of crucial prognostic importance for patients with completely resected esophageal adenocarcinoma, and lymph nodes are a common site for tumor recurrence [2]. We previously showed that in esophageal squamous cell carcinoma micrometastases can be detected by immunohistochemistry in approximately one-third of the cases in which the regional lymph nodes were free of tumor as shown by routine methods and that these newly detected tumor cells have a prognostic impact similar to that of metastases [28]. In comparison, nodal micrometastases from esophageal adenocarcinomas are much less common (only 7%) [29], perhaps owing to changes in esophageal lymphatic drainage resulting from fibrosis during the course of the chronic reflux esophagitis that precedes the development of Barrett's esophagus [30].

Conclusions

This brief overview of a few studies of the molecular biology of carcinoma development and progression in Barrett's esophagus demonstrates that we are beginning to understand a number of important biologic features of this tumor. New techniques (e.g., microarray technology) can accelerate this process still further. At present, the clinical approach to the detection and treatment of esophageal adenocarcinoma and its precursors is still determined by the histopathologic identification of dysplasia in endoscopic biopsy specimens and, once a carcinoma has developed, by histopathologically staging the tumor. It is only a matter of time, however, before molecular biologic findings begin to have a significant impact on clinical practice.

References

1. Williamson WA, Ellis FH Jr, Gibb SP, Shahian DM, Aretz HT, Heatley GJ, Watkins E Jr (1991) Barrett's esophagus: prevalence and incidence of adenocarcinoma. Arch Intern Med 151:2212–2216
2. Hölscher AH, Bollschweiler E, Bumm R, Bartels H, Siewert JR (1995) Prognostic factors of resected adenocarcinoma of the esophagus. Surgery 118:845–855
3. Hoff SJ, Sawyers JL, Blanke CD, Choy H, Stewart JR (1998) Prognosis of adenocarcinoma arising in Barrett's esophagus. Ann Thorac Surg 65:176–180
4. Chen MY, Ott DJ, Gelfand DW (1995) More evidence for the increasing prevalence of adenocarcinoma of the esophagus over an 18-year period. J Clin Gastroenterol 21:254–255
5. Levine DS, Haggitt RC, Blount PL, Rabinovitch PS, Rusch VW, Reid BJ (1993) An endoscopic biopsy protocol can differentiate high-grade dysplasia from early adenocarcinoma in Barrett's esophagus. Gastroenterology 105:40–50
6. Lewin K (1985) Barrett's esophagus, columnar dysplasia, and adenocarcinoma of the esophagus. In: Tumors of the esophagus and stomach, 2nd edn. Armed Forces Institute of Pathology, Washington, DC, p 99
7. Reid BJ, Haggitt RC, Rubin CE, Roth G, Surawicz CM, Van Belle G, Lewin K, Weinstein WM, Antonioli DA, Goldman H (1988) Observer variation in the diagnosis of dysplasia in Barrett's esophagus. Hum Pathol 19:166–178
8. Hagen JA (1997) Management of Barrett's esophagus with dysplasia. Semin Thorac Cardiovasc Surg 9:285–289
9. Weinstein WM, Ippoliti AF (1996) The diagnosis of Barrett's esophagus: goblets, goblets, goblets [editorial]. Gastrointest Endosc 44:91–95
10. Rusch VW, Levine DS, Haggitt R, Reid BJ (1994) The management of high grade dysplasia and early cancer in Barrett's esophagus: a multidisciplinary problem. Cancer 74:1225–1229
11. Pera M, Trastek VF, Carpenter HA, Allen MS, Deschamps C, Pairolero PC (1992) Barrett's esophagus with high-grade dysplasia: an indication for esophagectomy? Ann Thorac Surg 54:199–204
12. Hong MK, Laskin WB, Herman BE, Johnston MH, Vargo JJ, Steinberg SM, Allegra CJ, Johnston PG (1995) Expansion of the Ki-67 proliferative compartment correlates with degree of dysplasia in Barrett's esophagus. Cancer 75:423–429
13. Polkowski W, Baak JPA, Van Lanshot JJB, Meijer GA, Schuurmans LT, Ten Kate FJW, Obertrop H, Offerhaus GJA (1998) Clinical decision making in Barrett's oesophagus can be supported by computerized immunoquantitation and morphometry of features associated with proliferation and differentiation. J Pathol 184:161–168
14. Hamelin R, Flejou JF, Muzeau F, Potet F, Laurent-Puig P, Fekete F, Thomas G (1994) TP53 gene mutations and p53 protein immunoreactivity in malignant and premalignant Barrett's esophagus. Gastroenterology 107:1012–1018
15. Symmans PJ, Linehan JM, Brito MJ, Filipe MI (1994) P53 expression in Barrett's oesophagus, dysplasia, and adenocarcinoma using antibody DO-7. J Pathol 173: 221–226
16. Krishnadath KK, Tilanus HW, van Blankenstein M, Bosman FT, Mulder AH (1995)

Accumulation of p53 protein in normal, dysplastic, and neoplastic Barrett's oesophagus. J Pathol 175:175–180
17. Casson AG, Manolopoulos B, Troster M, Kerkvliet N, O'Malley F, Inculet R, Finley R, Roth JA (1994) Clinical implications of p53 gene mutation in the progression of Barrett's epithelium to invasive esophageal cancer. Am J Surg 167:52–57
18. Bailey T, Biddlestone L, Shepherd N, Barr H, Warner P, Jankowski J (1998) Altered cadherin and catenin complexes in the Barrett's esophagus-dysplasia-adenocarcinoma sequence: correlation with disease progression and dedifferentiation. Am J Pathol 152:135–144
19. Swami S, Kumble S, Triadafilopoulos G (1995) E-cadherin expression in gastroesophageal reflux disease, Barrett's esophagus, and esophageal adenocarcinoma: an immunohistochemical and immunoblot study. Am J Gastroenterol 90:1808–1813
20. Krishnadath KK, Tilanus HW, van Blankenstein M, Hop WC, Kremers ED, Dinjens WN, Bosman FT (1997) Reduced expression of the cadherin-catenin complex in oesophageal adenocarcinoma correlates with poor prognosis. J Pathol 182:331–338
21. Walch AK, Zitzelsberger HF, Bruch J, Keller G, Angermeier D, Aubele MM, Mueller JD, Stein H, Braselmann H, Siewert JR, Hofler H, Werner M (2000) Chromosomal imbalances in Barrett's adenocarcinoma and the metaplasia–dysplasia–carcinoma sequence. Am J Pathol 156:555–566
22. Cameron AJ, Lomboy CT, Pera M, Carpenter HA (1995) Adenocarcinoma of the esophagogastric junction and Barrett's esophagus. Gastroenterology 109:1541–1546
23. Siewert JR, Stein HJ (1996) Adenocarcinoma of the gastrointestinal junction: classification, pathology and extent of resection. Dis Esophagus 9:173–182
24. Van Dekken H, Geelen E, Dinjens WN, Wijnhoven BP, Tilanus HW, Tanke HJ, Rosenberg C (1999) Comparative genomic hybridization of cancer of the gastroesophageal junction: deletion of 14Q31–32.1 discriminates between esophageal (Barrett's) and gastric cardia adenocarcinomas. Cancer Res 59:748–752
25. Yanagi M, Keller G, Mueller JD, Walch AK, Werner M, Stein HJ, Siewert JR, Höfler H (2000) Comparison of loss of heterozygosity and microsatellite instability in adenocarcinomas of the distal esophagus and proximal stomach. Virchows Arch (in press)
26. Nekarda H, Schlegel P, Schmitt M, Becker K, Mueller JD, Fink U (1998) Strong prognostic impact of tumor-associated urokinase-type plasminogen activator in completely resected adenocarcinoma of the esophagus. Clin Cancer Res 4:1755–1763
27. Schmitt M, Harbeck N, Thomssen C, Wilhelm O, Magdolen V, Reuning U, Ulm K, Hofler H, Janicke F, Graeff H (1997) Clinical impact of the plasminogen activation system in tumor invasion and metastasis: prognostic relevance and target for therapy. Thromb Haemost 78:285–296
28. Natsugoe S, Mueller JD, Stein HJ, Feith M, Höfler H, Siewert JR (1998) Micrometastasis and tumor cell microinvolvement of lymph nodes in esophageal squamous cell carcinoma: frequency, associated tumor characteristics and impact on prognosis. Cancer 83:858–866
29. Mueller JD, Stein HJ, Ouyang T, Natsugoe S, Feith M, Werner M, Siewert JR (2000) Frequency and clinical impact of lymph node micrometastases and tumor cell microinvolvement in adenocarcinomas of the esophagogastric junction. Cancer 89:1874–1882
30. Rubio CA, Aberg B (1991) Further studies on the musculo-fibrous anomaly of the Barrett's mucosa in esophageal carcinomas. Pathol Res Pract 187:1009–1013

Q & A after Dr. Mueller's presentation

Dr. Rubio (Karolinska Institute, Sweden): There has been a lot of discussion about micrometastasis in the literature, especially warnings. Micrometastases are detected exclusively by molecular methods, implying that some may be macrophages. They are not really tumor cells. Do you have any comments on this?

Dr. Mueller: There are two aspects to that problem. First, many of the data on micrometastasis are based on the PCR, in which case there is no morphological control of what's being described. You do have to be wary of such descriptions. We have also seen in immunohistochemistry the cytological differences among macrophages in which some weak staining has been seen. When we identify we require micrometastasis or tumor cell microinvolvement, we require that the cells be cytologically consistent with tumor cells. It is an important aspect that needs to be controlled with the morphology.

Altered Expression of *FHIT* in Esophageal Neoplasm

MASAKI MORI[1], KOSHI MIMORI[1], HIROSHI INOUE[1], YOICHI TANAKA[2], KAY HUEBNER[3], and CARLO M. CROCE[3]

Introduction

The *FHIT* (fragile histidine triad) gene located at chromosome region 3p14 has been reported to be deleted in a variety of common tumors including esophageal carcinoma [1]. Previous studies clarified that the *FHIT* gene is inactivated by deletions in carcinoma cell lines and primary tumors of the lung, head and neck, breast, stomach, and colon and several others [2]. Few studies of the *FHIT* gene in esophageal carcinomas have been reported [3, 4]. Hence we studied the role of *FHIT* in human esophageal carcinomas at the levels of DNA, RNA, and protein.

Recent studies demonstrated that loss of *FHIT* expression is associated with exposure to environmental carcinogens [2]. In addition, loss of FHIT expression was detectable in precarcinomatous lesions of the lung [5, 6]. We thus studied whether similar findings could be seen in the human esophagus.

Materials and Methods

Clinical Cases

Forty-six Japanese patients with esophageal carcinoma were studied. The patients included 42 men and 4 women, whose ages ranged from 48 to 74 years (mean 60 years). Histologically, 44 of the lesions were squamous cell carcinomas, and 2 were small cell carcinomas. None of the 46 showed adenocarcinoma.

The clinical data for smoking and alcohol habits were obtained in 39 patients. Most patients were smokers, drinkers, or both. Only two patients were nonsmokers, and the other two were nondrinkers. The grade of smoking was classified by the Brinkman index: heavy ≥ 900 and light < 900 according to the median number. The grade of

[1]Department of Surgery, Medical Institute of Bioregulation, Kyushu University, 4546 Tsurumibaru, Beppu 874-0828, Japan
[2]Department of Surgery, Saitama Cancer Center, Saitama, Japan
[3]Kimmel Cancer Institute, Thomas Jefferson University, Philadelphia, PA 19107, USA

alcohol drinking was classified by the alcohol index (grams of alcohol/day × year): heavy ≥ 2300 and light < 2300 saccording to the median number.

Tissue Samples and DNA/RNA Extraction

Tumor tissue and its corresponding normal tissue were obtained from each patient. The tissue samples were excised and immediately stored at −80°C. DNA and RNA were extracted from each sample according to previously described methods [7, 8].

Loss of Heterozygosity Study

The loci examined were D3S1234, D3S1295, D3S1300, D3S1312, and D3S1313. D3S1300 is located in intron 5 of the *FHIT* gene locus, and D3S1234 is located in intron 7. D3S1295 and D3S1313 are telomeric to the gene, whereas D3S1312 is centromeric at 3p14.2. As described in a previous paper [9], cases were judged as loss of heterozygosity (LOH) when an allele peak signal from tumor DNA was reduced by 50% compared with the normal counterpart. Optimal conditions for amplification of those microsatellite loci are described elsewhere [1, 5, 6].

RT-PCR and DNA Sequencing

cDNA was synthesized from 2 μg of total RNA. Reverse transcriptase-polymerase chain reaction (RT-PCR) was performed according to a previously described protocol [10]. DNA bands corresponding to the normal- and abnormal-size *FHIT* transcripts were excised from the gel, purified, and sequenced.

Immunostaining

Expression of the *FHIT* protein in paraffin-fixed tumor sections was examined by immunohistochemical staining with a polyclonal serum specific for human FHIT [9, 10]. The detailed pathologic examination of the 46 resected esophageal samples disclosed that there were several kinds of premalignant lesion in addition to the primary malignant tumors. We selected several samples and studied them by immunohistochemical staining; they included 12 carcinomas in situ, 4 lesions with severe dysplasia, 8 with moderate dysplasia, and 9 with mild dysplasia.

Immunohistochemical staining was classified in the following two groups: negative, where no staining was present or when staining was detected in fewer than 10% of the cells; and positive, where more than 10% of the cells stained positively.

Clinical and Pathologic Comparison

FHIT-positive and FHIT-negative cases were compared with respect to age, gender, location of the tumor, histologic differentiation, depth of tumor invasion, lymphatic permeation, vascular vessel invasion, lymph node metastasis, stage of the disease, and prognosis.

Statistical Analysis

Fisher's exact test with a two-tailed *P* for analysis of statistical significance of correlation was used between clinicopathologic variables and FHIT expression. Survival curves were calculated by the Kaplan-Meier estimate, using log-rank testing to assess statistical significance.

Results

The correlation between FHIT reactivity and loss of heterozygosity of mRNA expression status was summarized in Table 1. The correlation between FHIT reactivity and smoking or alcohol habits is summarized in Table 2.

TABLE 1. Correlation among FHIT reactivity, loss of heterozygosity, and aberrant mRNA expression

	FHIT reactivity		
Parameter	Positive	Negative	*P*
Loss of heterozygosity			
Present	5	30	<0.01
Absent	9	2	
mRNA expression			
Normal	11	9	<0.01[a]
Normal + aberrant	3	15	
No expression	0	8	

[a] This is a comparison between the normal expression group and the other two groups

TABLE 2. Smoking and alcohol habits and FHIT reactivity

	FHIT reactivity		
Parameter	Positive	Negative	*P*
Smoking[a]			
Heavy	5	15	NS
Light or none	9	10	
Alcohol ingestion[b]			
Heavy	4	16	0.07
Light or none	10	9	
Smoking and alcohol ingestion			
Heavy	1	11[c]	<0.01
Light	8	5	

[a] The grade of smoking is classified by the Brinkman index: heavy ≥ 900 and light < 900

[b] The grade of alcohol drinking is classified by alcohol index (grams of alcohol/day × year): heavy ≥ 2300 and light < 2300

[c] Five of these eleven patients show negative FHIT reactivity in carcinomatous tissue and adjacent noncarcinomatous epithelium

LOH Study

The DNA analysis demonstrated that LOH was observed in 35 cases (76%). Seven patients showed homozygous deletion in exons of the *FHIT* gene with a presence of LOH. On the other hand, 11 non-LOH cases retained whole exons.

mRNA Expression

The RT-PCR study demonstrated that no FHIT products were recognized in 8 tumors, and aberrant products plus normal-sized FHIT RT-PCR product were seen in 17 tumors. One case showed only aberrant products. Sequence analysis of aberrant products showed the absence of coding and noncoding exons and nucleotide insertions. The remaining 20 showed normal-size product alone. All 46 samples from normal tissue showed normal-size product. Interestingly, however, aberrant products were also recognized in normal tissue samples in six patients, and these six were both heavy smokers and drinkers. The aberrant products were studied by sequence analysis, and the results showed an absence of coding and noncoding exons and nucleotide insertions. Five of the six showed negative FHIT staining in the normal (noncarcinomatous) tissues.

Immunostaining

The study demonstrated that 14 cases showed positive and 32 showed negative staining in carcinoma cells. As shown in Table 1, there was a significant correlation between LOH status and immunostaining status ($P < 0.01$). We next compared the results of RT-PCR with those of immunostaining. There was a significant correlation between mRNA expression status and immunostaining for FHIT ($P < 0.05$). All eight tumors with no RT-PCR products showed negative immunostaining.

Normal (noncarcinomatous) squamous epithelium showed positive FHIT reactivity in most cases, whereas five showed negative FHIT reactivity not only in the primary tumor but also in the normal squamous epithelium. Interestingly, all five patients were both heavy smokers and heavy drinkers, suggesting an association between FHIT protein loss and environmental carcinogens. Eight of twelve carcinomas in situ, two of four lesions with severe dysplasia, four of eight with moderate dysplasia, and three of nine with mild dysplasia showed negative FHIT reactivity.

Loss of FHIT Expression and Smoking and Drinking Habits

Altogether, 20 patients were heavy smokers, 17 were light smokers, and two were not smokers; 20 patients were heavy drinkers, 18 were light drinkers, and only one was not a drinker. The correlation between FHIT reactivity and smoking or alcohol habits is summarized in Table 2. Of the 12 patients who were both heavy smokers and drinkers, 11 had negative FHIT reactivity. On the other hand, 8 of 13 patients with both light or no smoking and drinking had positive FHIT reactivity. There was a significant difference between the two groups. Of the 12 patients with both heavy smoking and drinking, 5 had negative FHIT reactivity in the carcinomatous tissue and in normal tissue.

Clinical and Pathologic Comparison

There was no significant difference between FHIT-positive (n = 14) and FHIT-negative (n = 32) cases for any of the factors studied. The 5-year survival rate was 36% in FHIT-positive cases and 32% in FHIT-negative cases.

Discussion

Several investigators reported that loss of FHIT expression might be associated with carcinogen-induced damage. For example, in lung carcinomas the loss of FHIT expression was higher in tumors of smokers than in those of nonsmokers [5, 6, 11]. We studied the correlation between FHIT expression and a smoking or drinking habit (or both). The results showed there was no significant difference in loss of FHIT expression between heavy and light smokers or between heavy and light drinkers, although the heavy drinkers had a tendency to show a higher frequency of loss of FHIT expression ($P = 0.07$). If these two habits were combined, the patients with heavy degrees of both habits showed a significantly higher frequency of loss of FHIT expression than those with light degrees of both ($P < 0.01$). The findings support the hypothesis that loss of FHIT expression may be associated with environmental carcinogens.

The loss of FHIT expression was already detectable in precarcinomatous lesions of the lung [6]. Our present study also demonstrated that loss of FHIT expression was seen in 67% of carcinomas in situ (n = 12) and 43% of dysplasia lesions (n = 12).

There are two types of reduced FHIT expression in tumors. One occurs quite early in the development of carcinoma, as mentioned above and as seen in this study of esophageal carcinoma and other studies of lung carcinoma [5, 6, 11]. The other accompanies progression toward a more aggressive form of disease. In fact, loss of FHIT has been reported to correlate with more aggressive bladder, kidney [12], or breast [10] carcinomas. Our study of esophageal carcinoma demonstrated that there were no significant clinicopathologic differences between the cases with positive or negative FHIT reactivity.

Conclusions

We showed that loss of the FHIT protein occurred with most esophageal carcinomas, and the reduction of the protein was also detected in precarcinomatous conditions, such as dysplasia and carcinoma in situ. Interestingly, the reduction was also recognized in the surrounding normal-appearing squamous epithelium of some patients with high exposure to carcinogens. As esophageal carcinoma is one of the most aggressive diseases and has a poor prognosis [13], a new therapy such as *FHIT* gene therapy might be desirable for a breakthrough.

Acknowledgment. This work was supported in part by the Ministry of Education, Culture and Science of Japan.

References

1. Ohta M, Inoue H, Cotticelli MG, Kastury K, Baffa R, Palazzo J, Siprashvili Z, Mori M, McCue P, Druck T, Croce CM, Huebner K (1996) The FHIT gene, spanning the

chromosome 3p14.2 fragile site and renal carcinoma-associated t(3, 8) breakpoint, is abnormal in digestive tract cancers. Cell 84:587–597
2. Inoue H, Ishii H, Alder H, Snyder E, Druck T, Huebner K, Croce CM (1997) Sequence of the FRA3B common fragile region: implications for the mechanisms of FHIT deletion. Proc Natl Acad Sci USA 94:14584–14589
3. Mimori K, Druck T, Inoue H, Alder H, Berk L, Mori M, Huebner K, Croce CM (1999) Cancer-specific chromosome alterations in the constitutive fragile region FRA3B. Proc Natl Acad Sci USA 96:7456–7461
4. Michael D, Beer DG, Wilke CW, Miller DE, Glover TW (1997) Frequent deletions of FHIT and FRA3B in Barrett's metaplasia and esophageal adenocarcinomas. Oncogene 15:1653–1659
5. Nelson HN, Wiencke JK, Gunn L, Wain JC, Christiani DC, Kelsey KT (1998) Chromosome 3p14 alterations in lung cancer: evidence that FHIT exon deletion is a target of tobacco carcinogens and asbestos, Cancer Res 58:1804–1807
6. Morita M, Kuwano H, Ohno S, Sugimachi K, Seo Y, Tomoda H, Furusawa M, Nakashima T (1994) Multiple occurrence of carcinoma in the upper aerodigestive tract associated with esophageal cancer: reference to smoking, drinking and family history. Int J Cancer 58:207–210
7. Sozzi G, Pastorino U, Moiraghi L, Tagliabue E, Pezzella F, Ghirelli C, Tornielli S, Sard L, Huebner K, Pierotti MA, Croce CM, Pilotti S (1998) Loss of FHIT function in lung cancer and preinvasive bronchial lesions. Cancer Res 58:5032–5037
8. Mori M, Barnard GF, Staniunas RJ, Jessup JM, Steele GD, Jr, Chen LB (1993) Prothymosin-α mRNA expression correlates with that of c-myc in human colon cancer. Oncogene 8:2821–2826
9. Campiglio M, Pekarsky Y, Menard S, Tagliabue E, Pilotti S, Croce CM (1999) FHIT loss of function in human primary breast cancer correlates with advanced stage of the disease. Cancer Res 59:3866–3869
10. Ishi H, Baffa R, Numata S, Murakumo Y, Rattan S, Inoue H, Mori M, Fidanza V, Alder H, Croce CM (1999) The FEZ1 gene at chromosome 8p22 encodes a leucine-zipper protein, and its expression is altered in multiple human tumors. Proc Natl Acad Sci USA 96:3923–3933
11. Baffa R, Veronese ML, Santoro R, Mandes B, Palazzo JP, Rugge M, Santoro E, Croce CM, Huebner K (1998) Loss of FHIT expression in gastric carcinoma. Cancer Res, 58:4708–4714
12. Siprashvili Z, Sozzi G, Barnes LD, McCue P, Robinson AK, Eryomin V, Sard L, Tagliabue E, Greco A, Fusetti L, Schwartz G, Pierotti MA, Croce CM, Huebner K (1997) Replacement of FHIT in cancer cells suppress tumorigenicity. Proc Natl Acad Sci USA 94:13771–13776
13. Sugimachi K (1998) Advances in the surgical treatment of oesophageal Cancer. Br J Surg 85:289–290

Q & A after Dr. Mori's presentation

Dr. Shimada (Kyoto University, Japan): I have just published a paper in *Cancer* in which I recognized that in female patients with cancer there is a negative correlation between smoking and alcohol consumption and the FHIT protein. Do you have any data in that regard?

Dr. Mori: There were seven female patients in this series, so I have no data for a female-male comparison.

Dr. Kuwano (Gunma University, Japan): Concerning the intratumoral heterogeneity of expression or negative expression of FHIT proteins, what is the correlation between the FHIT positivity detected by immunostaining or RT-PCR and the prognosis?

Dr. Mori: There was a significant correlation between FHIT reactivity and LOH or the mRNA transcription level, although I didn't study heterogeneity or homogeneity of FHIT reactivity.

Dr. Kuwano: What was the staining pattern—diffuse or focal—for positive staining?

Dr. Mori: You mean the criteria for positive or negative? One-third of the examined area was positive, as we determined it.

Dr. Kuwano: What was the correlation between the positivity and prognosis of esophageal cancer?

Dr. Mori: There was no correlation.

Molecular Alterations in Dysplasia and Superficial Cancer of the Esophagus

Soji Ozawa, Yoshifumi Ikeda, Kazuo Koyanagi, Nobutoshi Ando, Yuko Kitagawa, Masakazu Ueda, and Masaki Kitajima

Introduction

Many molecular alterations may contribute to the pathogenesis of esophageal cancer. We reviewed the results of our molecular studies on dysplasia and cancer of the esophagus. In this paper we focus on expression of the oncogenes c-*erb*-B and *int-2/cyclin* D1, and telomerase activity in superficial esophageal cancer.

c-*erb*-B and *int-2/cyclin* D1 Oncogenes

It has been reported that oncogene c-erb-B, which codes for epidermal growth factor receptor (EGFR), is amplified (10%–12%) in advanced esophageal cancer [1]. This amplification is correlated with diminished survival after surgery and a high frequency of regional lymph node metastasis. Oncogene *int-2/cyclin* D1, which is an important cell cycle regulator, has also been reported to be amplified (25%–29%) in advanced esophageal cancer [2, 3]. This amplification was correlated with diminished survival after surgery and a high frequency of distant organ metastasis postoperatively. These two clinically important oncogene alterations were investigated in superficial esophageal cancer [carcinoma in situ (CIS) and T1a and T1b cancers] [4].

A total of 63 patients with superficial esophageal cancer who had undergone esophagectomy at Keio University Hospital between 1980 and 1991 were examined: 45 patients had undergone thoracotomy with esophagectomy, and 18 patients had undergone esophagectomy without thoracotomy. The Tl cases were divided into two groups: Tla cases, in which the tumor had invaded the lamina propria; and Tlb cases, in which the tumor had invaded the submucosa. CIS, Tla, and Tlb lesions were found in 6, 12, and 45 cases, respectively.

DNA was obtained from formalin-fixed, paraffin-embedded blocks of the primary tumor specimens and from normal tissue adjacent to the tumors (controls). The histopathologic findings in the tumor specimens obtained from the patients at operation were investigated by hematoxylin-eosin staining of sections prepared from the

Department of Surgery, School of Medicine, Keio University, 35 Shinanomachi, Shinjuku-ku, Tokyo 160-8582, Japan

paraffin blocks. Recurrence was diagnosed based on the results of diagnostic imaging, including routine chest roentgenograms, computed tomographic scans, and ultrasonography.

The tissue blocks were cut into five or more 20 μm thick sections. One section from each block was examined by hematoxylin-eosin staining to identify neoplastic and normal tissue areas. DNA from neoplastic and normal tissue was then extracted from the unstained sections in accordance with the method described by Dubeau et al. [5].

The probes used were pE7, a 2.4-kilobasepair (kbp) Cla I-Cla I fragment of the c-*erb*-B gene; 7C22, a 5.1-kbp EcoR I-EcoR I fragment of the pSP64 gene, SS6, a 0.9-kbp Sac I-Sac I fragment of the *int*-2 gene; and DRD2, a 1.6-kbp BamH I fragment of the dopamine receptor *D2* gene. The 7C22 and DRD2 probes were used as the internal control probes of chromosomes 7 and 11.

The extracted DNA (10 μg) was subjected to slot-blot hybridization analysis. Autoradiograms were evaluated quantitatively using a bioimage analyzer. Cases in which the gene copy numbers were more than threefold were believed to show gene amplification.

DNA was extracted from 54 of the 63 patients: 4 had CIS, 8 had Tla cancer, and 42 had Tlb cancer. Amplification of the c-*erb*-B gene was detected in 1 of the 8 patients with Tla cancer (12%) and 4 of the 42 with Tlb cancer (10%) (Table 1). Amplification of the *int*-2 gene was detected in 1 of the 4 cases with CIS (25%), 2 of the 8 cases with Tla cancer (25%), and 12 of the 42 cases with Tlb cancer (29%) (Table 2). Co-amplification of both c-*erb*-B and *int*-2 genes was detected in two patients with Tlb cancer.

Of the 12 Tlb patients showing *int*-2 amplification, 3 died of distant organ metastasis. The survival rate in the group showing *int*-2 amplification was significantly lower than that in the group not showing *int*-2 amplification. All four of the patients with Tlb cancer with c-*erb*-B amplification were found to have lymph node metastasis at operation.

Based on these results, it is evident that the incidence of c-*erb*-B and *int*-2 gene amplification in superficial esophageal cancer is not different from that reported for advanced esophageal cancer. In another of our studies, the *cyclin* D1 gene, which is located in the same amplicon as the *int*-2 gene, was not found to be overexpressed in dysplasia (data not shown). Thus, although the aforementioned gene amplifications in esophageal cancer may occur during the early stages of carcinogenesis, they probably do not occur in premalignant lesions (i.e., dysplasia).

TABLE 1. Histopathological findings and c-*erb*-B amplification

Histopathological findings	Amplification of c-*erb*-B		
	Positive	Negative	Total
CIS	0	4	4
T1a	1 (12%)	7	8
T1b	4 (10%)	38	42
Total	5 (9%)	49	54

CIS: carcinoma in situ; T1a: invasion of the lamina propria by the tumor; T1b: invasion of the submucosa by the tumor

TABLE 2. Histopathological findings and *int*-2 amplification

Histopathological findings	Amplification of *int*-2		
	Positive	Negative	Total
CIS	1 (25%)	3	4
T1a	2 (25%)	6	8
T1b	12 (29%)	30	42
Total	15 (28%)	39	54

Telomerase Activity

We also examined some other interesting molecular alterations in esophageal cancer. Telomerase is a ribonucleoprotein enzyme that adds telomeric repeats (TTAGGG)n onto chromosomal ends. Studies have demonstrated that, with few exceptions, telomerase is activated in tumor tissue but not in normal tissue adjacent to the primary tumor. We investigated telomerase activity in CIS and esophageal dysplasia. In this context, it has been demonstrated that whereas normal esophageal squamous epithelial cells produce glycogen that reacts with iodine, staining the normal epithelium brown, abnormal or immature epithelial cells produce less glycogen and do not stain with iodine; this forms the basis of the iodine-staining method introduced for diagnosis of carcinoma of the esophagus. It has been reported that CIS and dysplastic lesions also show iodine nonreactivity [6]. Thus, iodine-nonreactive lesions were selected to study the telomerase activity in dysplastic lesions and CIS of the esophagus [7].

A total of 18 iodine-nonreactive lesions were identified in regions located distal to the primary tumor in surgically resected specimens obtained from patients with esophageal cancer at Keio University Hospital between 1995 and 1997. The median age of these patients was 57 years. In addition, 55 endoscopic punch biopsy specimens of iodine-nonreactive lesions that were separate from the primary tumor were also obtained from 25 esophageal cancer patients (median age 64 years) and 30 patients who had undergone endoscopy for other reasons (median age 60 years).

Iodine staining was performed using a 3% iodine solution; the solution was sprayed onto the esophageal wall; and after allowing a reaction time of a little more than a minute, it was washed out with water. The iodine-nonreactive lesions were on average more than 5 mm in greatest dimension and were located more than 5 cm from the primary tumor.

Two sections were prepared from each sample, one of which was stained with hematoxylin-eosin for histopathologic examination and the other snap-frozen in liquid nitrogen and stored at −80°C until the time of the telomerase assay. According to the extent of the cellular deformity, the dysplastic lesions were classified into three subgroups: mild, moderate, severe. Those lesions in which the entire thickness of the epithelium was replaced by atypical basal cells were described as CIS. For the telomerase assay, the samples were treated according to the procedure described by Kim et al. [8]. Extracts were adjusted to 6.0 μg and 0.6 μg of the standard protein for each assay. Telomerase activity was measured by the polymerase chain reaction-based telomeric repeat amplification protocol (TRAP) and analyzed by electrophoresis as described previously. The extracts that produced 6-bp DNA ladders and were sensitive to RNAase were considered to be telomerase-positive.

Surgically Resected Specimens

Telomerase activity was detected in 10 of the 18 iodine-nonreactive lesions obtained from the surgically resected specimens. In all 10 telomerase-positive samples, CIS was observed by light microscopy in the iodine-nonreactive epithelium that was separate from the primary tumor; in contrast, no tumor cells were observed in any of the iodine-nonreactive lesions not showing telomerase activity. This group included one case with severe dysplasia and one with moderate dysplasia (Table 3). There was a significantly positive correlation between the presence of telomerase activity and the presence of tumor.

Endoscopic Punch Biopsy Samples

Telomerase activity was detected in 28 of the 55 specimens of iodine-nonreactive lesions obtained by endoscopic punch biopsy. CIS was observed in 25 of these 28 iodine-nonreactive lesions showing positive telomerase activity. However, no tumor cells were present in the 27 iodine-nonreactive lesions not showing telomerase activity, including 4 with moderate dysplasia and 23 specimens of normal epithelium (Table 4). There was again a significantly positive correlation between the presence of telomerase activity and the presence of tumor. Among the three telomerase-positive lesions in which no tumor tissue was observed, two were diagnosed as severe dysplasia and one as moderate dysplasia. Specimens of CIS showed strong 6-bp ladder signals when 0.6 μg of protein was used for the telomerase assay, whereas lesions showing severe dysplasia had weak signals. Moderately dysplastic lesions showed no ladder signals when 0.6 μg of protein was used (Table 5).

Strong telomerase activity was detected in all specimens of CIS and in some of dysplasia. Telomerase reactivation is reportedly observed in all cases of advanced esophageal cancer [9]. Demonstration of positive telomerase activity is thus essential

Table 3. Histopathological findings and telomerase activity in iodine-nonreactive lesions (obtained from surgically resected specimens)

Histopathological findings	Telomerase activity		
	Positive	Negative	Total
Normal	0	6	6
Dysplasia	0	2	2
Mild	0	0	0
Moderate	0	1	1
Severe	0	1	1
CIS	10 (100%)	0	10
Total	10 (56%)	8	18

From [7], with permission

TABLE 4. Histopathological findings and telomerase activity in iodine-nonreactive lesions (obtained from endoscopic punch biopsy specimens)

Histopathological findings	Telomerase activity		
	Positive	Negative	Total
Normal	0	23	23
Dysplasia	3 (43%)	4	7
Mild	0	0	0
Moderate	1 (20%)	4	5
Severe	2 (0%)	0	2
CIS	25 (100%)	0	25
Total	28 (51%)	27	55

From [7], with permission

TABLE 5. Detection of telomerase activity according to the standard protein concentration

Histopathological finding	Standard protein concentration[a]	
	6.0 μg	0.6 μg
Surgically resected specimens with CIS ($n = 10$)	10 (100%)	8 (80%)
Endoscopic punch biopsy specimens		
Moderate dysplasia ($n = 1$)	1 (100%)	0
Severe dysplasia ($n = 2$)	2 (100%)	1 (50%)
CIS ($n = 25$)	25 (100%)	20 (80%)

[a] Telomerase activity was detected when 6.0 or 0.6 μg of protein was used

From [7], with permission

for the diagnosis of carcinogenesis in the esophageal epithelium. In addition, dysplastic cells that show telomerase activity are also immortalized. Therefore, telomerase reactivation is an early event in carcinogenesis in the esophageal epithelium.

Conclusions

Based on the results of our studies, it is evident that amplification of the c-*erb*-B and *int-2/cyclin* D1 oncogenes and telomerase activation play important roles in esophageal carcinogenesis. Other molecular alterations may also contribute to carcinogenesis in the esophageal epithelium and must be investigated in the future.

References

1. Kitagawa Y, Ueda M, Ando N, et al (1996) Further evidence for prognostic significance of epidermal growth factor receptor gene amplification in patients with esophageal squamous cell carcinoma. Clin Cancer Res 2:909–914

2. Kitagawa Y, Ueda M, Ando N, et al (1991) Significance of int-2/hst-1 coamplification as a prognostic factor in patients with esophageal squamous carcinoma. Cancer Res 51:1504–1508
3. Shinozaki H, Ozawa S, Ando N, et al (1996) Cyclin D1 amplification as a new predictive classification for squamous cell carcinoma of the esophagus, adding gene information. Clin Cancer Res 2:1155–1161
4. Ikeda Y, Ozawa S, Ando N, et al (1996) Meanings of c-erbB and int-2 amplification in superficial esophageal squamous cell carcinomas. Ann Thorac Surg 62:835–838
5. Dubeau L, Chandler LA, Gralow JR, et al (1986) Southern blot analysis of DNA extracted from formalin-fixed pathology specimens. Cancer Res 46:2964–2969
6. Endo M, Takeshita K, Yoshida M (1986) How can we diagnose the early stage of esophageal cancer? Endoscopy 18(suppl 3):11–18
7. Koyanagi K, Ozawa S, Ando N, et al (2000) Telomerase activity as an indicator of malignant potential in iodine-nonreactive lesions of the esophagus. Cancer 88:1524–1529
8. Kim NW, Piatyszek MA, Prowse KR, et al (1994) Specific association of human telomerase activity with immortal cells and cancer. Science 266:2011–2015
9. Koyanagi K, Ozawa S, Ando N, et al (1999) Clinical significance of telomerase activity in the non-cancerous epithelial region of oesophageal squamous cell carcinoma. Br J Surg 86:674–679

Q & A after Dr. Ozawa's presentation

Dr. Sarbia (University of Düsseldorf, Germany): You investigated quite a number of dysplastic lesions by means of *p53* immunohistochemistry. Based on your results, would you judge *p53* immunohistochemistry to be useful for histopathological grading of dysplasia and carcinoma in situ?

Dr. Ozawa: For some of them the *p53* status helps partly but not definitively because *p53* status does not explain all of the carcinogenesis.

Dr. Sarbia: That was my impression. There is no clear cut-off point. There also seemed to be no clear cut-off point in your Ki-67 data to differentiate between lesions. Is that right?

Dr. Ozawa: Yes.

Anonymous (Japan): Do you have any ideas about telomerase analysis for early detection of esophageal cancer?

Dr. Ozawa: Telomerase provides us with a good differential diagnosis, that is, cancer or noncancer. Therefore, if the data indicate the presence of a telomerase-positive lesion, regardless of whether the pathological examination shows cancer, the lesion should be carefully followed endoscopically or resected by EMR.

Telomerase Activity and p53 Protein Accumulation in Lugol-Stained and Lugol-Unstained Esophageal Squamous Epithelia

YUTAKA SHIMADA[1], MAKI INAI[2], MASATO KANO[1], TAKAKI SAKURAI[3], TSUTOMU CHIBA[2], and MASAYUKI IMAMURA[1]

Introduction

Esophageal squamous cell carcinoma (ESC) is one of the most common cancers worldwide [1]. Its prognosis remains poor despite recent advances in both diagnosis and therapy. Moreover, multiple primary ESC is not uncommon [2, 3]. These reports support the concept that the entire esophagus may be considered as a single area of carcinogenesis. The elucidation of the carcinogenesis of ESC may have a considerable effect on early diagnosis and therapy.

Telomerase activity was detected in approximately 80% of the cases of advanced ESC, similar to other cancers, but it was also present in a considerable amount of normal esophageal epithelia [4–6]. To elucidate the meaning of telomerase activity in normal esophageal epithelium, we evaluated telomerase activity in both cancerous and noncancerous epithelia from the esophagus. For this purpose, we classified esophageal epithelium according to the results of Lugol's iodine staining. Lugol's iodine staining can be used for easy detection of abnormal squamous mucosa; normal mature squamous epithelium contains glycogen, which stains brown with iodine [7, 8]. In addition, because studies have shown that human telomerase reverse transcriptase (hTERT), a component of human telomerase, plays a key role in activation of telomerase in cancer cells [9, 10], we performed in situ hybridization for hTERT to clarify the localization of telomerase activity in various esophageal lesions and in Lugol-stained normal epithelia.

An absence of functional p53 allows cellular immortalization and predisposes cells to neoplastic transformation. In esophageal cancer, there is much evidence to suggest that p53 abnormality is linked with esophageal carcinogenesis [11–16]. Thus, the question raised was whether there is a similarity between telomerase activity and p53 in precancerous lesions of the esophagus. For this reason we also performed immunohistochemical analysis to detect p53 protein accumulation in Lugol-unstained epithelia and evaluated the relation to telomerase activity of these samples.

Departments of [1]Surgery and Surgical Basic Science, [2]Gastroenterology and Hepatology and [3]Laboratory of Anatomic Pathology, Kyoto University, Kawaharacho, Shogoin, Sakyo-ku, Kyoto 606-8507, Japan

Materials and Methods

Endoscopic Sampling

All tissue samples were obtained endoscopically at Kyoto University Hospital from July 1996 to April 1998. The study included 11 patients with advanced ESC and 35 patients who underwent routine endoscopic examination. We obtained written informed consent for Lugol's staining and endoscopic sampling before the endoscopic examination. Each tissue sample was obtained by biopsy or endoscopic mucosal resection. During endoscopic examination the esophagus was stained with 3% Lugol's solution, and two samples were obtained from the same Lugol-unstained lesion. Two Lugol-stained epithelial samples were also obtained from each patient at least 3 em distant from the lesions. If no focal lesion was found, a standard site in the mid-esophagus was sampled. One sample from each site was subjected to pathological examination and fixed in 10% buffered formalin embedded in paraffin, cut in 5 μm sections, and stained with hematoxylin and eosin (H&E). The other was immediately frozen and stored in liquid nitrogen for measurement of telomerase activity. If the Lugol-unstained lesion was too small to obtain two samples, only one sample was obtained for pathological examination.

Telomerase Activity

Telomerase activity was determined by a modified telomeric repeat amplification protocol (TRAP) assay combined with enzyme immunoassay (EIA) [17] and in situ hybrdization. Primer sequences were described by Krupp et al. [18, 19]. The relative specific telomerase activity of each sample was expressed as a corresponding amount of KYSE 273 protein.

p53 Immunohistochemical Procedure

Formalin-fixed, paraffin-embedded biopsy samples (Lugol-unstained lesion), which were a counterpart of the samples for telomerase activity measurement, were subjected to immunohistochemical staining using the avidin-biotin method as described previously [20]. The antibody for p53 used in this study was DO-7 (Dako, Tokyo, Japan). The unmasking of antigens was carried out by incubation in citrate buffer (pH 6.0) at 100°C for 2 min using five cycles (microwave). Sections were incubated overnight at 4°C with each antibody in phosphate-buffered saline containing 5% horse serum and were counterstained with Mayer's hematoxylin. The intensity of immunohistochemical staining was evaluated in all areas of the section for correlation with and confirmation of the tissue analysis. More than 10% positive staining in nuclei was defined as positive staining of p53 [21].

Results

Telomerase Activity in Tissue Samples

Tissue samples were obtained from 46 patients. Nine patients had a history of reflux esophagitis, but none was involved with an active phase of inflammation at the time of the endoscopic examination. We collected 46 samples of Lugol-stained epithelia, 31 samples of Lugol-unstained lesions (14 esophagitis, 7 mild dysplasia, 5 severe dysplasia, 5 intramucosal ESC), and 9 samples of advanced ESC tissue. We first evaluated telomerase activity limited to the Lugol-stained epithelia because it was in a common normal physiological state and contained enough glycogen for Lugol's staining.

We divided these Lugol-stained epithelia into five groups based on their accompanying lesions: group A (control group), no Lugol-unstained lesion or advanced ESC; group B, Lugol-unstained epithelia diagnosed as esophagitis; group C, Lugol-unstained epithelia diagnosed as mild dysplasia; group D, Lugol-unstained epithelia diagnosed as severe dysplasia or intramucosal ESC; group E, advanced ESC. We considered severe dysplasia and intramucosal ESC to be in the same group (i.e., early ESC). One Lugol-stained epithelium sample (group E) was excluded owing to a lack of protein concentration.

Telomerase activity in the Lugol-stained epithelia increased with the abnormal progression of the esophageal lesions (Fig. 1). Indeed, the mean telomerase activity in group E was the highest of the five Lugol-stained epithelial groups. All four groups of Lugol-stained epithelia with lesions exhibited significantly higher telomerase activity than that in the control group (group A).

Figure 2 shows the telomerase activity in various Lugol-unstained lesions and advanced ESC. There was virtually no difference between the severe dysplasia group and the intramucosal ESC group. The telomerase activity in these two groups was

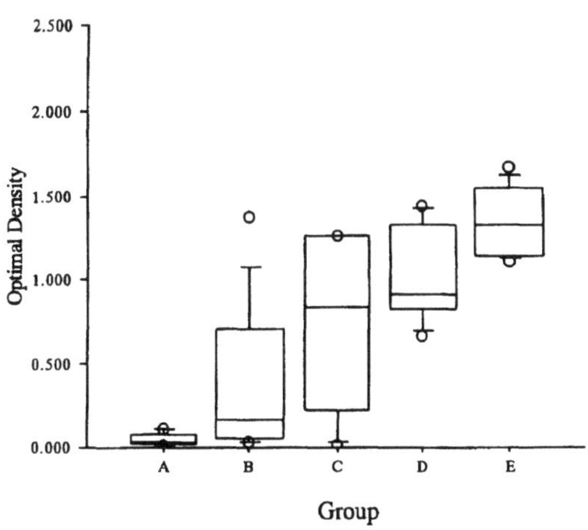

FIG. 1. Box-and-whisker plot of telomerase activity in esophageal samples. Telomerase activities were determined by telomeric repeat amplification protocol–enzyme-linked immunosorbent assay (TRAP-EIA). *Bottom and top edges* of the box mark the 25th and the 75th percentiles. The *center horizontal line* is drawn at the sample median. *Center vertical lines* drawn from the boxes extend to the 10th or 90th percentiles. Telomerase activity of the Lugol-stained epithelia is classified by the accompanying lesions: group A, no Lugol-unstained lesion or advanced esophageal squamous cell carcinoma (ESC); group B, esophagitis; group C, mild dysplasia; group D, early ESC (severe dysplasia or intramucosal ESC); group E, advanced ESC. There was statistical significance in the comparison of A to D,E ($P < 0.05$) (Steel Dwass test)

significantly higher than in noncancerous lesions and significantly lower than in advanced ESC. The mean telomerase activity of Lugol-stained epithelium compared with that in Lugol-unstained lesions in each group was significantly higher in the Lugol-unstained lesions with the exception of group C. In addition, almost all of the telomerase activity was up-regulated in each Lugol-unstained lesion compared with the Lugol-stained epithelium obtained from the same patient.

Expression of hTERT mRNA in Esophageal Tissues

In situ hybridization for hTERT revealed that it was expressed not only in cancer tissues but also in Lugol-stained normal esophageal tissues, where it was mainly observed in the basal and parabasal layers of the mucosa. Among stromal cells, only lymphocytes expressed the hTERT signal. These basal and parabasal layer cells in the Lugol-stained normal mucosa and lymphocytes showed a similar, relatively weak intensity. On the other hand, almost all the advanced cancer cells clearly showed higher intensity. The signal intensity of hTERT in the cytoplasm of cancer cells varied [22].

In an analysis of the relation between the hTERT signal and histological examination, there appeared to be a trend toward an increase in the intensity of the hTERT signal with an increase in the severity of the cellular atypia in Lugol-unstained lesions and advanced ESC. We found no significant correlation between the signal intensity of hTERT and the telomerase activity in any case (data not shown).

Relation Between hTERT Expression and p53 Protein Accumulation

In this series lesions with p53 protein accumulation had a high level of telomerase activity, although it was not significantly different from that in the controls ($P = 0.188$)

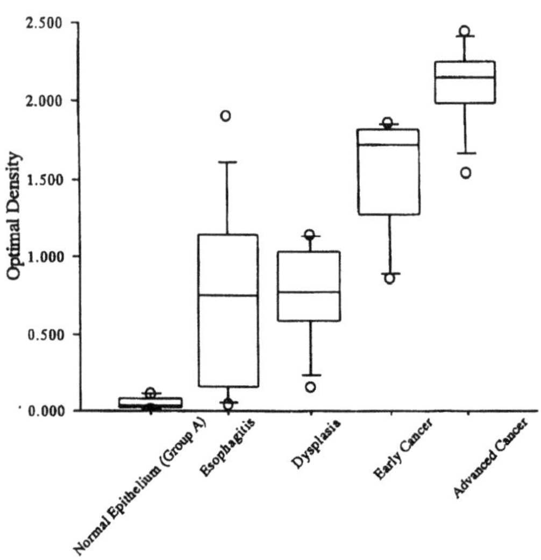

FIG. 2. Telomerase activity of Lugol-stained normal epithelia (group A), Lugol-unstained epithelia (esophagitis, mild dysplasia, severe dysplasia, intramucosal ESC), and advanced ESC. There was statistical significance in the comparison of normal epithelia to esophagitis, dysplasia, early cancer, and advanced cancer ($P < 0.05$) (Steel Dwass test)

(Fig. 3). When the mucosal carcinoma was included in the evaluation, there was a significant correlation between p53 protein accumulation and telomerase activity ($P = 0.024$).

Discussion

We semiquantified telomerase activity in cancerous and various noncancerous epithelia of the esophagus using TRAP-EIA to elucidate the meaning of telomerase activity in various states of the esophagus. Interestingly, we found that the level of telomerase activity in the Lugol-stained normal epithelia accompanied by ESC was high, and the telomerase activity in the Lugol-stained epithelia increased with progression of the accompanying esophageal lesions. These findings indicated that telomerase in the Lugol-stained epithelia may be up-regulated by risk factors for carcinogenesis. With this in mind, it is important to emphasize that the hTERT signal was detected even in the basal and parabasal layers of Lugol-stained epithelia. Thus, considering that hTERT plays a key role in the activation of telomerase, high telomerase activity would be derived from basal and parabasal layer cells in the normal esophagus. Because there are many reports that telomerase activity is absent in most normal human somatic tissues, it is unexpected that the Lugol-stained normal epithelia with accompanying ESC would exhibit such a high level of telomerase activity. Koyanagi et al. [23]. reported that 10% of normal esophageal tissue accompanied by advanced ESC showed telomerase activity derived from the microinvasion of cancer cells. We detected no cancer cells in the Lugol-stained epithelia with H&E staining. Of course, it is difficult to rule out completely the presence of cancer cells in entire samples, but it is unlikely because almost all the telomerase activity in the Lugol-stained epithelia with accompanying ESC was high in this study.

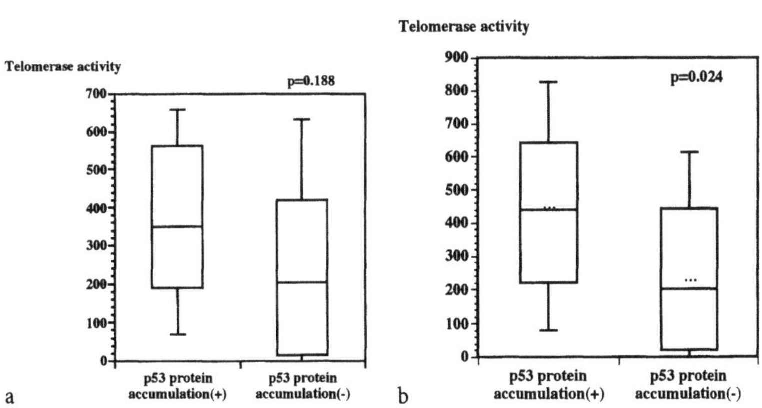

FIG. 3. **a** Relation of telomerase activity and p53 protein accumulation in Lugol-stained lesions and dysplasia. There was no significant difference between them ($P = 0.188$). **b** When the mucosal carcinoma was included in the analysis, there was a significant correlation between p53 protein accumulation and telomerase activity ($P = 0.024$)

The up-regulation of telomerase in Lugol-stained epithelia may be due to an acceleration of cell cycle reproduction of normal epithelial cells because telomerase is regarded as a biomarker of cell proliferation. Based on these results, telomerase activity in Lugol-stained epithelium may show the stability of the cells, which is influenced by the process of carcinogenesis or reproduction. According to the Lugol-unstained lesions and advanced ESC, telomerase activity increased relative to the severity of the disease. Similar results were recently reported concerning Lugol-unstained lesions, but there were no evaluation of esophagitis and advanced ESC [24]. In this study, telomerase activity in mild dysplasia was significantly higher than that in the Lugol-stained normal control group A, but there was no appreciable difference between mild dysplasia and esophagitis. Moreover, the signal intensity of dysplastic cells was relatively weak. This finding suggests that mild dysplasia is immature epithelium in the middle of normal reproduction or a neoplastic epithelium that grows slowly. Severe dysplasia exhibited higher telomerase activity than did mild dysplasia, and there was no significant difference between severe dysplasia and intramucosal ESC, although additional up-regulation of telomerase was seen in advanced ESC. A similar tendency was revealed by in situ hybridization. These data suggest that telomerase activity is up-regulated during the early stage of esophageal carcinogenesis and may play a critical role in the progression of ESC. Figure 2 shows that telomerase activity was elevated in ESC compared with that in Lugol-stained epithelia in groups D and E. The regulatory mechanism of telomerase activity is not known.

There was no clear correlation between telomerase activity and the intensity of hTERT expression. Nakano et al. [25]. obtained similar results and suggested that additional regulation, such as modulation of the hTERT gene production or coordination with other unknown proteins, may participate in the activation of telomerase.

With regard to the relation between telomerase activity and p53 protein accumulation, our results suggested that there may be an association between telomerase activity and p53 abnormalities in precancerous lesions of the esophagus. Our data are strongly supported by recent reports that telomerase activity was controlled by wild-type p53 [26–28]. However, no report has indicated a relation of telomerase activity and *p53* gene status in precancerous lesions of the esophagus. When we included mucosal lesions in the analysis, there was a significant correlation between p53 protein accumulation and telomerase activity. Taken together, our data suggest that p53 may take part in the control of telomerase activity during esophageal carcinogenesis, but further large-scale analysis is needed in this matter.

Conclusions

Telomerase activity in Lugol-stained areas may predict the development of esophageal abnormal mucosa, especially cancer. There is a possibility that high telomerase activity in normal esophageal epithelium leads to a tendency of cancerization in which the entire esophagus may be considered as a single area of carcinogenesis. Therefore, high telomerase activity in the Lugol-stained areas cannot be used as a diagnostic marker for ESC but may be a marker of high risk for ESC.

References

1. Parkln DM, Prsani P, Feriay J (1999) Estimates of the worldwide incidence of 25 major cancers in 1990. Int J Cancer 80:827–841
2. Kuwano H, Ohno S, Matsuoka H, et al (1988) Serial histologic evaluation of multiple primary squamous cell carcinomas of the esophagus. Cancer 61:1635–1638
3. Pesko P, Rakic S, Milicevic M, et al (1994) Prevalence and clinicopathological features of multiple squamous cell carcinoma of the esophagus. Cancer 73:2687–2690
4. Takubo K, Nakamura K, Izumiya N, et al (1997) Telomerase activity in esophageal carcinoma. J Surg Oncol 66:88–92
5. Bachor C, Bachor OA, Boukamp P (1999) Telomerase is active in normal gastrointestinal mucosa and not up-regulated in precancerous lesions. J Cancer Res Clin Oncol 125:453–460
6. Ikeguchi M, Unate H, Maeta M, et al (1999) Detection of telomerase activity in esophageal squamous cell carcinoma and normal esophageal epithelium. Langenbecks Arch Surg 384:550–555
7. Dawsey SM, Fleischer DE, Wang GQ, et al (1998) Mucosal iodine staining improves endoscopic visualization of squamous dysplasia and squamous cell carcinoma of the esophagus in Linxian, China. Cancer 83:220–231
8. Mori M, Adachi Y, Matsushima T, et al (1993) Lugol staining pattern and histology of esophageal lesions. Am J Gastroenterol 88:701–705
9. Takakura M, Kyo S, Kanaya T, et al (1998) Expression of human telornerase subunits and correlation with telomerase activity in cervical cancer. Cancer Res 58:1558–1561
10. Kiaris H, Schally AV (1999) Decrease in telomerase activity in U-87MG human glioblastomas after treatment with an antagonist of growth hormone-releasing hormone. Proc Natl Acad Sci USA 96:226–231
11. Tian D, Feng Z, Hanley NM, et al (1998) Multifocal accumulation of p53 protein in esophageal carcinoma: evidence for field cancerization. Int J Cancer 78:568–575
12. Shi ST, Feng B, Yang GY, et al (1996) Immunohistoselective sequencing (IHSS) of p53 tumor suppressor gene in human oesophageal precancerous lesions. Carcinogenesis 17:2131–2136
13. Parenti AR, Rugge M, Frizzera E, et al (1995) P53 overexpression in the multistep process of esophageal carcinogenesis. Am J Surg Pathol 19:1418–1422
14. Volant A, Nousbaum JB, Giroux MA, et al (1995) P53 protein accumulation in oesophageal squamous cell carcinomas and precancerous lesions. J Clin Pathol 48:531–534
15. Wang LD, Hong JY, Qiu SL, et al (1993) Accumulation of p53 protein in human esophageal precancerous lesions: a possible early biomarker for carcinogenesis. Cancer Res 53:1783–1787
16. Bennett WP, Hollstein MC, Metcalf RA, et al (1992) P53 mutation and protein accumulation during multistage human esophageal carcinogenesis. Cancer Res 52:6092–6097
17. Cheng AJ, Tang R, Wang JY, et al (1999) Polymerase chain reaction-based enzyme immunoassay for quantitation of telomerase activity: application to colorectal cancers. Jpn J Cancer Res 90:280–285
18. Kruppe G, Kuhne K, Tamm S, et al (1997) Molecular basis of artifacts in the detection of telomerase activity and a modified primer for a more robust "TRAP" assay. Nucleic Acids Res 25:919–921
19. Klapper W, Singh KK, Heidorn K, et al (1998) Regulation of telomerase activity in quiescent immortalized human cells. Biochim Biophys Acta 1442:120–126
20. Uchida S, Shimada Y, Watanabe G, et al (1998) In oesophageal squamous carcinoma vascular endotherial growth factor is associated with p53 mutation, advanced stage and poor prognosis. Br J Cancer 77:1704–1709

21. Casey G, Lopez ME, Ramos JC, et al (1996) DNA sequence analysis of exon 2 through 11 and immunohistochemical staining are required to detect all known p53 alterations in human malignancies. Oncogene 13:1971–1981
22. Inai M, Kano M, Shimada Y et al (2001) Telomerase activity of the lugol-stained and unstained squamous epithelia in process of the oesophageal carcinogenesis, Br J Cancer (in press)
23. Koyanagi K, Ozawa S, Ando N, et al (1999) Clinical significance of telomerase activity in the non-cancerous epithelial region of oesophageal squamous cell carcinoma. Br J Surg 86:674–679
24. Koyanagi K, Ozawa S, Ando N, et al (2000) Telomerase activity as an indicator of malignant potential in iodine-nonreactive lesions of the esophagus. Cancer 88:1524–1529
25. Nakano K, Watney E, McDougall JK (1998) Telomerase activity and expression of telomerase RNA component and telomerase catalyiic subunit gene in cervical cancer. Am J Pathol 153:857–864
26. Xu D, Wang Q, Gruber A, et al (2000) Downregulation of temolerase reverse transcriptase mRNA expression by wild type p53 in human tumor cells. Oncogene 19:5123–5133
27. Kanaya T, Kyo S, Hamada K, et al (2000) Adenoviral expression of p53 represses telomerase activity through down-regulation of human telomerase reverse transcriptase transcription. Clin Cancer Res 6:1239–1247
28. Kusumoto M, Ogawa T, Mizumoto K, et al (1999) Adenovirus-mediated p53 gene transduction inhibits telomerase activity independent of its effects on cell cycle arrest and apoptosis in human pancreatic cancer cells. Clin Cancer Res 5:2140–2147

Q & A after Dr. Shimada's presentation

Dr. Jankowski (Bermingham University, UK): Your most interesting finding was the increased telomerase activity in esophagitis. It would be interesting to follow these individuals and see what happens to telomerase activity after esophagitis because that is perhaps the key.

Dr. Shimada: It may be infiltrating lymphocytes or other mesenchymal cells that express telomerase activity. We checked hTERT signals, but they are not as strong. I guess other epithelial cells are stimulated by mesenchymal cells.

Dr. Jankowski: Is there any other analogy between inflammatory situations? What happens to telomerase activity in inflammatory bowel disease, for example, or *Helicobacter*-associated gastritis?

Dr. Shimada: There are no data on *Helicobacter pylori.*

Dr. Ozawa (Keio University, Japan): Did you evaluate the telomerase activity during the healing process of the esophagitis?

Dr. Shimada: No, not during the active stage in this group selected by iodine staining.

Dr. Rubio (Karolinska Institute, Sweden): We have learned about the biology of esophageal cancer by studying biomarkers, but biomarkers are just that—indicators, not diagnostic procedures. The correlation between biomarkers and histology depends on the reliability of the classification of the histological preparations used by pathologists. This histological classification varies among institutions throughout the world, so the correlation between biomarkers and histology may vary among these institutions. Histology, with all its pitfalls, will remain the gold standard for choosing treatments for some time. The challenge in the future will be to close the gap among pathologists throughout the world, perhaps by using the Vienna classification internationally.

Part 6
Less-Invasive Treatment of Superficial Esophageal Neoplasms

Laparoscopy- and Thoracoscopy-Assisted Esophagectomy for Squamous Cell Carcinoma of the Esophagus

Haruhiro Inoue[1], Tatsuya Yoshida[1], Shinsuke Usui[1], Shin-ei Kudo[1], Tatsuyuki Kawano[2], and Mitsuo Endo[2]

Introduction

The laparoscopic procedure has already been accepted as the gold standard for cholecystectomy and has several major advantages. One is the small surgical wound, which reduces postoperative wound pain and postoperative respiratory dysfunction. Another advantage is that it maintains a better endoscopic magnified view of the surgical field, which enables fine surgical manipulation with less bleeding when hemostatic procedures are performed meticulously.

Recently there have been reports on the application of thoracoscopic and/or laparoscopic procedures in esophagectomy in advanced-stage esophageal cancer [1–7]. We have also attempted to apply endoscopic surgical techniques in esophagectomy, intending to establish a novel surgical procedure resulting in less surgical stress. In our initial experience, we attempted to perform the abdominal phase of this procedure using a purely laparoscopic approach, but that proved frustrating and time-consuming. Therefore, we changed from the pure laparoscopic approach to hand-assisted laparoscopic surgery (HALS) [8]. The abdominal phase of this surgery is a faster and more reliable procedure when HALS is utilized.

Procedures

Laparoscopy- and Thoracoscopy-Assisted Esophagectomy Utilizing HALS Techniques

In the abdominal and neck phases of surgery, the patient is fixed on the operating table in the lithotomy position. Cervical esophageal dissection is carried out through an open incision in the left neck. The cervical esophagus is exposed and divided in the neck. Simultaneously, the abdominal surgical team performs gastric mobilization utilizing HALS techniques.

[1]Digestive Disease Center, Showa University Northern Yokohama Hospital, Yokohama 224-8503, Japan
[2]Department of Surgery, Tokyo Medical and Dental University, Tokyo, Japan

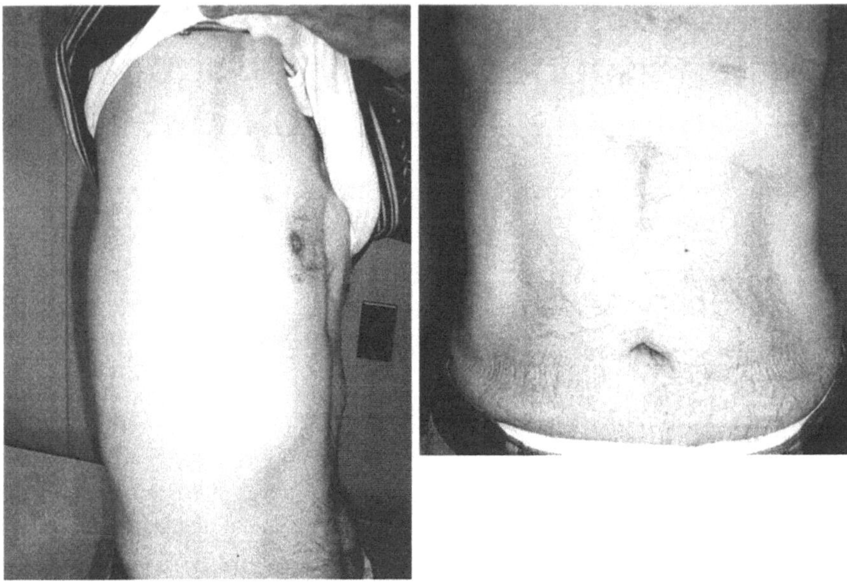

a b

FIG. 1. Surgical wounds after hand-assisted laparascopic surgery for esophageal cancer. **a** Right chest wall. Small incision scars are observed. **b** Abdominal wall. A 6.5-cm upper midline incision and some small incision scars are observed

First, a 6.5-cm midline incision is made in the upper abdomen (Fig. 1). The left hand of the first surgeon is inserted into the abdominal cavity through that small incision. Pneumoperitoneum is maintained at approximately 12 mmHg. Three ports are inserted into the abdominal cavity in the left upper quadrant of the abdomen. Gastric mobilization begins at the lesser omentum of the stomach, mainly utilizing ultrasonic coagulating scissors. The abdominal esophagus is dissected and divided using a mechanical stapler. After dissecting the short gastric vessels, the dissection proceeds to the greater curvature of the stomach. The right gastroepiploic artery and vein are preserved as feeding vessels of the gastric tube. The left gastric artery and vein are laparoscopically dissected and divided using a mechanical stapler.

After completing laparoscopic mobilization of the upper two-thirds of the stomach, the mobilized stomach is removed from the abdominal cavity through the small HALS incision. A gastric tube is created with open surgical techniques outside the abdominal cavity. A retrosternal route is also created by blunt dissection with the first surgeon's left hand. In the neck, a pulled-up gastric tube is anastomosed with the previously divided cervical esophagus using a mechanical circular stapler. This completes the reconstructive process with the gastric tube.

In the thoracic phase of the surgery, the patient's position is changed to the left lateral. Single-lung ventilation after collapsing the right lung is carried out by an anesthetist to obtain a better thoracoscopic view. Dissection of the isolated thoracic esophagus starts by dividing the azygos arch. Dissection of the upper thoracic esophagus is completed, with preservation of the bilateral recurrent laryngeal nerves. The middle and lower thoracic esophagus is dissected along the esophagus. Lymph nodes along the thoracic esophagus are also resected when total esophagectomy is intended. The resected thoracic esophagus and lymph nodes are removed through a small thoracic incision. After achieving complete hemostasis, the entire procedure is completed.

Indications

When we began to use this procedure in 1997, we limited the indications to T1N0 lesions, because the level of lymph node dissection during this procedure had not yet reached the level possible during open surgery. After our initial experience, we extended the indications to T2 and T3 lesions with lymph node metastasis. In addition, when difficulties are encountered in achieving optimum lymph node dissection during endoscopic surgery we do not hesitate to convert to an open procedure.

Results

Twenty-five patients with squamous cell carcinoma of the esophagus have undergone endoscopic esophagectomy by our team. (Twenty cases in Tokyo Medical and Dental University, five cases in Showa Univeristy Northern Yokohama Hospital). Thirteen had T1 carcinomas, and the other seven had T2, T3 lesions. Laparo- and thoracoscopic esophagectomy was successful in 16 patients. In the remaining four endoscopic surgery was converted to an open procedure: one patient with chronic cholecystitis required open laparotomy because of a severe adhesion; two with T3, T4 lesions needed open thoracotomy to resect the tumor in an en-bloc manner; and in one injury to the right lung was repaired through open thoracotomy.

The mean postoperative hospital stay was 25.5 days. There have been no fatal complications. Two patients developed temporary laryngeal nerve palsy. During the maximum 4-year follow-up period, two patients died of liver, bone, and skin metastases with mediastinal tumor recurrences.

Discussion

The prognosis of advanced-stage esophageal cancer remains poor. According to the comprehensive registry in Japan, the 5-year overall survival rate is approximately 35%. The prognosis of esophageal cancer patients is mainly decided by disease stage. In particular, the number of lymph node metastases affects prognosis.

Open esophagectomy is one of the most invasive types of surgery, requiring three-field lymph node dissection in the neck, thorax, and abdomen. To reduce the invasiveness of esophageal surgery, we developed an endoscopic procedure utilizing the HALS technique in 1997 for the treatment of esophageal cancer. The small surgical wound minimizes the injury to the chest and abdominal walls, with less impairment of respiratory function.

The abdominal and neck phases of this technique are well established. In the thoracic phase, dissection along the esophagus is sometimes complicated and time-consuming, particularly when a patient has pleural adhesions. With further improvement of the procedure during the thorax phase, we believe that this surgery will becomes the standard procedure for advanced esophageal cancer surgery.

References

1. McAnena OJ, Rojers J, Williams NS (1994) Right thoracoscopically assisted esophagectomy for cancer. Br J Surg 81:236–238
2. Law S, Fok M, Chu KM, Wong J (1997) Thoracoscopic esophagectomy for eosphageal cancer. Surgery 122:8–14
3. Robertson GM, Lloyd DM, Wicks AC, Veich PS (1996) No obvious advantages for thracoscopic two-stage oesophagectomy. Br J Surg 83:675–678
4. Jagot P, Sauvanet A, Berthoux L, Belghiti J (1996) Laparoscopic mobilization of the stomach for replacement. Br J Surgery 83:675–678
5. Akaishi T, Kaneda I, Higuchi N, et al (1996) Thoracoscopic en bloc total esophagectomy with radical mediastinal lymphadenectomy. J Thorac Cardiovasc Surg 112:1533–1541
6. DePaula AL, Hashiba K, Ferreira EA et al (1995) Laparoscopic transhiatal esophagectomy with esophagogastroplasty. Surg Laparosc Endosc 5:1–5
7. Swanstrom LL, Hansen P (1997) Laparoscopic total esophagectomy. Arch Surg 132: 943–949
8. Kusminsky RE, Boland JP, Tiley EH et al (1995) Hand-assisted laparoscopic splenectomy. Surg Laparosc Endosc 5:463–467

Q & A after Dr. Inoue's presentation

Dr. Udagawa (Toranomon Hospital, Japan): The quality of LN dissection is far from that seen with thoracotomy. This kind of effort is necessary if there is to be further advancement in this area. What are your indications for this procedure?

Dr. Inoue: We limit the procedure to T1 and T2 lesions with no LN involvement based on our preoperative evaluation of the patient.

Dr. Hölscher (University of Cologne, Germany): I agree with Dr. Udagawa. At the moment I don't see where this procedure stands in our armamentarium, especially as you have to perform one-lung ventilation to these patients, don't you? In my opinion, you could also do blunt dissection without thoracotomy because most of the LNs we remove during en bloc esophagectomy (for example, bifurcational LNs) remain with this procedure. The clear dissection you perform does not seem risky. The extent of the lymphadenectomy seems more similar to a transhiatal dissection than to a transthoracic dissection.

Dr. Inoue: For now, the quality of LN dissection during my procedure is limited. I therefore select patients whose tumors are limited to the esophageal wall, not exposed to the adventitia, and with no evidence of LN involvement. That's the reason we have so far performed only 25 of these procedures. With some refinement of the device (for example, the lung retractor) I believe we could obtain a better endoscopic view; and if we had better hemostatic devices, we could perform a much better lymphadenectomy. At the moment, I think this procedure will be accepted as one of the standard techniques for esophageal cancer patients. Of course, I know that many doctors perform laparoscopic transhiatal resection, as started by Depaula in Brazil. With the transhiatal procedure, lymphadenectomy is extremely limited in the lower third or middle third of the esophagus. With our procedure, we can probably approach the paratracheal LNs, so I would like to improve the procedure.

Dr. Bumm (Technische University, München, Germany): Have you seen any port-site metastases in your patients?

Dr. Inoue: So far we have not experienced any port-site metastases. One of the reasons, I think, is that among our 25 cases only 10 had LN metastases, and in those cases there was only one LN involved. Moreover, cancer infiltration was limited to T2 at worst. We have also started to use a special device for a hand-assisted procedure, and I have started to use hand-ports that cover the open wound to avoid port-site recurrence of the tumor.

Benefits and Limitations of Mediastinal Endodissection During Radical Transhiatal Esophagectomy

RUDOLF BUMM and J. RÜDIGER SIEWERT

Introduction

Transhiatal esophagectomy (THE) is used in many centers to remove the thoracic esophagus. This one-cavity procedure has theoretical advantages in terms of reducing the operative risk but has been described as a nonradical operation with limited control of mediastinal resection margins because of the blunt dissection.

The concept of THE was proposed during the early twentieth century by Denk [1] in Austria, and the operation was first performed by Turner [2] and Fischer [3]. In recent decades THE was rediscovered by several groups and was made popular by Orringer and Sloan [4–6].

In 1990 Buess and coworkers described an endoscopic technique for dissecting the thoracic esophagus from the neck under direct vision [7–9]. To improve the THE technique we modified, evaluated, and applied it clinically in larger series [10, 11]. We defined the mediastinoscopic dissection of the thoracic esophagus as "endodissection" and added extensive regional lymphadenectomy and radical transhiatal en bloc resection of the primary tumor to our standard procedure. A similar modification (transhiatal en bloc resection of the primary tumor) has been reported by Alderson et al. [12].

The natural history, risk pattern, prognosis, and local tumor spread differ for adenocarcinoma and squamous cell carcinoma of the esophagus [13, 14]. Therefore, our institution has defined precise surgical strategies for both subtypes.

Radical THE combined with endodissection is routinely used in our institution for esophagectomy in patients with adenocarcinoma of the distal esophagus [13]. In more recent years, transthoracic en bloc esophagectomy with intrathoracic anastomosis (TIA) and limited resection of the distal esophagus and interposition of a jejunal segment (LIM, also called Merendino's procedure) are alternatives in selected patients. TIA is used in patients with an adenocarcinoma and enlarged mediastinal lymph nodes. LIM can be offered for early adenocarcinoma of the distal esophagus and high-grade dysplasia. In turn, transthoracic en bloc esophagectomy (TTE) with gastric interposition and cervical esophagogastrostomy is used primarily for

Department of Surgery, TU Munich, Ismaningerstrasse 22, D-81675 Munich, Germany resectable squamous cell carcinoma. This paper describes the benefits and limitations of endodissection during radical transhiatal esophagectomy.

Technique

The technique for radical transhiatal esophagectomy with endodissection has been reported in several recent publications. In short, the operation begins with bringing the patient into a supine position and disinfecting the skin. We usually have two operating teams, as outlined in Fig. 1. The esophagus should be intubated with a rigid rubber tube. The cervical team mobilizes the esophagus via a left cervical access (Fig. 2) and performs mediastinal endodissection; the other (abdominal) team performs en bloc resection of the primary tumor with lymphadenectomy and preparation of the gastric tube.

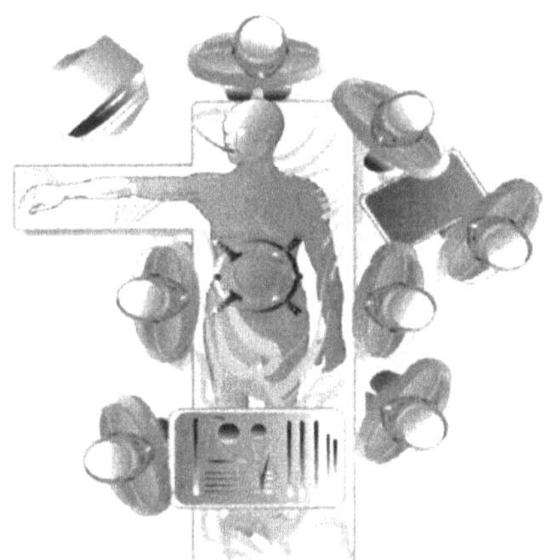

FIG. 1. Position of the operating team. (From [11], with permission)

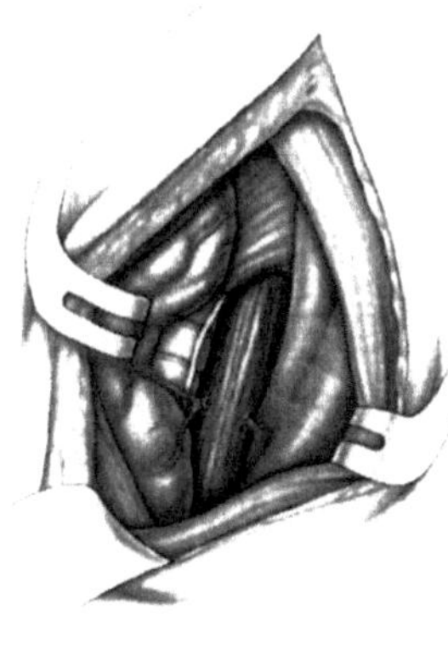

FIG. 2. Cervical access showing the carotid artery and jugular vein (right), esophagus and left recurrent nerve. (Modified from [11], with permission)

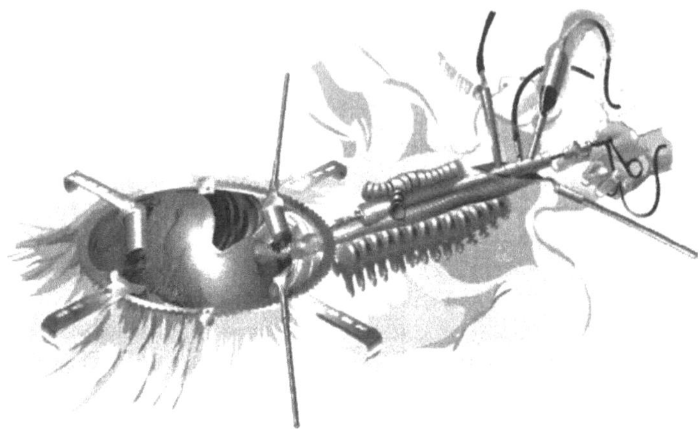

FIG. 3. En bloc resection of the primary tumor, combined with simultaneous endodissection

Cervical Procedure and Endodissection

The cervical incision (Fig. 2) is made at the anterior edge of the sternocleidomastoids muscle. The cervical esophagus is dissected after division of the omohyoid muscle and the inferior thyroid artery. The recurrent laryngeal nerve must be identified and carefully preserved.

The mediastinal endodissector (Fig. 3) is then assembled and inserted into the upper mediastinum. This instrument (Storz, Tuttlingen, Germany) features a tissue dilator at the tip, a 15° Hopkins fiberoptic device, and a working channel for one 5-mm laparoscopic instrument. The tissue dilator is anatomically designed so it can "ride" on the esophageal surface and opens an anterograde dissection space of 2–3 cm in the mediastinum. The tissued dilator of the mediastinoscope can be freely rotated 360°. For full operation the mediastinoscope is connected to a video camera (Storz endocamera), a xenon light source, and a flushing/suction device.

It is normal that the first steps of endoscopic dissection of the retrotracheal space are difficult owing to the limited initial vision and the anatomical narrowing behind the jugulum. Microinstruments such as scissors, forceps, or a coagulation/suction instrument can be used through the working channel of the mediastinoscope. The retrotracheal tissues are divided by pushing the tissue with the coagulation/suction device followed by application of a short "coagulation" impulse. Direct dissection with the scissor is also possible but not often recommended owing to the risk of damage to the mediastinal structures such as the trachea. The anterior surface of the esophagus is subsequently dissected to 2–3 cm below the tracheal bifurcation, which can be easily identified. With retraction of the mediastinoscope there is an excellent view of the back wall of the trachea and the tracheal bifurcation (Fig. 4). Visible lymph nodes should be totally removed and lymph node biopsy specimens attained. The tissue dilator at the tip of the instrument is then rotated anteclockwise so all surfaces of the esophagus can be dissected. The problematic area of the dissection is the left main

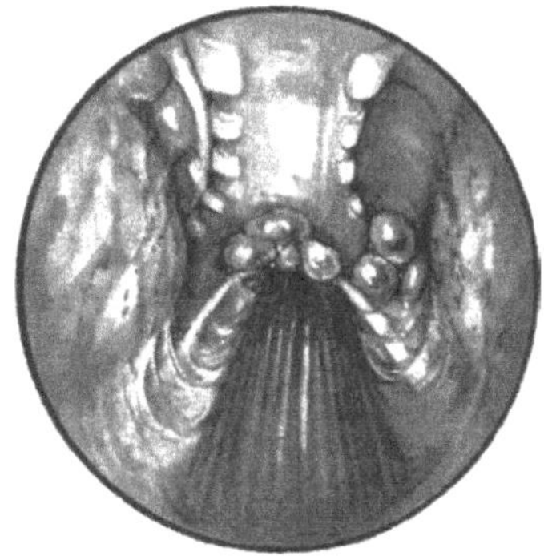

FIG. 4. Endodissection. Anterior view with tracheal bifurcation (*middle*) and mediastinal lymph nodes, left recurrent nerve and anterior surface of the esophagus (*below*) (From [11], with permission)

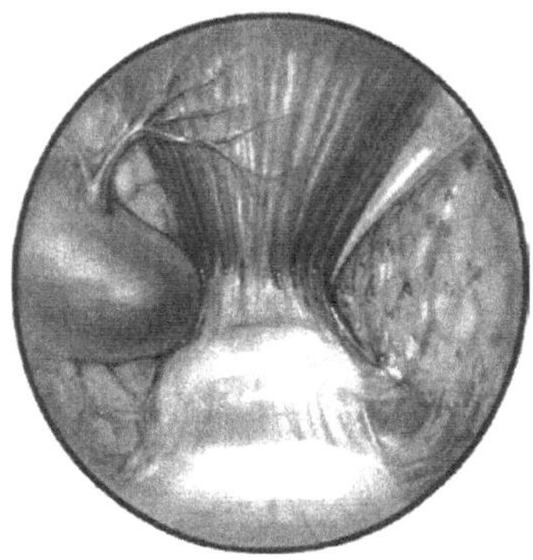

FIG. 5. Endodissection. Posterior view with esophageal back wall (*top*), spine (*below*), and pleural layers as well as a direct nutritional artery from a bronchial artery. (From [11], with permission)

bronchus, where one often finds physiologic embryonic adhesions/ligaments. Care must be taken not to divide the longitudinal muscle layer of the esophagus. The back wall (Fig. 5) and the right surface of the esophagus usually present no major difficulties, and opening the mediastinal pleura is not critical. It is advisable for the abdominal team (see below) to keep the hiatus closed during mediastinal dissection to avoid flooding the mediastinum with lavage fluids. At the end of the mediastinal dissection, contact between the cervical and abdominal teams should be made. The cervical team assists during the phase of en bloc dissection of the infracarinal esophagus (Fig. 4) by providing light and suction from above. This can be helpful especially with large tumors. Finally, the cervical esophagus is divided by a longitudinal stapling device and is retracted into the abdominal cavity. The mediastinal procedure is completed by controlling hemorrhage and removing the visible lymph nodes to provide supplementary staging information.

Abdominal Procedure

The abdominal team performs an inverse-T laparotomy. The routine replacement for the resected esophagus is a gastric tube. The duodenum is well mobilized in an extended Kocher procedure, and the gastrocolic ligaments are divided, carefully preserving the gastroepiploic arcade.

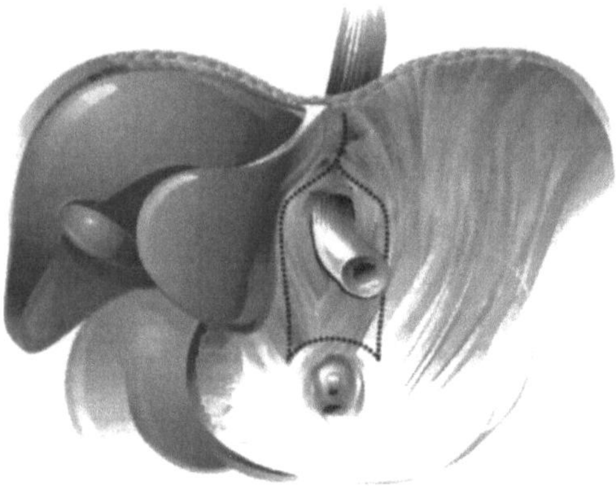

FIG. 6. Excision of the crura of the diaphragm and hiatal incision line during transhiatal esophagectomy

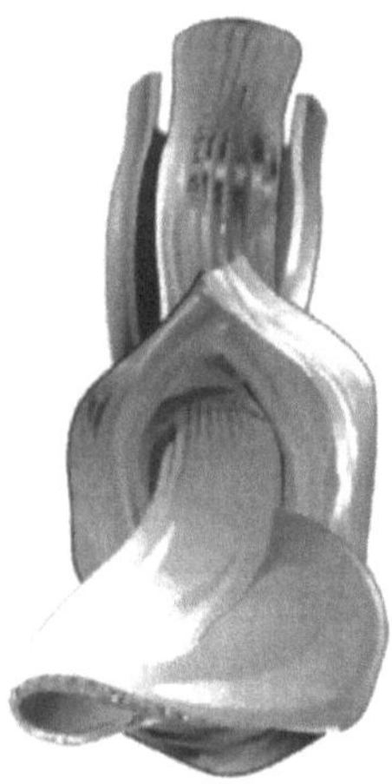

FIG. 7. Tumor in the distal esophagus, both pleural layers, crura of the diaphragm, and fundus. All should be resected during radical transhiatal esophagectomy

When endodissection is nearly completed, the abdominal team opens the hiatus widely by excising portions of the crura of the diaphragm (left adherent to the specimen) (Fig. 6) and dividing the diaphragmatic vein between clamps. Palpation of the lower mediastinum establishes that the primary tumor is located in the infracarinal segment of the esophagus. The periesophageal mediastinal fat and lymphatic tissue is dissected from the pericardium and remains adherent to the specimen in en bloc fashion (Fig. 7). The primary tumor should not be exposed during the operation. Both visceral layers of the pleura may be resected without a problem if necessary. Figure 8 shows a final view into the lower mediastinum.

When the specimen is completely mobilized, the cervical team divides the cervical esophagus with a linear stapler, and the esophagus is retracted into the abdominal cavity. Finally, abdominal lymphadenectomy is performed involving the lymph nodes along the hepatic artery, splenic artery, and upper margin of the pancreas.

A narrow gastric tube is constructed using a linear stapling device. Finally, the gastric tube is retracted into the posterior mediastinum to the cervical incision, where

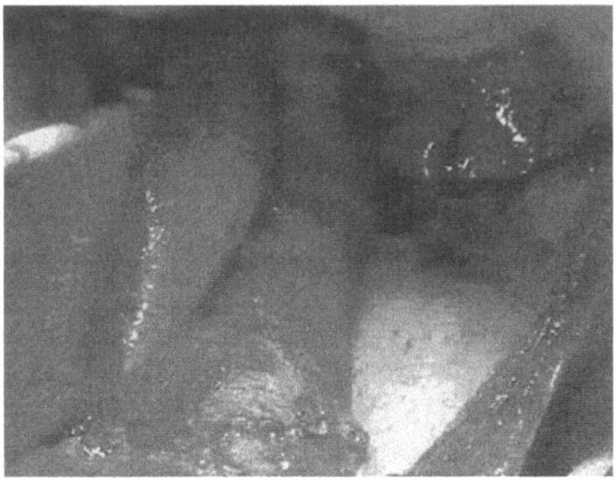

FIG. 8. Final transhiatal view from the abdominal position after radical transhiatal esophagectomy

a esophagogastrostomy is performed end to end or end to side by single sutures. The anterior reconstruction route is sometimes used when there is an extensive tumor to ensure uncomplicated postoperative irradiation of the posterior mediastinum.

Results

Between July 1982 and December 1999 a total of 304 patients [266 men (87.5%) and 38 women (12.5%), with a median age of 60 years] underwent THE in our department. Most of these patients suffered from adenocarcinoma of the esophagus (n = 259, 85.2%). The other patients had squamous cell carcinoma (n = 32, 10.5%) or other reasons for esophagectomy such as f.e. acid ingestion or spontaneus perforation (n = 13, 4.3%). Altogether, 74 patients were subjected to a neoadjuvant treatment protocol prior to esophagectomy (24.3%). The frequency of esophagectomy being performed in our department increased over the years. Micro- and macroscopically complete tumor resection (R0 resection according to the UICC was recorded in 80% of all patients. There was a 4.9% (n = 15) overall hospital mortality, with an overall decreasing tendency over the years, and a 37.5% overall complication rate (excluding minor cervical fistulas) in the total cohort.

A prospective study [5] revealed that addition of en bloc resection and endodissection techniques (radical transhiatal esophagectomy, or RTE) improved the short-term and long-term results. Patients after RTE suffered from fewer pulmonary (18.9% vs. 27.9%) and cardiac (2% vs. 12%) complications. In addition, we were able to demonstrate a prognostic benefit for patients after RTE over THE (5-year survival: 40% vs. 20%, [4]) and a larger number of resected mediastinal and abdominal lymph nodes than with the standard THE.

Benefits of Endodissection

Endodissection is an excellent supplementary technique during RTE, mainly for the following reasons: First, endodissection can be performed independently of the abdominal team, which is a time-saver during the procedure because the abdominal team is presented with a predissected mediastinum when opening the hiatus. Second, visual control of the mediastinal dissection can be indispensable in patients with large tumors or after neoadjuvant radiation therapy, when mediastinal tissue resistance is abnormal. Third, endodissection offers mediastinal lymph node sampling, which adds valuable information for the overall tumor staging of the patient. Fourth, at the end of the transhiatal esophagectomy, assistance of the cervical team (suction, light source) can ease the critical transhiatal en bloc resection of the distal esophagus.

Limitations of Endodissection

The current technique of endodissection is limited by the following facts. The oncological part of the operation must be done transhiatally by an open classical dissection technique. Currently, endodissection is used to dissect the healthy esophagus. Because of the construction of the mediastinoscope, there can be only one instrument in the working channel, which makes the dissection cumbersome. The mediastinoscope is a rigid instrument that is limited in its "angle of attack," especially farther down in the mediastinum. En bloc resection of the suprabifurcational thoracic esophagus is not possible with endodissection for anatomical reasons: The esophagus should always be in sight during the whole dissection. Furthermore, our clinical data have not demonstrated fewer recurrent nerve palsies when endodissection is accomplished.

Conclusions

Endodissection is an excellent supplementary technique during THE. As the incidence of adenocarcinoma arising from Barrett's epithelium increases worldwide, there is a need for a standard surgical procedure in these patients. As noted before, radical THE combined with endodissection may be a major candidate for this procedure during the next decade. Endodissection can be further improved technically by allowing multiple instruments to be used at the same time, bipolar electrocoagulation, and an ultrasound knife. A combination of endodissection and laparoscopic abdominal dissection is a true minor-access procedure that should be evaluated.

References

1. Denk W (1913) Zur Radikaloperation des Ösophaguskarzinoms. Zentralblatt Chir 40:1065–1069
2. Turner GG (1933) Excision of the thoracic esophagus for carcinoma with construction of an extrathoracic gullet. Lancet 2:13–15
3. Fischer AW (1937) Erfolgreiche Entfernung eines Krebses der Speiseröhre nach dem abdominocollaren Durchzugsverfahren. Laugenbeck, Arch Chir 189:498–503
4. Orringer MB (1984) Transhiatal esophagectomy without thoracotomy for carcinoma of the thoracic esophagus. Ann Surg 200:282–288
5. Orringer MB (1985) Transhiatal esophagectomy for benign disease. J Thorac Cardiovasc Surg 90:649–655

6. Orringer MB, Marshall B, Iannettoni MD (1999) Transhiatal esophagectomy: clinical experience and refinements. Ann Surg 230:392–403
7. Buess G, Becker HD, Mentges R, Teichmann R, Lenz G (1990) Die endoskopisch-mikrochirurgische Dissektion der Speiseröhre. Chirurg 61:308–311
8. Kipfmüller K, Buess G, Nahrun M, Bätz W (1990) Die endoskopisch-mikrochirurgische Dissektion der Speiseröhre: eine tierexperimentelle Studie. Chirurg 61:187–191
9. Kipfmüller K, Duda D, Kessler S, Melzer A, Buess G (1990) Die endoskopische-mikrochirurgische Dissektion der Speiseröhre: ein Beitrag zur Reduzierung pulmonaler Komplikationen nach Ösophagusresektion? Eine vergleichende tierexperimentelle Studie. Langenbecks Arch Chir 375:11–18
10. Bumm R, Hölscher AH, Feussner H, Tachibana M, Bartels H, Siewert JR (1993) Endodissection of the thoracic esophagus: technique and clinical results in transhiatal esophagectomy. Ann Surg 218:97–104
11. Bumm R, Hölscher AH, Siewert JR (1994) Transmediastinal endodissection. In: Peters JH, DeMeester TR (eds) Minimally invasive surgery of the foregut. Quality Medical Publishing, St. Louis, pp 250–261
12. Alderson D, Courtney SP, Kennedy RH (1994) Radical transhiatal oesophagectomy under direct vision. Br J Surg 81:404–407
13. Siewert JR, Hölscher AH, Horvath OP (1986) Transmediastinale Ösophagektomie. Langenbecks Arch Chir 367:203–213
14. Siewert JR, Hölscher AH, Roder J, Bartels H (1988) En bloc Resektion der Speiseröhre beim Ösophaguskarzinom. Langenbecks Arch Chir 373:367–376
15. Bumm R, Feussner H, Bartels H, Stein H, Dittler HJ, Höfler H, Siewert JR (1997) Radical transhiatal esophagectomy with two field lymphadenectomy and endodissection for distal esophageal adenocarcinoma. World J Surg 21:822–831

Q & A after Dr. Bumm's presentation

Dr. Aikou (Kagoshima University, Japan): Which LN is the sentinel node for type 1 tumors? When you find the involved node in the upper mediastinum, do you open the chest? Do you perform conventional lymphadenectomy in such a case?

Dr. Bumm: We usually perform your kind of lymph node sampling, sending the nodes to the pathologist and changing the strategy of the operation depending on the results. We try en bloc removal of the inferior esophagus and the lower mediastinum. Only if we have the impression when we open the diaphragm or when we do the dissection with endoscopy, that there are many LNs that may be tumor-invaded do we switch to thoracotomy. That does not happen frequently. Usually we do the operation we planned.

Dr. Udagawa (Toranomon Hospital, Japan): You concluded that upper mediastinal LNs were not particularly important in your series based on your limited sampling of LN data, but your No patients still had a 50%–60% five-year survival rate. This low rate may be the result of remaining metastatic LNs. What is the main pattern of recurrence? How do you plan to improve your results?

Dr. Bumm: I think that the low rate is not due only to upper mediastinal LNs and that it is not a big problem. If there are positive LNs in that position, the disease becomes systemic somehow and you cannot improve the survival of people with this disease only by surgery. Maybe we should have included more tumors with wall penetration. We couldn't show you all of our results, but we also had many T3 tumors in our series, which may be one reason for these results. In the future we must think about how to treat not adenocarcinoma of the esophagus as a whole but how to threat the very early one, the intermediate one, and the late one. We will have to do several operations. Even now, this is not the only technique we use. In some cases we also perform transthoracic resection for adenocarcinoma with intrathoracic anastomosis, so it's not as easy as it was about 5 years ago when we only had two operating techniques available. Now, we have about five, and it becomes more difficult to choose the right patient for the right operation.

Dr. Udagawa: As you just said, the patients must be stratified according to the tumor infiltration depth. The location of the tumor is important too.

Dr. Merigliano (University of Padova School of Medicine, Italy): What are the indications for the transhiatal and transthoracic approaches? Which is your choice?

Dr. Bumm: We use the transthoracic approach in all patients with an SCC. If the patient with an SCC is very old and has high risk factors, sometimes we use the technique I just described, but normally we use the transthoracic approach. For adenocarcinomas, we mainly use the trans-hiatal approach and sometimes the transthoracic approach.

Dr. Hagen (University of Southern California, USA): One of the advantages you listed for transhiatal esophagectomy was the shorter operating time. It seems that addition of this endo-dissection technique would add significantly to the operating time compared to the transhiatal approach. Can you give us information about that? You also listed as one of the disadvantages of the transhiatal esophagectomy that it is a less radical procedure. This operation is intended to improve the radicality of the resection. Could you can give us information on LN yield of this operation compared to your standard transhiatal resection.

Dr. Bumm: Regarding your first question: I start with the esophagus portion of the operation, and the abdominal team starts dissecting the stomach and performing the lymphadenectomy. Hence there is no time loss with the operation. I think we even save some time because when the abdominal team open the hiatus and dissects the mediastinum they meet the predissected space, which is then easier to deal with. To answer the second question: The criticism of transhiatal esophagectomy previously was that it is not a radical operation. However, for selected tumors of the lower esophageal or infracarinal tumors, you can perform a radical operation. We have analyzed all the LNs from the operation and found the same dependencies; for example, in gastric cancer you also have the high impact of the LN ratio, which is also true for these tumors, indicating that we can sufficiently improve the results with transhiatal esophagectomy.

Mediastinoscopy-Assisted Transhiatal Esophagectomy: A Safe Technique for Squamous Cell Carcinoma of the Esophagus

Akira Tangoku, Shigefumi Yoshino, Toshihiro Abe, Katuhiko Morita, Takashi Ueno, Hideto Hayashi, and Masaaki Oka

Introduction

Esophagectomy with lymphadenectomy has improved the survival of patients with esophageal cancer [1, 2]. The morbidity and mortality associated with transthoracic (abdominothoracic) esophagectomy (TTE) is substantial, despite improvements in perioperative support, including anesthesia and postoperative intensive care [3, 4]. To decrease the complications of TTE, transhiatal esophagectomy (THE) has been adopted [5–8]. The disadvantages of THE are blind manipulation of the esophagus and the inability to perform lymph node dissection. With mediastinoscopy, THE decreased morbidity because of direct visualization of the mediastinal structures.

Indication

Transthoracic en bloc esophagectomy (TTE) [1, 2] is indicated to cure advanced tumors of the esophagus. Endoscopic mucosal resection (EMR) has been adopted for localized, superficial esophageal cancers (ep, m1, m2; invasion of the lamina propria) in which no lymphatic metastases are expected [9, 10]. Because widespread and multiple mucosal lesions require wider EMR, postoperative stenosis or perforation of the esophagus may result. Therefore mediastinoscopy assisted transhiatal esophagectomy (MATHE) is recommended in these cases. Patients with esophageal cancer are often elderly with many preoperative risks, such as diabetes mellitus, heart disease, liver cirrhosis, and pulmonary dysfunction. Because TTE causes too great surgical stress for these patients, MATHE should be selected (Fig. 1).

Mediastinoscope

A 5 mm diameter mirror scope attached to a flat retractor (Subcu-dissector, Endopath saphenous vein harvest tray; Ethicon Endosurgery, Cincinnati, OH, USA) (Fig. 2) was

Department of Digestive Surgery and Surgical Oncology, Yamaguchi University School of Medicine, 1-1-1 Minami Kogushi, Ube, Yamaguchi 755-8505, Japan

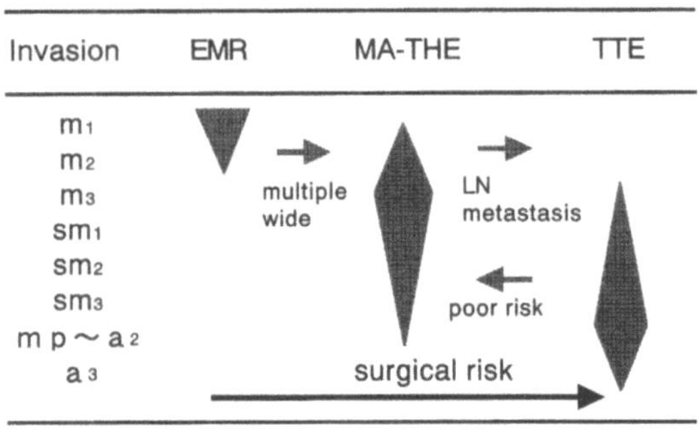

FIG. 1. Indications for mediastinoscopy-assisted transhiatal esophagectomy (*MA-THE*). Endoscopic mucosal resection (*EMR*) is selected for localized, superficial esophageal cancer (ep, m1, m2; invasion within the lamina propria). MATHE is recommended for patients with widespread and multiple lesions and for patients with preoperative risks

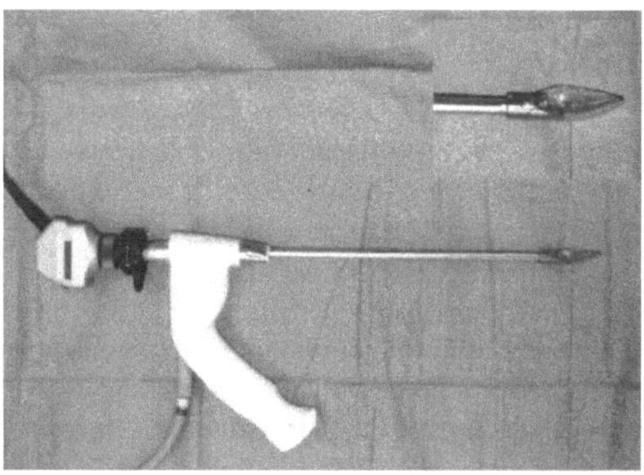

FIG. 2. Mediastinoscope. A 5 mm diameter mirror scope was used. The flat transparent retractor was necessary to create a mediastinal operating space

the mediastinoscope used. This instrument, which has no channels or openings, is necessary to create a mediastinal operating space.

Surgical Technique

The patient was placed in the supine position on the operating table with both arms tucked. One surgeon and an assistant performed MATHE via the neck while the others prepared the interposition graft and dissected the abdominal lymph nodes, terminal esophagus, and lower esophageal nodes using the mediastinoscope (Fig. 3). MATHE was started via a left cervical approach. A collar incision was made in the left anterior neck. The anterior edge of the sternocleidomastoid muscle and the anterior cervical muscles were divided. The cervical esophagus was circumferentially exposed and elevated with a rubber tube. The mediastinoscope was inserted carefully from the left side of the esophagus and pushed gently into the mediastinum. The thoracic duct was then easily retrieved on the left side of the esophagus (Fig. 4). The lymphatic and blood vessels were safely exposed and coagulated with laparosonic coagulating shears (LCS) (Harmonic Scarpel; Ethicon Endosurgery) and a coagulator, which suctioned and irrigated simultaneously (Endopath Probe Plus II; Ethicon Endosurgery). On the right side the esophagus was dissected gently with LCS, and the azygos arch and

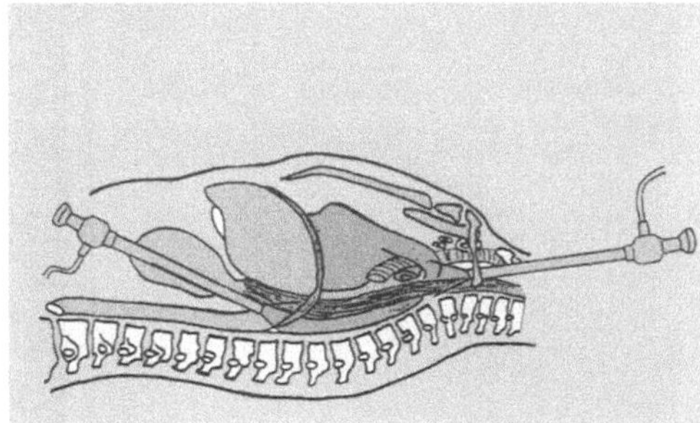

FIG. 3. Method. The mediastinoscope was inserted into the mediastinum via the neck and the hiatus. The esophagus was dissected under vision

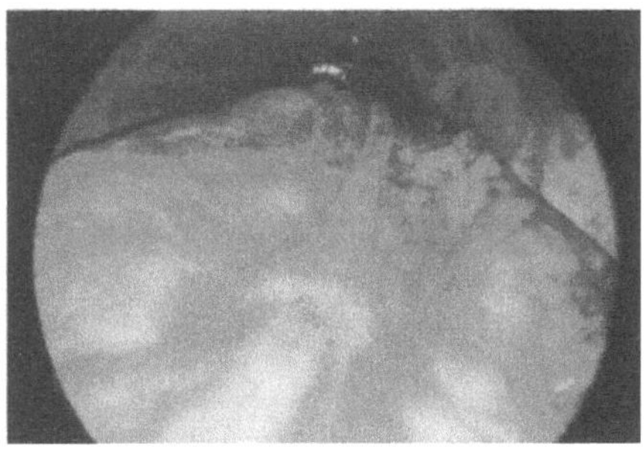

FIG. 4. Thoracic duct was easily retrieved on the left side of the esophagus

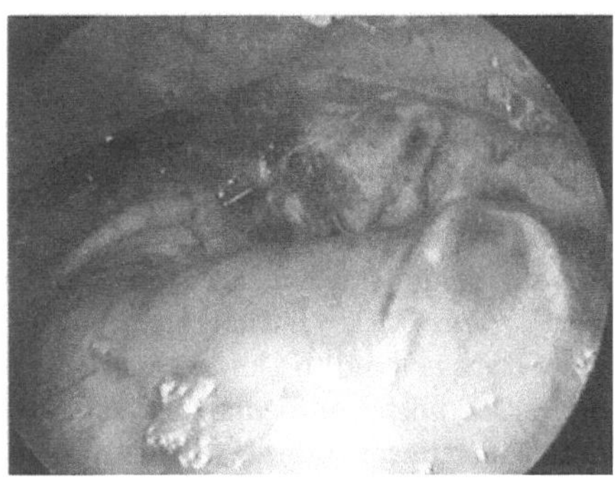

FIG. 5. Azygos arch and the bronchial artery were observed

bronchial artery were clearly exposed (Fig. 5). On the anterior side of the esophagus the tracheoesophageal ligament was divided sharply, and the tracheal bifurcation and pulmonary hilar nodes were then visible. The heart, the azygos vein, and vagal nerve were also visible. The left recurrent nerve was seen under the aortic arch and the left side of the trachea. The pararecurrent nerve nodes were carefully dissected with the LCS without damage to the recurrent nerves. After dissection the left recurrent nerve was visualized clearly (Fig. 6). The right recurrent nerve was also observed under the right edge of the trachea, and the nodes were dissected (Fig. 7). The upper thoracic

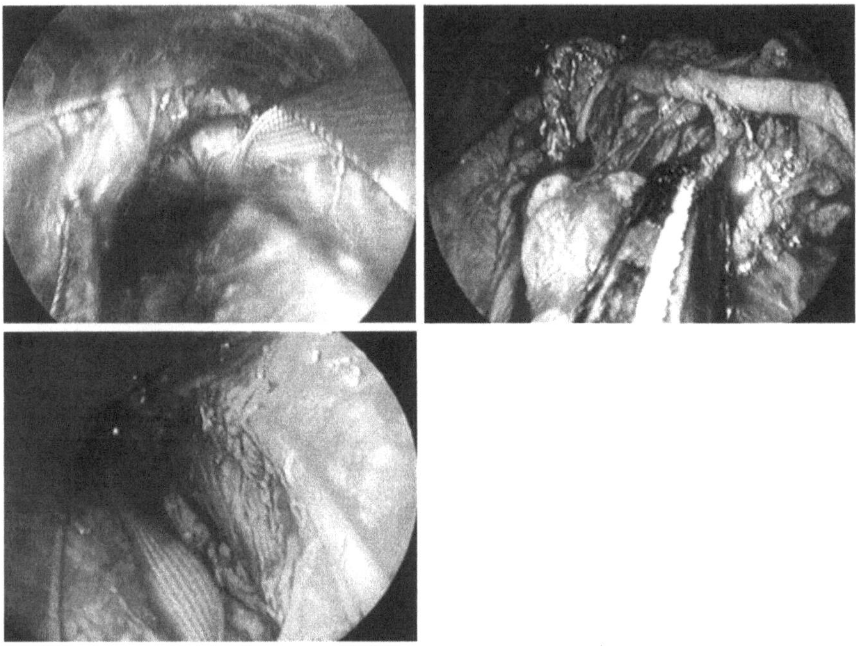

a b c

FIG. 6. Under the aortic arch the left main bronchus and left recurrent nerve were clearly observed (**a**). The left recurrent nerve is seen under the left side of the trachea. The pararecurrent nerve nodes were carefully dissected with laparosonic coagulating shears (LCS) (**b**). After dissection the left recurrent nerve was visualized clearly (**c**)

paraesophageal and lower paraesophageal lymph nodes were exposed and dissected together with the esophagus (Fig. 8). During this procedure by the cervical team, the abdominal team prepared the interposition graft. The stomach was used in all but three patients who had previously undergone gastrectomy and two patients with gastric cancer. The gastric lymph nodes (right cardiac, left cardiac, lesser curve, left gastric artery) and the lower thoracic paraesophageal lymph nodes, diaphragmatic nodes, and posterior mediastinal nodes were dissected. The esophagus was cut in the neck with a linear cutter (Proximate Linear Cutter; Ethicon Endosurgery). The esophagus was pulled through from the mediastinum toward the abdomen as the dissection was completed. The mediastinoscope was inserted again to confirm hemostasis and to dissect the remnant lymph nodes. The gastric tube or colon graft was pulled up to the neck. The anastomosis was performed using a detachable circular stapler (Endopath ILS; Ethicon Endosurgery).

Patients

Between November 1993 and July 2000 a series of 32 patients (24 men, 8 women) ranging in age from 50 to 82 years (mean 68 years) with squamous cell carcinoma of the esophagus underwent MATHE. MATHE was employed in 11 patients with a pre-

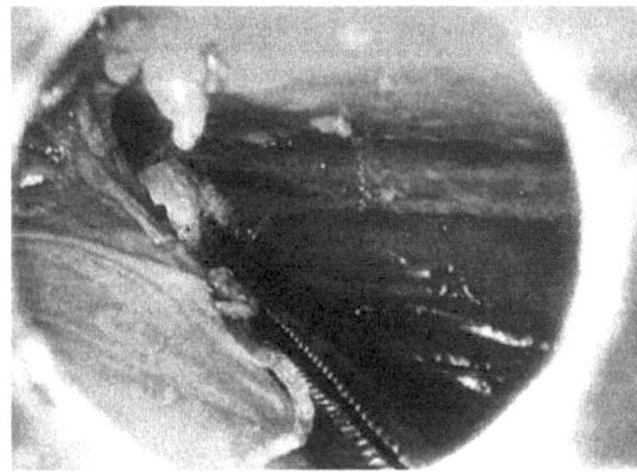

FIG. 7. Right recurrent nerve is observed under the right edge of the trachea. The nodes were dissected

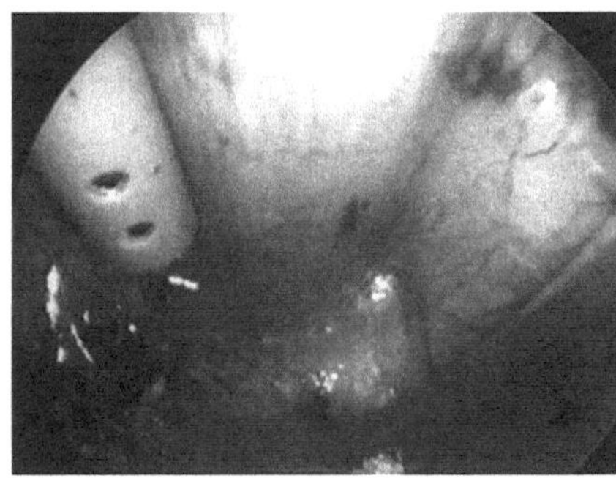

FIG. 8. Upper thoracic paraesophageal and lower paraesophageal lymph nodes were exposed and dissected together with the esophagus

operative diagnosis of superficial cancer that had been established by endoscopy and endoscopic ultrasonography. It was also employed in 28 patients with medical risk factors (7 of whom had superficial tumors). The main risks were old pulmonary tuberculosis (including patients who had undergone thoracoplasty), emphysema, and pulmonary dysfunction defined as a vital capacity (VC) less than 2.5 L. The other risks were heart disease, liver cirrhosis, aged, diabetes mellitus, malnutrition, poor performance status, history of neurovascular disease, thrombocytopenia, and cancer (synchronous hypopharyngeal cancer, gastric cancer with a liver tumor, tongue cancer, pancreatic tumor). EMR had been performed in three patients preoperatively in whom residual cancer was noted. The preoperative diagnosis, risks, and postoperative complications were recorded. These patients were compared with 68 patients who synchronously underwent TTE. TTE was performed by two-field dissection in 43 cases and three-field dissection in 25 cases [1, 2].

Results

Preoperative VC and forced expiratory volume in 1 s (FEV_1) were significantly worse in MATHE patients (Table 1). The tumor location, depth of tumor invasion, stage, intent of resection, and type of interposition graft were no different for the MATHE and TTE groups.

TABLE 1. Preoperative pulmonary function

Measurement	MATHE ($n = 32$)	TTE ($n = 68$)	P
VC (L)	2.89 ± 0.18	3.60 ± 0.10	<0.01
FEV_1 (L)	2.02 ± 0.13	2.76 ± 0.07	<0.01

VC, vital capacity; FEV_1, forced expiratory volume in 1 s; MATHE, mediastinoscopy-assisted transhiatal esophagectomy; TTE, transthoracic esophagectomy

TABLE 2. Postoperative morbidity and mortality

Parameter	MATHE ($n = 32$)	TTE ($n = 68$)	P
Operation time (min)	203 ± 8.5	365 ± 6.2	<0.01
Blood loss (g)	321 ± 42	449 ± 25	<0.01
Pulmonary failure (%)	1 (3.1%)	11 (16.2%)	<0.1
Pneumonia (%)	8 (25%)	17 (25%)	<0.1
Hospital death (%)	1 (3.1%)	4 (5.8%)	<0.05
Pulmonary failure death (%)	0	2 (2.9%)	<0.05

The average operating time was 203 min (range 118–295 min), and the total blood loss was 321 g (range 50–600 g), which were less than for TTE (Table 2). Most patients were extubated on the first or second postoperative day and spent only 1–3 days in the intensive care unit. Eight patients had pulmonary infiltration; seven of them recovered with antibiotics and chest physiotherapy. Only one patient required reintubation and tracheostomy for repeated aspiration pneumonia. None of the others developed respiratory failure. There was one hospital death due to cerebral infarction on the 29th postoperative day. No pulmonary mortality was recognized after MATHE; this compares favorably with TTE, following which two patients died of pulmonary complications (Table 2).

One patient, a 54-year-old woman, was diagnosed as having a lesion with a IIC and IIA; preoperative endoscopic ultrasonography demonstrated tumor invasion in the lamina propria, but the dysplasia lesion was widespread. Her past history revealed an episode of cerebral hemorrhage that resulted in left hemiplegia. Therefore, MATHE was selected. During the operation the slightly swollen pararecurrent nerve nodes were observed. They were sampled carefully and were noted to be positive by pathologic examination. The operation was converted to TTE with radical lymphadenectomy. Three metastases in the pararecurrent nerve nodes and massive lymph vessel involvement were found despite the fact that thin-slice specimen examination showed the tumor infiltration to be m2 (in the lamina propria) (Fig. 9).

The overall survival rate did not differ between the two groups. The 5-year survival rates were 66.6% (MATHE) and 62.7% (TTE).

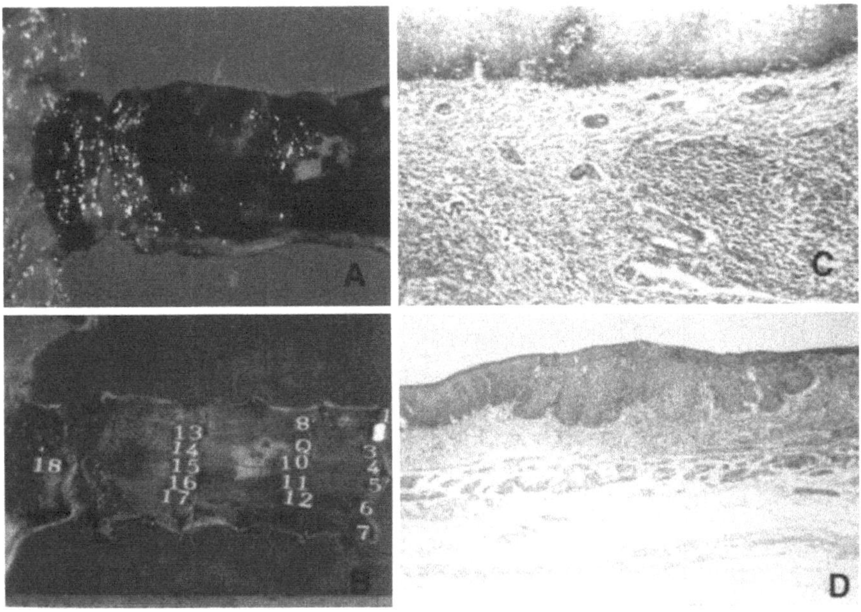

FIG. 9. Specimen of case 13 showed superficial widespread tumor (**A**). Thin-sliced pathological examination (**B**). Massive lymph vessel involvement was found pathologically (**D**), despite the tumor infiltration being rated m2 (**C**)

Discussion

Radical en bloc resection of the esophagus is the treatment of choice for squamous cell carcinoma [1–4]. The long-term results of surgical treatment of esophageal cancer continue to be the poorest of all digestive tract surgery [5]. The patients are often elderly with many risk factors, and curative therapy usually is not possible [5–8]. Transhiatal esophagectomy with a cervical anastomosis, avoiding the need for thoracotomy, appears to reduce the incidence of major pulmonary complications because of the shorter operating time [5–8]. However, the complications of blind dissection of the thoracic esophagus make the overall advantages difficult to demonstrate [5, 6]. Because of its limited access, radical lymphadenectomy, which provides more information for pathologic staging, cannot be performed. Minimally invasive surgery has been proposed to improve the quality of life of patients with esophageal cancer but has failed to reduce the rates of pulmonary complications and in-hospital mortality [9, 10]. Other complications also have been reported, including vascular laceration [11], bronchial injury [12], and port-site recurrence [9, 13]. Videoscopy also appears to reduce the incidence of major complications in THE [14–17]. The advantages include safe handling of the mediastinal structures under direct vision and the ability to dissect the lymph nodes. Lymph node sampling is also feasible.

TABLE 3. Preoperative and pathological diagnosis

Preoperative	Pathological infiltration											
diagnosis	m1	m2	m3	sm1	sm2	sm3	m	sm	Unknown	Total	Accuracy (%)	Underestimated %
m1	203	*27*	*27*	*4*	*8*	*12*	59	13	11	283	71.7	*27.6*
m2	80	107	*39*	*13*	*12*	*0*	26	26	9	261	71.6	*10.2*
m3	29	30	97	*28*	*26*	*19*	56	74	2	232	67.2	*31.5*
sm1	24	25	49	73	*57*	*41*	98	172	1	271	26.9	*36.2*
sm2	6	12	25	50	99	*63*	43	214	4	261	37.9	*24.1*
sm3	3	3	7	27	80	188	13	298	4	315	60.0	
mp	2	4	8	21	37	164	14	242	1	257		
m	322	169	171	48	50	23	677	133	24	834	81.2	
sm	36	43	88	157	252	327	175	788	3	976	80.7	
Unknown	52	27	46	29	62	70	134	200	16	350		
Total	412	243	313	255	401	584	1000	1364	54	2418		

The 49th Japanese Association for Esophageal Diseases (1995)

TABLE 4. Pathological infiltration and n, ly, and v factors

Pathological infiltration	n (+)	%	ly (+)	%	v (+)	%
m1	0/199	0.0	4/381	1.0	1/379	0.3
m2	*5/153*	*3.3*	*15/231*	*6.5*	*1/231*	*0.4*
m3	28/230	12.2	70/303	23.1	13/300	4.3
sm1	58/219	26.5	101/248	40.7	32/248	12.9
sm2	133/372	35.8	209/396	52.8	88/397	22.2
sm3	260/567	45.9	391/581	67.3	191/581	32.9
m	34/611	5.6	93/946	9.8	15/941	1.6
sm	498/1270	39.0	766/1340	57.0	366/1340	25.0
Total	532/1880	28.2	859/2280	37.5	351/2280	15.4

The 49th Japanese Association for Esophageal Diseases (1995)

Postoperative therapy can be guided with pathologic staging information. The maximal direct vision was supplied with accompanying mediastinoscopy [14, 15] or laparoscopy [16, 17]. Insertion of the mediastinoscope via the neck has been advocated by Buess et al. [14] and Bumm et al. [15]. It allows visualization of upper mediastinal structures where lymph node recurrences are often recognized in patients with squamous cell carcinoma. They used a bulky dissector with a working channel through which the esophagus was dissected with monopolar thermocautery, biopsy forceps, and microscissors. Vision was restricted, and anatomic orientation was difficult. We used a 5-mm laparoscope with a sharp, transparent dissector as the mediastinoscope. All manuevers were performed with ease under wide visualization. There was little postoperative morbidity, including pulmonary failure.

The absolute indication for this procedure is attempted cure in patients with superficial cancer without metastasis [18, 19]. However, preoperative diagnosis is difficult despite the recent advances in endoscopic ultrasonography. The sensitivity and specificity of endoscopic ultrasonography for nodal evaluation have been reported to be 65% and 66%, respectively. The sensitivity is decreased to 40% for lymph node metastases less than 1 cm in diameter [20]. A national questionnaire distributed by the Japanese Society for Esophageal Diseases reported in 1995 a preoperative diagnostic precision of 70%. About 30% of tumors had been underestimated with respect to infiltration (Table 3). In 5 of 153 (3.3%) cases, metastases were reported in patients with m2 lesions (infiltration in the lamina propria). In these cases no lymph node metastases had been expected (Table 4) [19]. MATHE can salvage these patients with preoperatively underestimated disease and exceptional metastasis by sampling the lymph nodes.

It is easy to convert MATHE to TTE if the patient's risk allows. In one case we found upper mediastinal lymph node metastasis during MATHE and converted the operation to TTE plus radical lymphadenectomy.

It is difficult to perform en bloc lymph node dissection because the mediastinum is narrow and movement of the equipment is limited. We should develop our technique and the equipment with which radical lymph node dissection can be performed because MATHE is the only operation for cure in patients with high medical risks.

Conclusions

MATHE allows clear visualization of the mediastinal structures, so it is safer than traditional transhiatal esophagectomy. In addition to reducing the risk of tissue damage, clear visualization of the lymph nodes allows easier sampling and dissection, resulting in radicality.

References

1. Akiyama H, Tsurumaru M, Udagawa H, et al (1994) Radical lymph node dissection for cancer of the thoracic esophagus. Ann Surg 220:364–373
2. Nishihira T, Hirayama K, Mori S (1998) A prospective randomized trial of extended cervical and superior mediastinal lymphadenectomy for carcinoma of the thoracic esophagus. Am J Surg 175:47–51
3. Nagawa H, Kobori O, Muto T (1994) Prediction of pulmonary complications after transthoracic oesophagectomy. Br J Surg 81:860–862
4. Boyle MJ, Franceschi D, Livingstone AS (1999) Transhiatal versus transthoracic esophagectomy: complication and survival rates. Am Surg 65:1137–1142
5. Jauch KW, Bacha EA, Denecke H, et al (1992) Esophageal carcinoma: prognostic features and comparison between blunt transhiatal dissection and transthoracic resection. Eur J Surg Oncol 18:553–562
6. Terz JJ, Beatty JD, Kokal WA, et al (1987) Transhiatal esophagectomy. Am J Surg 154:42–48
7. Wong J (1987) Esophageal resection for cancer: the rationale of current practice. Am J Surg 153:18–24
8. Orringer MB, Marshall B, Iannettoni MD (1999) Transhiatal esophagectomy: clinical experience and refinements. Ann Surg 230:392–403
9. Law S, Fok M, Chu KM, et al (1997) Thoracoscopic esophagectomy for esophageal cancer. Surgery 122:8–14
10. Robertson GSM, Lloyd DM, Wicks ACB, et al (1996) No obvious advantages for thoracoscopic two-stage oesophagectomy. Br J Surg 83:675–678
11. Collard J, Lengele B, Otte J, et al (1993) En bloc and standard esophagectomies by thoracoscopy. Ann Thorac Surg 56:675–679
12. Cuschieri A, Shimi S, Banting S (1992) Endoscopic oesophagectomy through a right thoracoscopic approach. J R Coll Surg Edinb 37:7–11
13. Segalin A, Bonavina L, Rosati R, et al (1994) Parietal seeding of esophageal cancer after thoracoscopic resection. Dis Esophagus 7:645
14. Buess G, Kaiser J, Manncke K, et al (1997) Endoscopic microsurgical dissection of the esophagus (EMDE). Intern Surg 82:109–112
15. Bumm R, Feussner H, Bartels H, et al (1997) Radical transhiatal esophagectomy with two-field lymphadenectomy and endodissection for distal esophageal adenocarcinoma. World J Surg 21:822–831
16. DePaula AL, Hashiba K, Ferreira EAB, et al (1995) Laparoscopic transhiatal esophagectomy with esophagogastrostroplasty. Surg Laparosc Endosc 5:1–5
17. Swanstrom LL, Hansen P (1997) Laparoscopic total esophagectomy. Arch Surg 132: 943–948
18. Yoshida M, Hanashi T, Momma K, et al (1995) Endoscopic mucosal resection for radical treatment of esophageal cancer. Jpn J Cancer Chemother 22:847–854
19. Makuuchi H, Shimada H, Mizutani K, et al (1997) Endoscopic criteria for invasive depth of superficial esophageal cancer. Dig Endosc 9:110–115
20. Luketich JD, Schauer P, Landreneau R, et al (1997) Minimally invasive surgical staging is superior to endoscopic ultrasound in detecting lymph node metastases in esophageal cancer. J Thorac Cardiovasc Surg 114:817–823

Q & A after Dr. Tangoku's presentation (video presentation)

Dr. Bumm (Technishe University, München, Germany): This is an interesting technique. I saw that you use several instruments through the working channel and that you inflate the mediastinum. Do you have a balloon at the top?

Dr. Tangoku: No, there is no inflation, just retraction. We make the space.

Dr. Bumm: You open the mediastinal scope?

Dr. Tangoku: No, we just push the esophagus with the retractor.

Dr. Hagen (University of Southern California, USA): It is appropriate that we finished this symposium with three interesting presentations that are looking toward the future of esophageal surgery as we focus on trying to reduce the extent of the insult to the patients but maintain prospects of cure through an adequate resection. I think that all of the presenters would agree, however, that it is a bit premature to entertain application of these techniques until it can be shown that they reduce the mortality and morbidity associated with the operation compared with standard techniques. Perhaps it is even more important that results show the same cure rates.

Subject Index

FSC
www.fsc.org
MIX
Papier aus verantwortungsvollen Quellen
Paper from responsible sources
FSC® C105338

If you have any concerns about our products,
you can contact us on
ProductSafety@springernature.com

In case Publisher is established outside the EU,
the EU authorized representative is:
Springer Nature Customer Service Center GmbH
Europaplatz 3, 69115 Heidelberg, Germany

Printed by Libri Plureos GmbH
in Hamburg, Germany